Pharmacy Technician Exam
Certification and Review

NOTICE

Pharmacy Technician Exam Certification and Review

Jodi Dreiling, PharmD, BCPS
Pharmacotherapy Specialist
Medical Intensive Care Unit
Akron General Medical Center
Akron, Ohio

Kristy Malacos, MS, CPhT
Pharmacy Administrator
Magruder Hospital–Pharmacy Systems, Inc.
Port Clinton, Ohio
Former Program Director of Pharmacy Technology
Sanford-Brown College
Cleveland, Ohio

Allison Cannon, PharmD
Pharmacy Manager
Cleveland Clinic Foundation
Cleveland, Ohio

Eric Schmidt, PharmD
Pharmacy Manager Coverage Determinations
EnvisionRx
Twinsburg, Ohio

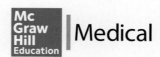

New York   Chicago   San Francisco   Athens   London   Madrid
Mexico City   Milan   New Delhi   Singapore   Sydney   Toronto

Pharmacy Technician Exam Certification and Review

1 2 3 4 5 6 7 8 9 0   CTP/CTP   18 17 16 15 14

Set ISBN 978-0-07-182689-1
Set MHID 0-07-182689-0
Book ISBN 978-0-07-183701-9
Book MHID 0-07-183701-9
CD ISBN 978-0-07-183703-3
CD MHID 0-07-183703-5

This book was set in Avenir by Cenveo Publisher Services.
The editors were Michael Weitz and Robert Pancotti.
The production supervisor was Richard Ruzycka.
Project management was provided by Shruti Awasthi, Cenveo Publisher Services.
The text designer was Dream It!, Inc.; the cover designer was Anthony Landi.
China Translation & Printing Services, Ltd. was the printer and binder.

Library of Congress Cataloging-in-Publication Data

Dreiling, Jodi, author.
  Pharmacy technician exam certification and review / Jodi Dreiling, Kristy Malacos, Allison R. Cannon, Eric Schmidt.
      p. ; cm.
  Includes index.
  ISBN 978-0-07-182689-1 (alk. paper)—ISBN 0-07-182689-0 (alk. paper)
  I. Malacos, Kristy, author. II. Cannon, Allison, author. III. Schmidt, Eric (Pharmacist), author. IV. Title.
  [DNLM: 1. Pharmacy—Examination Questions. 2. Pharmaceutical Preparations—Examination Questions. 3. Pharmaceutical Services—Examination Questions. 4. Pharmacists' Aides. QV 18.2]
  RM301.13
  615.1076—dc23
                                                                                            2014018054

Dedication

We would like to dedicate this book to our families.
Thank you for allowing us to put countless hours into
this book and supporting us throughout. We would
also like to thank Michael, Robert, and Shruti for their
assistance during this process.
Finally, this book is dedicated to pharmacy technicians.
Your hard work and dedication to the profession of
pharmacy is invaluable and often underappreciated.

Jodi, Kristy, Allison, Eric

Key Features of
Pharmacy Technician Exam Certification and Review

- **Organized** to mimic the outline of the Pharmacy Technician Certification Board test
  - ◆ Chapters mirror the Pharmacy Technician Certification Exam Knowledge domains

- **Patient cases and real pharmacy examples** are integrated throughout the book to make information more applicable

- **CD-ROM** allows you to create an endless number of PTCE tests
  - ◆ Question bank with more than 2,000 questions
  - ◆ Each test is a timed, 90-question test that follows the exact PTCE content
  - ◆ The test is presented in similar format to that of the Pearson Vue testing center to help you feel at ease during the actual PTCE

- **Extra chapter on pharmacy math**—includes step-by-step instructions and explanations of answers

- **Key terms** at the beginning of each chapter highlight unfamiliar terms

- **Check point review questions** throughout the chapter to assess your learning

- **Chapters contain "Tech Alerts"** to highlight facts that may be applicable to pharmacy practice.

- End of each chapter contains **50 test questions**

- **Appendices highlight the Top 200 medications**, over-the-counter medications, and herbal products

> Chapters mirror **outline of Pharmacy Technician Certification Board test**
>
> **Key terms** highlighting new terms at beginning of every chapter

---

Sterile and Nonsterile Compounding

CHAPTER
3

PTCB KNOWLEDGE AREAS

3.1 Infection control (eg, hand washing PPE)
3.2 Handling and disposal of hazardous waste (eg, receptacle, waste streams)
3.3 Documentation (eg, batch preparation, compounding record)
3.4 Selection and use of compounding equipment and supplies
3.5 Determination of compounded product stability (eg, beyond-use dating, signs of incompatibility)
3.6 Selection and use of equipment and supplies
3.7 Sterile compounding processes
3.8 Nonsterile compounding processes

KEY TERMS

Analytical balance: Uses electronic calibrations to determine the weight of a product

Aseptic technique: Technique necessary to minimize the risk of microbial contamination of a sterile product

Compounding: The act of reconstituting, mixing, or otherwise preparing a medication into a dosage form usable by the patient

Drip rate: The rate at which an intravenous (IV) medication is infused

Epidural: Injection of a medication directly into the epidural space, or the outermost part, of the spinal canal

Extemporaneous compounding: The preparation of pharmaceuticals in a nonsterile environment

Gauge (G): Thickness or diameter of a needle bore

Geometric dilution: A process in which ingredients are mixed together in equal proportions to ensure that the compounded substance results in an evenly mixed substance

Graduate: A cylindrical or conical-shaped container with clearly defined calibrations used for measuring liquids

Heterogeneous: A mixture that does not contain uniformly mixed ingredients

Homogeneous: A mixture of uniformly distributed ingredients. Homogeneous mixtures are the goal in pharmaceutical compounding

Intramuscular (IM): Medications administered into the muscle

Intravenous (IV): Medications administered into a vein

143

Rewrite the equation using a common denominator for all the fractions.
1, 5, and 15 have a common denominator of 15.

$$\frac{3}{1} \times \frac{15}{15} = \frac{45}{15}$$

$$\frac{1}{5} \times \frac{3}{3} = \frac{3}{15}$$

$$\text{and, } \frac{16}{15}$$

So, $3 + \frac{1}{5} + 1\frac{1}{15}$ becomes $\frac{45}{15} + \frac{3}{15} + \frac{16}{15}$

$$\frac{45}{15} + \frac{3}{15} + \frac{16}{15} = \frac{64}{15}$$

Next, reduce to lowest terms by dividing the numerator (64) by the denominator (15).

$64 \div 15 = 4$ with a remainder of 4 so, $\frac{64}{15} = 4\frac{4}{15}$

Subtraction: $3 - \frac{1}{5} - 1\frac{1}{15}$

Convert the whole number 3 to an improper fraction: $3 = \frac{3}{1}$

$\frac{1}{5}$ is a proper fraction and does not need to be changed.

Convert the mixed number $1\frac{1}{15}$ to an improper fraction: $1\frac{1}{15} = \frac{16}{15}$

Rewrite the equation using a common denominator for all the fractions.
1, 5, and 15 have a common denominator of 15.

$$\frac{3}{1} \times \frac{15}{15} = \frac{45}{15}$$

$$\frac{1}{5} \times \frac{3}{3} = \frac{3}{15}$$

$$\text{and, } \frac{16}{15}$$

So, $3 - \frac{1}{5} - 1\frac{1}{15}$ becomes $\frac{45}{15} - \frac{3}{15} - \frac{16}{15}$

$$\frac{45}{15} - \frac{3}{15} - \frac{16}{15} = \frac{26}{15}$$

Next, reduce to lowest terms by dividing the numerator (26) by the denominator (15).

$26 \div 15 = 1$ with a remainder of 11 so, $\frac{26}{15} = 1\frac{11}{15}$

Multiplying Fractions

When multiplying fractions, the numerators and denominators are multiplied separately.

 EXAMPLE

$\frac{1}{2} \times \frac{3}{4}$

$\frac{1}{2} \times \frac{3}{4} = \frac{(1 \times 3)}{(2 \times 4)} = \frac{3}{8}$

CASE STUDY

You are working in a retail pharmacy store that you have never worked at before, covering a shift as requested by your district manager. The pharmacy phone is ringing as a new patient, Kim Thomas, brings in 3 new prescriptions. She is talking on her cell phone and appears to be rushed. The patient does not have her prescription insurance card with her and would like you to call the local competitor to obtain the information. She also informs you that she takes 2 other medications, "one blue pill, and one little white pill." When you ask her if she knows what the prescriptions are for, she shakes her head, no (Figure 4-1).

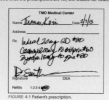

TMD Medical Center

Name _____ Date _____

Address _____

Rx: _____

Signature _____   DEA _____

Refills   1234

FIGURE 4-1 Patient's prescription.

As you work through this chapter, keep the above case study in mind. After completing this chapter you should be able to answer the following self-assessment questions.

Self-Assessment Questions
- What are the distractions occurring in the pharmacy?
- What elements of the prescriptions could potentially lead to an error?
- Are there any safety strategies that the pharmacy can utilize to help prevent errors with these prescriptions?

INTRODUCTION

In 2006, Emily Jerry began her last chemotherapy treatment. She had just turned 2 years old. Unfortunately, her chemotherapy had been prepared with 23.4% concentrated sodium chloride instead of 0.9% sodium chloride, a concentration error which would be fatal for an adult or a child. This chemotherapy was prepared by a pharmacy technician and double checked by a pharmacist. Emily Jerry died as a result of an avoidable medication error. As a result of this and other serious and fatal errors, laws, regulations, and safety efforts have been put in place to help identify and prevent system or process breakdowns which can lead to medication errors and negative patient outcomes. This chapter discusses the critical responsibility of medication safety required of all personnel working in the practice of pharmacy.

TABLE 1-10 Examples of Fluoroquinolones

Generic	Brand	Form	Strengths
Ciprofloxacin	Cipro	Injection	200 mg/100 mL, 400 mg/200 mL
		Suspension	250 mg/5 mL, 500 mg/5 mL
		Tablet	100 mg, 250 mg, 500 mg, 750 mg
		Tablet, XR	500 mg, 1000 mg
Levofloxacin	Levaquin	Injection	250 mg/50 mL, 500 mg/100 mL, 750 mg/150 mL
		Solution	25 mg/mL
		Tablet	250 mg, 500 mg, 750 mg
Moxifloxacin	Avelox	Injection	400 mg/250 mL
		Tablet	400 mg

- Gastrointestinal toxicity occurs most commonly with erythromycin, then clarithromycin, and then azithromycin.

Fluoroquinolones

MOA: Prevent bacteria growth by inhibiting protein replication

Indication: Utilized in multiple different types of infections (ie, abdominal infections, skin infections, pneumonia, sinusitis, UTI)

ADRs: Diarrhea, gastrointestinal upset, nausea, dizziness

Additional notes:

- Medications have a common ending of "-oxacin" (Table 1-10).
- Administer quinolones either 2 hours before or 6 hours after calcium (including dairy products), iron, or zinc.
- There have been reports of tendon inflammation or rupture with quinolones, thus they should not be used in children and have a black box warning for this use.

Tetracyclines

MOA: Inhibit protein synthesis within cell wall

Indications: Acne, bronchitis, malaria, **periodontitis**, pneumonia, **rosacea**, sexually transmitted diseases

ADRs: Gastrointestinal upset, **phototoxicity**

Additional notes:

- Medications have a common ending of "-cycline" (Table 1-11).
- Enters developing bone and teeth causing weakness, thus should be avoided in children and pregnant women.
- Tetracycline should be taken on an empty stomach and antacids should be avoided. Minocycline and doxycycline can be taken without regards to meals or antacids.

Contents

Reviewers

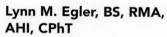

Lynn M. Egler, BS, RMA, AHI, CPhT
Author, Consultant
LME Solutions
Saint Clair Shores, Michigan
Adjunct Faculty
Baker College
Clinton Township, Michigan

Samantha Milakovich, BSPS, CPhT
Pharmacy Technology Instructor
Sanford-Brown College
Cleveland, Ohio

Denise Propes, CPhT
Senior Technician
Research Pharmacy Lead
Technician
University of Michigan Hospital
and Health Systems
Research Pharmacy
(Investigational Drug Service)
Ann Arbor, Michigan

Brigid Whelan, BS, CPhT
Pharmacy Technology Instructor
Sanford-Brown College
Cleveland, Ohio

Preface

Pharmacy technicians play a large role in the practice of pharmacy. Job duties may include helping a pharmacist prepare prescription medications, maintain patient profiles, prepare insurance claims, interact with customers, and various other duties (ie, answer phones, ordering stock, restocking medications). Pharmacy technicians may practice in a variety of settings: community (retail) pharmacies, inpatient and outpatient hospital pharmacies, mail-order facilities, or government settings. According to the Bureau of Labor and Statistics, employment of pharmacy technicians is expected to increase by 32% between 2010 and 2020.

Certified Pharmacy Technicians

The National Association of Boards of Pharmacy has recommended that all pharmacy technicians become certified pharmacy technicians by 2015. Pharmacy technicians who meet all eligibility requirements and who pass a national examination are considered certified pharmacy technicians (CPhT).

Pharmacy Technician Examination Options

The **Pharmacy Technician Certification Examination (PTCE)** is the only competency-based examination that is valid nationwide and is endorsed by major national pharmacy organizations. It was established in 1995 by the Pharmacy Technician Certification Board and has certified more than 400,000 pharmacy technicians. This test is the gold standard for certifying pharmacy technicians.

The **Examination for the Certification of Pharmacy Technicians (ExCPT)** is another pharmacy technician examination. However, it is not valid nationwide.

Features of This Book

This book is presented to match the blueprint for the PTCE that was implemented November 1, 2013. It exactly mimics the knowledge domains, knowledge areas, and percentage of content. Each chapter covers one knowledge domain, with the knowledge areas of the domain listed at the beginning of each chapter. This format will help you study and pass the examination. Each chapter also contains a patient case to help you relate the information that you are learning to real world experiences. A list of key terms is included at the beginning of each chapter to help you understand unfamiliar vocabulary. The "Tech alert" boxes in the side columns of the pages highlight important points that will be helpful during your training. Each chapter also contains quick quizzes to check your knowledge throughout the lesson. At the end of each chapter, there are 50 test questions. In addition, the book is packaged with a CD that contains more than 2000 unique test questions. The tests on the CD exactly mimic the PTCE. Each test contains 90 questions from the 9 knowledge domains. The test is presented in similar format to the Pearson Vue testing center to help you feel at ease during the actual PTCE. The questions are randomly selected for each test so you will have an unlimited number of tests available. We have also included a math review chapter to help you teach and refresh your comprehension of pharmacy math.

Blueprint Domains for PTCE

Knowledge Domains	Domain Description	% of PTCE Content	Knowledge Areas
1	Pharmacology for Technicians	13.75	6
2	Pharmacy Law and Regulations	12.5	15
3	Sterile and Nonsterile Compounding	8.75	7
4	Medication Safety	12.5	6
5	Pharmacy Quality Assurance	7.5	5
6	Medication Order Entry and Fill Process	17.5	7
7	Pharmacy Inventory Management	8.75	5
8	Pharmacy Billing and Reimbursement	8.75	5
9	Pharmacy Information System Usage and Application	10.00	2

Pharmacy technician candidates should use this guide to help assist in studying for the PTCE. In addition, candidates should refer to the Pharmacy Technician Certification Board website for more details: www.ptcb.org

About the Authors

Jodi Dreiling, PharmD, BCPS

Jodi Dreiling graduated from Ohio Northern University with her Doctor of Pharmacy degree. She went on to pursue a pharmacy practice residency at Duke University Medical Center. She currently is a critical care pharmacotherapy specialist at Akron General Medical Center. Dr. Dreiling is actively involved in the education of health care professionals including pharmacy technicians. In her free time, Jodi loves spending time with her family and enjoys watching college athletics.

Kristy Malacos, MS, CPhT

Kristy obtained her Master of Science degree from Kent State University in Biomedical Science and Pharmacology. She is a certified pharmacy technician and has practiced as a technician in both retail and institutional settings. She worked as a program director for an ASHP-accredited pharmacy technician training program and was responsible for preparing students for the Pharmacy Technician Certification Examination. Kristy is currently employed with Pharmacy Systems, Inc. as the pharmacy administrator for Magruder Hospital. In her free time, Kristy enjoys spending time with family and watching the Reds and Bengals.

Allison Cannon, PharmD

Allison obtained her Doctor of Pharmacy degree from The University of Toledo. In her career, she has worked closely with pharmacy technicians in both retail and health-system pharmacy settings. Prior to becoming a pharmacist, she worked as a pharmacy technician in a hospital pharmacy. Dr. Cannon is currently an Inpatient Pharmacy Manager at Cleveland Clinic and is pursuing her Master of Science in Health-System Pharmacy Administration at Northeast Ohio Medical University. In her free time, Allison enjoys spending time with her husband and their 2 dogs, listening to live music, and traveling.

Eric Schmidt, PharmD

Eric obtained his Doctor of Pharmacy degree from Ohio Northern University. He has had the opportunity to work closely with many technicians as a peer, clinical pharmacist, manager, and director. Dr. Schmidt is currently the Pharmacy Manager of Coverage Determinations at EnvisionRx. He is formerly the Director of Pharmacy in a speciality setting at the Medical Service Company. In his free time, Eric spends time with his family, plays golf, and loves to travel.

Test-Taking Strategies

Prior to the Test

- Review the content outline. Understand what you should study for the test.
- Develop a study plan. Review for the test over an extended period of time so that you will not have to cram at the last minute.
- Make flash cards to remember key facts (ie, brand/generic drugs).
- Review practice tests several times.
- Maintain healthy living habits prior to the test by minimizing alcohol use and maintaining a healthy diet and exercise schedule.
- Get a good night's sleep the night before the test. Pulling an all-nighter studying will negatively affect your score.
- Know the location of your testing site and how long it will take to get there. Allow for extra time in case of traffic.

Day of the Test

- Eat a good breakfast that includes protein and minimizes sugar.
- Arrive at the testing site 30 minutes prior to your scheduled appointment.
- Make sure to bring government-issued identification as directed by the testing site.
- Visit the bathroom 15 to 30 minutes prior to the test in order to minimize testing interruptions.
- Wear comfortable clothing and consider dressing in layers to account for indoor temperature variations. Coats and jackets are not permitted inside the testing site and must be left inside a locker.

- Personal items cannot be brought into the testing area. All items must be placed inside a locker, including cell phones, hats, purses, wallets, pens, paper, food, and drinks.

During the Test

- Read each question carefully, paying attention to key words and ignoring distractors.
- Pay attention to the time. The test consists of 90 questions over 1 hour and 50 minutes.
- If you are struggling to answer a question, skip it and come back to it at the end.
- When guessing to answer a question, try to eliminate one or more of the answers and then make an educated guess.
- If you have time remaining at the end of the test, review your answers. Don't second guess yourself, just check for careless errors and unanswered questions.
- Remember to answer all questions. You are scored on all questions, even those you don't answer. A blank answer will count negatively against your score.
- Try not to get distracted by other testers in the room.
- Remember, if others are leaving before you, the testing site is used for multiple different tests that vary in length.
- Don't panic. If you start to get nervous, take some slow deep breaths.

Math Review

KNOWLEDGE AREAS

Upon completion of this chapter, the student will understand:

1. Roman numerals
2. Interpretation and use of decimals and fractions
3. Cross multiplication to solve for an unknown variable in a proportion
4. Conversion between units of measure common in pharmacy practice
5. Interpretation of concentration in ratios and percentage format

KEY TERMS

Apothecary system: An antiquated system of measurement used in pharmacy

Avoirdupois (household) system: A system of measurement commonly used in daily life in the United States

Denominator: The bottom number in a fraction that represents the total number of equal parts that make up the whole

International units (IU): Standardized and specific units of measure unique to each medication

Leading zero: A zero written before the decimal point. The leading zero ensures that the decimal point is not overlooked

Metric system: The most common system of measurement used in medicine

Milliequivalent (mEq): A measurement of the combining power of one chemical ion with another

Numerator: The top number in a fraction that represents a specific number of equal parts

Percentage: Parts per 100

Proportion: An equation that states 2 ratios are equal

Ratio: A statement of how 2 numbers compare

Trailing zero: Extra zeroes written after a decimal number. Trailing zeroes are forbidden to limit the chance and magnitude of an error

Unit: The quantity of a medication necessary to produce a specific effect

CASE STUDY

You are working as a pharmacy technician in a community retail pharmacy. While you are helping customers at the prescription drop-off window, a mother hands you the following prescription (Figure MR-1):

Patient: *Anthony Miller*
Address: *3333 Elm Street   Springfield, OH 43215*

Weight: *33 lb.*   DOB: *1/1/2010*

Amoxicillin oral suspension 125 mg/5 mL
25 mg/kg PO bid x 7d

Refills: 0   *D Smith, MD*
                                      Dr. David Smith, MD

FIGURE MR-1 Sample prescription.

After completing the math review, you will be able to answer the following questions:
- What dose has been prescribed for Anthony?
- How much liquid will be needed in order for him to take the medication for the prescribed 7 days?

INTRODUCTION

Pharmacy technicians are expected to perform dosage calculations in everyday practice with 100% accuracy. This section reviews math skills commonly performed by a pharmacy technician. After completing the math review section, you should be able to confidently work with fractions, decimals, ratios and proportions, percentages, and metric conversions. These skills will be utilized in chapters throughout this book.

ROMAN NUMERALS

Roman numerals are sometimes used as an alternative way to designate quantities in pharmacy practice. Many prescribers often use Roman numerals to denote quantities on a prescription. For example, rather than writing directions as "2 tablets every 8 hours," many prescribers may write "ii tabs q8h." The Roman numeral ii is used in place of the number 2. Table MR-1 lists commonly used Roman numerals and the numerical equivalents.

Roman numerals can be written and read by the following 4 basic rules:

1. Understand the numerical value of each base letter (see the highlighted rows in Table MR-1).
2. If Roman numerals are arranged from left to right by descending value (the letter to the left is larger in value), the values are added to each other (eg, XV = 10 + 5 = 15).
3. If Roman numerals are arranged from left to right by ascending value (the letter to the left is smaller in value), the value of the first Roman numeral is subtracted from the second (eg, XL = 10 − 50 = 40).

TABLE MR-1. **Roman Numerals**	
Roman Numeral	*Numerical Equivalent*
i, I	1
ii, II	2
iii, III	3
iv, IV	4
v, V	5
vi, VI	6
vii, VII	7
viii, VIII	8
ix, IX	9
x, X	10
xv, XV	15
xx, XX	20
xxv, XXV	25
xxx, XXX	30
xl, XL	40
l, L	50
c, C	100
d, D	500
m, M	1000

4. A Roman numeral written 2 or 3 times repeats its value that many times (eg, XX = 10 + 10 = 20, or CCC = 100 + 100 + 100 = 300).
   a. A Roman numeral cannot be used more than 3 consecutive times. If a number is too large to describe using a Roman numeral 3 times, the next larger Roman numeral should be used (eg, the number 4 is written IV rather than IIII).

DECIMALS

Many medications are written, dosed, and dispensed using decimals. A decimal is a value that is not a whole number. Examples of decimals are 0.25 and 1.5. In pharmacy practice, it is very important that a zero placeholder, called a **leading zero**, is written before the decimal point, as in 0.25. The leading zero ensures that the decimal point is not overlooked, reducing the chance of a medication dosing error. It is equally important that no extra zeroes, called a **trailing zero**, are written after a number.

EXAMPLE: Leading zero
If a provider writes a dose as .25 mg, a leading zero should be added to ensure that the dosage is interpreted correctly as 0.25 mg as opposed to 25 mg.

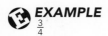 **EXAMPLE:** **Trailing zero**
If a provider writes a dose as 1.50 mg, it may accidentally be misinterpreted as 150 mg. The dose should be written 1.5 mg to reduce the chance of an error occurring.

FRACTIONS

Fractions are another means to express a value that is not a whole number. Although fractions are not commonly used to write medication dosages, understanding how to work with fractions is essential to pharmacy calculations. A fraction is made up of 2 numbers separated by a fraction bar, one on top and one on the bottom. The top number is called the **numerator** and the bottom number is called the **denominator**. These terms will be used throughout this chapter in describing calculations with fractions.

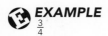 **EXAMPLE**
$\frac{3}{4}$

$$\frac{3}{4} \begin{array}{l} \rightarrow 3 \text{ is the numerator} \\ \rightarrow 4 \text{ is the denominator} \end{array}$$

The numerator (in this example 3) represents the number of equal parts and the denominator (in this example 4) represents how many of those equal parts make a whole. The concept of fractions can be visualized by dividing a whole circle into equal parts. The whole circle in Figure MR-2 is divided into 4 equal parts. The fraction 3/4 represents 3 of the 4 equal parts.

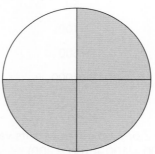

FIGURE MR-2 Representation of 3 of 4 equal parts.

There are 3 types of fractions:

1. Proper fractions: Have a numerator that is smaller than the denominator.
2. Improper fractions: Have a numerator that is larger than the denominator.
3. Mixed numbers: Combine a whole number with a proper fraction.

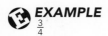 **EXAMPLE:** **Proper fraction**
$\frac{3}{4}$

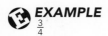 **EXAMPLE:** **Improper fraction**
$\frac{4}{3}$

Improper fractions can be converted to mixed numbers easily by dividing the numerator by the denominator.

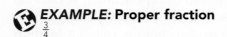

$$4 \div 3 = 1 \text{ } with \text{ } a \text{ } remainder \text{ } of \text{ } 1$$

The remainder is then placed over the denominator to create a mixed number.

So, the improper fraction of $\frac{4}{3}$ converts easily to the proper fraction of $1\frac{1}{3}$, which would be considered a mixed number because it combines a whole number and a fraction.

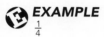 **EXAMPLE: Mixed number**
$1\frac{1}{3}$

A mixed number can also be converted into an improper fraction by multiplying the whole number by the denominator and adding the numerator. This value is then placed over the original denominator. So in the example above the whole number = 1 and the denominator = 3. $1 \times 3 = 3$, then add the numerator = 4 and place this value over the denominator = $\frac{4}{3}$.

A fraction can also be converted to a decimal by dividing the numerator by the denominator.

EXAMPLE
$\frac{1}{4}$

$$\frac{1}{4} = 1 \div 4 = 0.25$$

Improper factions can also be converted to a decimal by dividing the numerator by the denominator in the same fashion.

$$\frac{9}{5} = 9 \div 5 = 1.8$$

Adding and Subtracting Fractions

When adding and subtracting fractions, convert all whole numbers and mixed numbers to improper fractions and ensure they have common denominators, then simply add or subtract.

Always convert your answers to proper fractions or mixed numbers unless directed otherwise.

EXAMPLE: Adding and subtracting proper fractions with common denominators

Addition: $\frac{1}{5} + \frac{3}{5} = \frac{4}{5}$

Subtraction: $\frac{4}{5} - \frac{1}{5} = \frac{3}{5}$

Note: To add or subtract fraction, they must have a common (the same) denominator.

EXAMPLE: Adding and subtracting fractions, whole numbers and mixed numbers

Addition: $3 + \frac{1}{5} + 1\frac{1}{15}$

Convert the whole number 3 to an improper fraction: $3 = \frac{3}{1}$

$\frac{1}{5}$ is a proper fraction and does not need to be changed.

Convert the mixed number $1\frac{1}{15}$ to an improper fraction: $1\frac{1}{15} = \frac{16}{15}$

Rewrite the equation using a common denominator for all the fractions.

1, 5, and 15 have a common denominator of 15.

$$\frac{3}{1} \times \frac{15}{15} = \frac{45}{15}$$

$$\frac{1}{5} \times \frac{3}{3} = \frac{3}{15}$$

$$and, \frac{16}{15}$$

So, $3 + \frac{1}{5} + 1\frac{1}{15}$ becomes $\frac{45}{15} + \frac{3}{15} + \frac{16}{15}$

$$\frac{45}{15} + \frac{3}{15} + \frac{16}{15} = \frac{64}{15}$$

Next, reduce to lowest terms by dividing the numerator (64) by the denominator (15).

$64 \div 15 = 4$ *with a remainder of* 4 so, $\frac{64}{15} = 4\frac{4}{15}$

Subtraction: $3 - \frac{1}{5} - 1\frac{1}{15}$

Convert the whole number 3 to an improper fraction: $3 = \frac{3}{1}$

$\frac{1}{5}$ is a proper fraction and does not need to be changed.

Convert the mixed number $1\frac{1}{15}$ to an improper fraction: $1\frac{1}{15} = \frac{16}{15}$

Rewrite the equation using a common denominator for all the fractions.

1, 5, and 15 have a common denominator of 15.

$$\frac{3}{1} \times \frac{15}{15} = \frac{45}{15}$$

$$\frac{1}{5} \times \frac{3}{3} = \frac{3}{15}$$

$$and, \frac{16}{15}$$

So, $3 - \frac{1}{5} - 1\frac{1}{15}$ becomes $\frac{45}{15} - \frac{3}{15} - \frac{16}{15}$

$$\frac{45}{15} - \frac{3}{15} - \frac{16}{15} = \frac{26}{15}$$

Next, reduce to lowest terms by dividing the numerator (26) by the denominator (15).

$26 \div 15 = 1$ *with a remainder of* 11 so, $\frac{26}{15} = 1\frac{11}{15}$

Multiplying Fractions

When multiplying fractions, the numerators and denominators are multiplied separately.

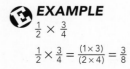 **EXAMPLE**

$\frac{1}{2} \times \frac{3}{4}$

$\frac{1}{2} \times \frac{3}{4} = \frac{(1 \times 3)}{(2 \times 4)} = \frac{3}{8}$

When multiplying a whole number and a fraction, the whole number can be thought of as the numerator divided by 1. In the following example, the whole number 5 can be written as 5 over 1, and then multiplied by the fraction as shown previously. When working with fractions in a pharmacy setting, always reduce your answers to lowest terms and always list your answer as a proper fraction unless directed otherwise.

EXAMPLE

$5 \times \frac{2}{3}$

$$\frac{5}{1} \times \frac{2}{3} = \frac{(5 \times 2)}{(1 \times 3)} = \frac{10}{3}$$

To reduce the improper fraction $\frac{10}{3}$ to a proper fraction in lowest terms, divide the numerator (10) by the denominator (3).

Therefore, $\frac{10}{3} = 3\frac{1}{3}$.

Dividing Fractions

When dividing fractions, invert (flip) the second fraction and then simply multiply the numerators and the denominators.

EXAMPLE

$\frac{1}{2} \div \frac{3}{4}$

Invert the second fraction. So $\frac{3}{4}$ becomes $\frac{4}{3}$.
Set up the new equation and multiply.

$$\frac{1}{2} \times \frac{4}{3} = \frac{(1 \times 4)}{(2 \times 3)} = \frac{4}{6}$$

Reduce to lowest term. Both 4 and 6 are divisible by 2, so $\frac{4}{6}$ reduces to $\frac{2}{3}$.

QUICK QUIZ MR-1

1. $\frac{3}{4} \times \frac{4}{5} =$

2. $6 \times \frac{2}{5} =$

3. Convert the answer from question 2 to a decimal.

4. Multiply the equation; **do not reduce** to lowest terms.

$$120 \times \frac{1}{30} =$$

5. Reduce the answer from question 4 to lowest terms.

RATIOS AND PROPORTIONS

A **ratio** is a statement of how 2 numbers compare. For example, if you have a bowl of fruit containing 3 apples and 4 oranges, the ratio of apples to oranges is 3/4. Likewise, since there are 7 total pieces of fruit in the bowl, the ratio of apples to total fruit is 3/7 and the ratio of oranges to total fruit is 4/7. Ratios are written using a colon (:) and can also be written as fractions; 3/4 is the same as 3:4. This ratio can be read as "the ratio of 3 to 4" or "3 is to 4."

A **proportion** is an equation that states 2 ratios are equal. Proportions can be written using fractions or ratios. The fraction proportion expressing the equality of the fractions $\frac{3}{4}$ and $\frac{9}{12}$ is written as $\frac{3}{4} = \frac{9}{12}$. The ratio proportion expressing the equality of the ratios 3:4 and 9:12 is written 3:4::9:12. This can be read as 3 is to 4 as 9 is to 12. Proportions are most often used to solve for an unknown value when given one value and the equivalent ratio.

Let us use the previous example. You have a bowl of fruit containing 3 apples and 4 oranges. Suppose you also have a second larger bowl and want to have the same ratio of apples to oranges in it as in the first bowl. Suppose you have 12 apples to put in the large bowl, how many oranges should you put in to maintain the same ratio of apples to oranges?

SOLUTION

$$\frac{3 \text{ apples}}{4 \text{ oranges}} = \frac{12 \text{ apples}}{X \text{ oranges}}$$

Since these are whole numbers, you may be able to solve this without using any sophisticated calculations. But what if the numbers were not as simple? A technique known as cross multiplication is used to solve for the unknown variable in a proportion.

Cross multiplication is a mathematical technique used to solve for an unknown variable. If the relationship is known between 2 quantities (the ratio), and are given the value of one quantity, we can solve for the missing quantity.

The most important step in cross multiplication is setting up ratios correctly. Make sure that the numerators and denominators of each ratio have the same units. This is the most important step to cross multiplication as it ensures the ratios are set up appropriately to yield the correct answer.

EXAMPLE

$$\frac{3 \text{ apples}}{4 \text{ oranges}} = \frac{12 \text{ apples}}{X \text{ oranges}}$$

The next step is to multiply the numerator of the first ratio by the denominator of the second ratio. This is where the term "cross" multiplying comes from.

$$\frac{3 \text{ apples}}{4 \text{ oranges}} = \frac{12 \text{ apples}}{X \text{ oranges}}$$

$3 \times X$. This is one side of your equation.

Then multiply the other 2 numbers, the denominator of the first ratio and the numerator of the second ratio.

$$\frac{3 \text{ apples}}{4 \text{ oranges}} = \frac{12 \text{ apples}}{X \text{ oranges}}$$

4×12. This is the other side of your equation.

Now set the 2 sides of the equation equal to each other.

$3 \times X = 4 \times 12$

The next step is to multiply the numbers on both sides.

$3 \times X = 3X$

$4 \times 12 = 48$

So, $3X = 48$

Next, divide both sides by the number associated with X in order to solve for X.

$$\frac{3X}{3} = \frac{48}{3}$$

The 3's cancel out on the left side, leaving your unknown X by itself.

$$\frac{\cancel{3}X}{\cancel{3}} = \frac{48}{3}$$

Now solve for X. $X = 48 \div 3 = 16$

$X = 16$

So, X = 16 oranges.

Now, let us try a situation that you could see in pharmacy practice.

🔵 EXAMPLE

You have a stock bottle of morphine sulfate that has a solution strength of 20 mg in each 5 mL. A doctor has written a prescription to dispense 60 mL of morphine sulfate solution. How many milligrams will be in the 60-mL bottle of morphine you dispense?

🔵 SOLUTION

First, identify the unit of the unknown value. In this example, we are looking for milligram, so X = milligram.

Next, set up the ratios with like units in the numerator and denominator.

$$\frac{20 \text{ mg}}{5 \text{ mL}} = \frac{X \text{ mg}}{60 \text{ mL}}$$

(stock bottle)　　(dispensed bottle)

Now cross multiply.

$$\frac{20 \text{ mg}}{5 \text{ mL}} ✕ \frac{X \text{ mg}}{60 \text{ mL}}$$

Next, set the 2 sides of the equation equal to each other.

$20 \times 60 = 5 \times X$

Multiply the numbers on both sides.

$20 \times 60 = 1200$
$5 \times X = 5X$

So, $1200 = 5X$.

Divide both sides by the number associated with X to solve for X.

$$\frac{1200}{5} = \frac{5X}{5}$$

The 5's cancel out on the right side, leaving your unknown X by itself.

$$\frac{1200}{5} = \frac{\cancel{5}X}{\cancel{5}}$$

Now solve for X. $X = 1200 \div 5 = 240$

So, $X = 240$ mg.

QUICK QUIZ MR-2

Solve for the unknown variable, X, in the following questions:

1. $\dfrac{4}{8} = \dfrac{5}{X}$

2. $\dfrac{X}{27} = \dfrac{8}{9}$

3. $\dfrac{3}{36} = \dfrac{X}{12}$

4. $\dfrac{6}{X} = \dfrac{40}{60}$

5. You are filling a prescription written for 30 mg of dextromethorphan every 8 hours, dispense a 7-day supply. The concentration of your stock bottle of dextromethorphan liquid is 10 mg per 15 mL. The patient wants to know how many milliliters of solution he will have to swallow for each dose.

★ *TECH ALERT: Do not be confused by extra information in a question! First read the question to figure out what it is asking for, then read it again and extract only the necessary information.*

MEASUREMENT SYSTEMS

There are several different measurement systems used in pharmacy practice. One measurement system is the **household system**, also known as the **avoirdupois system**. The household system is commonly used in daily life in the United States.

TABLE MR-2. **Metric System Conversions**				
Prefix	*Abbreviation*	*Value*	*Use in Pharmacy*	*Important Notes*
Kilo	k	1000	Kilogram (kg)	
	1		Gram (g) Liter (L)	1000 g = 1 kg
Milli	m	0.001	Milligram (mg) Milliliter (mL)	1000 mg = 1 g 1000 mL = 1 L
Micro	μ	0.00001	Microgram (μg)	1000 μg = 1 mg

Some units of measure used frequently from this system include *teaspoon*, *tablespoon*, *pound*, and *ounce*. An additional measurement system used in pharmacy practice is the **apothecary system**. The most common units still used from this system are *grains* and *drams*. Although this is an archaic system, there are still several medications that are measured and prescribed this way. The most frequent measurement system used in pharmacy practice and throughout the world is the **metric system**. Table MR-2 displays the common units of measurement in the metric system and their relationship to each other.

As described in the "Important Notes" column of Table MR-2, the most common metric system units used in pharmacy are all related to each other by a power of 1000. That is, a kilogram is 1000 times heavier than a gram. And a gram is 1000 times heavier than a milligram. Likewise, a milligram is 1000 times heavier than a microgram. Figure MR-3 depicts this relationship.

To convert between metric system value places manually, you can simply move your decimal point 3 places.

⭐ *TECH ALERT: In the apothecary system, the unit of measure is written before the value. The value is always written as a Roman numeral. For example, 2 grains is written as gr ii.*

🔄 **EXAMPLE**

To convert 0.75 g to milligrams, move the decimal point 3 places to the right.

0.75 g = 750 mg, we simply moved the decimal 3 places to the right.

To convert 42.5 mg to grams, move the decimal point 3 places to the left.

42.5 mg = 0.0425 g, we simply moved the decimal 3 places to the left.

It is essential for a pharmacy technician to be able to convert quickly and correctly from other measurement systems into the metric system. Tables MR-3 and MR-4 display the conversion factors from household and apothecary measurements

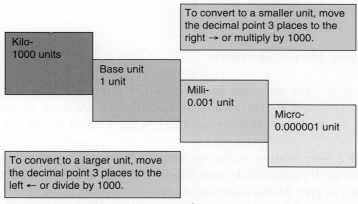

FIGURE MR-3 Metric conversion chart.

TABLE MR-3. Fluid Measurement Conversions			
Volume Measurement Unit	Abbreviation	Metric Conversion	Important Notes
Dram	dr, Ʒ	5 mL	
Drop	gtt	0.05 mL	
Teaspoon	tsp	5 mL	3 tsp = 1 tbsp
Tablespoon	tbsp	15 mL	
Fluid ounce	fl oz	30 mL	16 fl oz = 1 pt
Pint	pt	480 mL	2 pt = 1 qt
Quart	qt	946 mL (~1 L)	4 qt = 1 gal
Gallon	gal	3785 mL	

TABLE MR-4. Solid Measurement Conversions			
Weight Measurement Unit	Abbreviation	Metric Conversion	Important Notes
Grain	gr	60 mg	
Ounce	oz	28.349 g	16 oz = 1 lb
Pound	lb	454 g	2.2 lb = 1 kg

to metric units. It is important to note that some conversions listed are approximate measurements. These measurements are widely accepted in pharmacy practice and are acceptable to use on technician certification examinations.

Medical Measurement Systems

★ TECH ALERT: Units should not be abbreviated. Both u and un are on The Joint Commission's forbidden abbreviation list. They can easily be mistaken for zeroes if handwriting is not clear, creating risk for a 10- or 100-fold overdose.

There are some measurement systems that are unique to medicine. A **unit** is the quantity of a medication necessary to produce a specific effect. Insulin, heparin, penicillin, and many vaccines are commonly dosed in units. **International units (IU)** are standardized and specific for each medication. International units are often used to measure vitamins, such as vitamin D. **Milliequivalent (mEq)** is a measurement of the combining power of one chemical ion with another. Electrolytes, such as sodium and potassium, are often measured in milliequivalent because the individual electrolyte ion is therapeutically active.

Temperature Measurements

Many medications are sensitive to temperature fluctuations. It is important for pharmacy technicians to be aware of appropriate storage temperatures for medications, as noted on the manufacturer's packaging or on the medication label.

There are 2 temperature scales commonly used in pharmacies in the United States. Fahrenheit (F) is the traditional household measurement, and thus is sometimes included as part of the avoirdupois system. Celsius (C) is commonly used in science and is often included as part of the metric system.

Conversion between the temperature scales is as follows:

$$(°F − 32) ÷ 1.8 = °C$$
$$(°C × 1.8) + 32 = °F$$

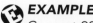 **EXAMPLE**
Convert 99.6°F to °C.

$(°F − 32) ÷ 1.8 = °C$

First subtract 32 from 99.6°F.

$99.6 − 32 = 67.6$

Then divide the above answer by 1.8.

$67.6 ÷ 1.8 = 37.55$, *which rounds to 37.6°C*

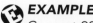 **EXAMPLE**
Convert 12°C to °F.

$(°C × 1.8) + 32 = °F$

First multiply 12°C by 1.8.

$12 × 1.8 = 21.6$

Then add 32 to the above answer.

$21.6 + 32 = 53.6°F$

Conversion Between Units

When filling a prescription, it is important to pay close attention to the units of measure noted on the prescription and the manufacturer's medication label. Similarly, you should pay close attention to the units stated in each question on the certification examination. The first step in every calculation should be to convert all information to the same unit of measure. Since the metric system is the most common system used in pharmacy practice, you will most often convert all necessary information to metric units.

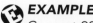 **EXAMPLE**
560 g equals how many kilograms?

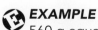 **SOLUTION USING CROSS MULTIPLICATION**
When setting up your cross-multiplication fractions, be sure to set them up with like units in both the numerator and the denominator.

$$\frac{1\,kg}{1000\,g} = \frac{X\,kg}{560\,g}$$

Cross multiply.

$1 × 560 = X × 1000$

Divide.

560 ÷ 1000 = X

And solve.

X = 0.56

So, 560 g equals 0.56 kg.

⊛ SOLUTION USING THE DIMENSIONAL ANALYSIS METHOD (ALSO KNOWN AS THE CANCEL OUT METHOD)

The dimensional analysis (cancel out) method can be used to convert between as many units as necessary with one equation. The key to the cancel out method is that the equation must be set up so that like units cancel. The equation should be set up so that your desired (unit you are converting to) unit is in the numerator, and your given unit (unit you are converting from) is in the denominator.

⊛ EXAMPLE

Convert 560 g to kilograms.

The desired unit (unit you are converting to) is kilogram and the given unit (unit you are converting from) is gram. Set up your conversion factor fraction with kilogram as the numerator and gram as the denominator.

$$560 \; \cancel{g} \times \frac{1 \, kg}{1000 \; \cancel{g}} = 0.56 \; kg$$

The unit gram cancels out, and you are left with your desired unit of measure, kilogram. So, 560 g equals 0.56 kg.

⊛ EXAMPLE

How many milliliters are in 4 fl oz?

⊛ SOLUTION USING CROSS MULTIPLICATION

When setting up your cross-multiplication fractions, be sure to set them up with like units in the numerator and like units in the denominator.

This can be thought of as, if there are 30 mL in each 1 fl oz, how many milliliters are there in 4 fl oz?

$$\frac{30 \, mL}{1 \, fl \, oz} = \frac{X \, mL}{4 \, fl \, oz}$$

Cross multiply.

30 × 4 = X × 1

Divide.

120 ÷ 1 = X

And solve.

X = 120

So, there are 120 mL in 4 fl oz.

🄢 *SOLUTION USING DIMENSIONAL ANALYSIS (CANCEL OUT METHOD)*

When setting up your equation using the cancel out method, be sure to set it up so that like units cancel out. The conversion fraction should be set up so that your desired unit (in this case, milliliter) is in the numerator and your given unit (in this case, fluid ounce) is in the denominator.

$$4 \; \cancel{\text{fl. oz.}} \times \frac{30 \text{ mL}}{1 \; \cancel{\text{fl. oz.}}} = 120 \text{ mL}$$

The unit fluid ounce cancels out, and you are left with your desired unit of measure, milliliter.

So, there are 120 mL in 4 fl oz.

QUICK QUIZ MR-3

1. _____ °C = 98°F

2. How many kilograms does a 185-lb man weigh?

3. A medication label on a manufacturer's bottle indicates that each tablet contains 117 µg of levothyroxine. How many milligrams of levothyroxine are in each tablet?

4. You receive a prescription written for hydrocortisone 2% ointment dispenses 2 oz. What size hydrocortisone ointment tube (in grams) will you dispense?

5. How many kilograms are in 16 lb?

~~~~~~

CONCENTRATIONS

In pharmacy, concentrations of drugs are often expressed as ratios. When a concentration is written as a ratio, it is describing the amount of active drug per amount of total product. In this type of ratio, the first number is almost always in grams since most drugs are solids, even if they are suspended in solution. If the final product is a solid (or a semisolid like an ointment or cream), the second number is also in grams. If the final product is a liquid (like a solution or suspension), the second number represents milliliters. For example, an ointment that is 1:100 hydrocortisone contains 1 g of hydrocortisone per every 100 g of ointment. Epinephrine intravenous solution 1:1000 contains 1 g of epinephrine per every 1000 mL of solution.

Another common way of expressing drug concentration is by **percentage**. It is important to remember that percentages are defined as parts per hundred. For example, 2% = 2 parts per 100, or 2:100. This can also be written as a fraction, 2/100. Just like in ratios, the units associated with the numerator and the denominator of a percentage depend on if the ingredient and final product are solids or liquids.

If the ingredient is a solid and is in a solution, then the percentage can be expressed as **weight per volume**, or w/v. In this case, 2% would be 2 g per 100 mL. This is the most common percentage used in pharmacy practice. Some examples

TABLE MR-5. Summary of Drug Concentration by Percentage		
Weight per volume	w/v	g/100 mL
Weight per weight	w/w	g/100 g
Volume per volume	v/v	mL/100 mL

of w/v calculations are compounded intravenous solutions, oral suspensions, and ophthalmic and otic solutions. If the ingredient is a solid and the final product is a solid, then the percentage can be expressed as **weight per weight**, or w/w. In this case, 2% means 2 g per 100 g. An example of w/w percentages is when an active ingredient cream is mixed with other creams to make a final product. If the ingredient is a liquid and is in a solution, then the percentage can be expressed as **volume per volume**, or v/v. In this case, 2% means 2 mL per 100 mL. An example of v/v percentages is when oral solutions are mixed together to get a final compounded product. Table MR-5 lists the summary of drug concentrations by percentage.

It is often required to convert from a concentration expressed as a ratio or percentage to a concentration expressed in metric units. This can be done by first converting the concentration into a fraction, and then multiplying through your conversion factors as needed. Let us try a few examples.

Converting a Ratio Into a Metric Concentration

🔅 EXAMPLE
You receive a prescription written for an EpiPen (epinephrine 1:1000). The directions read, "inject 0.3 mL as needed for allergic reaction." How many milligrams will the patient inject with each dose?

First, convert the ratio 1:1000 into a fraction using metric units.

$$1:1000 = \frac{1 \text{ g of active drug (epinephrine)}}{1000 \text{ mL of injectable solution}}$$

Then use cross multiplication or the cancel out method to determine how many milligrams are in each 0.3-mL dose.

🔄 SOLUTION USING CROSS MULTIPLICATION
Remember to set up your proportion with like units in the numerator and like units in the denominator.

$$\frac{1 \text{ g}}{1000 \text{ mL}} = \frac{X \text{ g}}{0.3 \text{ mL}}$$

Cross multiply.

$$1 \text{ g} \times 0.3 = 1000 \times X \text{ g}$$

Divide.

$$0.3 \text{ g} \div 1000 = X$$

And solve.

$$X = 0.0003 \text{ g}$$

But wait! What unit of measure was your unknown variable (X) in your original proportion? Grams. What unit is the question asking you for? Milligrams. That means you need to do one more conversion. Again, this could be done using cross multiplication or the cancel out method. The cross-multiplication method is used as follows.

$$\frac{1000\ mg}{1\ g} = \frac{X\ mg}{0.0003\ g}$$

Cross multiply.

$1000 \times 0.0003 = 1 \times X$

Divide.

$0.3 \div 1 = X$

And solve.

$X = 0.3\ mg$

So, there is 0.3 mg of epinephrine in 0.3 mL of 1:1000 epinephrine injection.

💲 SOLUTION USING DIMENSIONAL ANALYSIS (CANCEL OUT METHOD)
First, convert the ratio 1:1000 into a fraction using metric units.

$$1:1000 = \frac{1\ g\ of\ active\ drug\ (epinephrine)}{1000\ mL\ of\ injectable\ solution}$$

Then set up your equation. Remember to set it up so that like units cancel out.

$$0.3\ \cancel{mL} \times \frac{1\ g}{1000\ \cancel{mL}} = 0.0003\ g$$

The unit milliliter cancels out, and you are left with grams.
Again, what unit of measure is the question asking you for? Milligrams. That means you need to do one more conversion. Again, this could be done using cross multiplication or the cancel out method. The cancel out method is used below.

$$0.0003\ \cancel{g} \times \frac{1000\ mg}{1\ \cancel{g}} = 0.3\ mg$$

So, there is 0.3 mg of epinephrine in 0.3 mL of 1:1000 epinephrine injection.

Converting a Percentage Into a Metric Concentration

📝 EXAMPLE
You have a stock bottle of 1% viscous lidocaine oral solution. How many grams of lidocaine are in each 30-mL bottle?

First, convert the percentage into a fraction using metric units.

$$1\% = \frac{1 \text{ g of active drug (lidocaine)}}{100 \text{ mL of solution}}$$

Then use cross multiplication or the cancel out method to determine how many grams of lidocaine are in each 30-mL bottle.

⊜ SOLUTION USING CROSS MULTIPLICATION

Remember to set up your proportion with like units in the numerator and like units in the denominator.

$$\frac{1 \text{ g}}{100 \text{ mL}} = \frac{X \text{ g}}{30 \text{ mL}}$$

Cross multiply.

$$1 \times 30 = 100 \times X$$

Divide.

$$30 \div 100 = X$$

And solve.

$$X = 0.3 \text{ g}$$

So, there is 0.3 g of lidocaine in a 30-mL bottle of 1% viscous lidocaine oral solution.

⊜ SOLUTION USING THE CANCEL OUT METHOD

First, convert the percentage into a fraction using metric units.

$$1\% = \frac{1 \text{ g of active drug (lidocaine)}}{100 \text{ mL of solution}}$$

Then set up your equation. Remember to set it up so that like units cancel out.

$$30 \; \cancel{\text{mL}} \times \frac{1 \text{ g}}{100 \; \cancel{\text{mL}}} = 0.3 \text{ g}$$

The unit milliliter cancels out, and you are left with grams.

So, there is 0.3 g of lidocaine in a 30-mL bottle of 1% viscous lidocaine oral solution.

Converting a Metric Concentration Into a Percentage

⊕ EXAMPLE

Dextrose 50% injectable syringes are on national shortage. As an IV room technician, you have been tasked with compounding a solution of dextrose from raw material. Before beginning compounding, you want to double-check the pharmacist's calculations. He has asked you to make a 500-mL bag of dextrose solution by adding 250 g of dextrose to 500-mL sterile water. Will this make a 50% injectable dextrose solution? Percentages are expressed in grams per 100 mL of solution. So, a 50% dextrose solution contains 50 g dextrose in 100 mL.

⊖ SOLUTION USING CROSS MULTIPLICATION

Remember to set up your proportion with like units in the numerator and like units in the denominator.

$$\frac{50 \text{ g}}{100 \text{ mL}} = \frac{X \text{ g}}{500 \text{ mL}}$$

Cross multiply.

$50 \times 500 = 100 \times X$

Divide.

$25{,}000 \div 100 = X$

And solve.

$X = 250 \text{ g}$

Yes, 250 g of dextrose in 500 mL of sterile water will create a 50% dextrose solution.

⊖ SOLUTION USING THE CANCEL OUT METHOD

Remember to set up your equation so that like units cancel out.

$$500 \text{ m\cancel{L}} \times \frac{50 \text{ g}}{100 \text{ m\cancel{L}}} = 250 \text{ g}$$

The unit milliliter cancels out, and you are left with grams.

Yes, 250 g of dextrose in 500 mL of sterile water will create a 50% dextrose solution.

QUICK QUIZ MR-4

1. An ointment contains 5% hydrocortisone. How many grams of hydrocortisone are in a 30-g tube of ointment?

2. There are 5 g of magnesium sulfate in each 10-mL injectable syringe. What is the percentage of this magnesium sulfate injectable solution?

3. How many milligrams are in 5 mL of epinephrine 1:10,000 solution?

4. How many milligrams of drug are in 15 mL of a 1:100 solution?

5. What is the concentration in mg/mL of sodium chloride 7% solution for inhalation?

CASE STUDY REVIEW

You are working as a pharmacy technician in a community retail pharmacy. While you are helping customers at the prescription drop-off window, a mother hands you the following prescription:

```
Patient: Anthony Miller
Address: 3333 Elm Street  Springfield, OH 43215

      Weight: 33 lb.        DOB: 1/1/2010
Amoxicillin oral suspension 125 mg/5 mL
25 mg/kg PO bid x 7d


Refills: 0                          D Smith, MD
                              Dr. David Smith, MD
```

Self-Assessment Questions
This chapter has reviewed all of the mathematical skills necessary to solve the 2 questions posed in the case at the beginning of the chapter.
- What dose has been prescribed for Anthony?
  - Dose prescribed: 375 mg twice daily
- How much liquid will be needed in order for him to take the medication as prescribed for 7 days?
  - How much liquid needed: 15 mL per dose × 2 doses per day × 7 days = 210 mL

More advanced pharmacy calculations will be introduced in later chapters. You must be familiar with the conversions defined in this chapter in order to swiftly and accurately solve pharmacy math problems. If you are comfortable with the math reviewed in this section, you will be able to easily apply it to any pharmacy calculation required on the pharmacy technician certification examination and in your career as a pharmacy technician.

CHAPTER SUMMARY

- Decimals should always be written with a leading zero (as in 0.25) and never with a trailing zero (as in .250). Proper writing of decimals helps minimize the risk of errors.
- Proportions are most often used to solve for an unknown value when given one value and the equivalent ratio. Cross multiplication is a mathematical technique used to solve for an unknown variable in a proportion.
- The first step in every pharmacy calculation is to convert all information to the same unit of measure. Since the metric system is the most common system used, it is essential to be able to quickly and accurately convert to and within the metric system.
- Concentrations of drugs are often expressed as ratios. When a concentration is written as a ratio, it is describing the amount of active drug per amount of total product. The first number in a ratio is always grams. The number after the colon in a ratio is either grams or milliliters, depending on the physical state of the product.
- Concentrations expressed in percentage are parts per hundred. Again the units are always grams or milliliters.

ANSWERS TO QUICK QUIZZES

Quick Quiz MR-1

1. 12/20, which reduces to $\frac{3}{4}$ **2.** 12/5, which reduces to $2\frac{2}{5}$ **3.** 2.4 **4.** 120/30 **5.** 4

Quick Quiz MR-2

1. 10 **2.** 24 **3.** 1 **4.** 9 **5.** 45 mL

Quick Quiz MR-3

1. 36.6°C **2.** 84 kg **3.** 0.117 mg **4.** 56.698, or round to 56.7 g **5.** 7.27 kg

Quick Quiz MR-4

1. 1.5 g **2.** 50% **3.** 0.5 mg **4.** 150 mg **5.** 70 mg/mL

CHAPTER QUESTIONS

1. You receive a prescription written for phenobarbital gr i. Which strength of phenobarbital tablets (in milligrams) should be dispensed?
a. 15 mg
b. 30 mg
c. 60 mg
d. 90 mg

2. The manufacturer produces dopamine intravenous solution in the concentration of 1600 µg/mL. How many milligrams of dopamine are in the 250-mL stock bag?
a. 160 mg
b. 400 mg
c. 800 mg
d. 1600 mg

3. What is the weight in pounds of a 14-kg child?
a. 6.4 lb
b. 12.6 lb
c. 26.4 lb
d. 30.8 lb

4. What number does the Roman numeral xlv represent?
a. 40
b. 45
c. 50
d. 55

5. How many teaspoons are in 4 tablespoons?
a. 1.3
b. 2
c. 8
d. 12

6. $\frac{15}{20} \times \frac{2}{3} =$
a. 17/23
b. 40/45
c. 45/40
d. 30/60

7. Express your answer to #6 as a decimal (round to 1 decimal place).
a. 0.7
b. 0.9
c. 1.1
d. 0.5

8. How many fluid ounces are there in 360 mL?
a. 8 fl oz
b. 12 fl oz
c. 16 fl oz
d. 36 fl oz

9. How many milligrams of clindamycin are in a 30-g tube of 1% clindamycin topical gel?
   a. 0.3 mg
   b. 30 mg
   c. 300 mg
   d. 3000 mg

10. How many milliliters does an 8-dram amber vial hold?
    a. 24 mL
    b. 32 mL
    c. 40 mL
    d. 80 mL

11. What types of drugs are typically expressed in milliequivalent?
    a. Insulin
    b. Narcotics
    c. Electrolytes
    d. Topical preparations

12. You receive an order for fentanyl 12 µg/h transdermal patch: replace patch every 72 hours. The physician is concerned about the potential for abuse and only wants you to dispense enough for 2 weeks. How many patches should you dispense?
    a. 4 patches
    b. 5 patches
    c. 6 patches
    d. 12 patches

13. You receive a prescription written as "ampicillin 0.5 g PO qid × 10 days." You only have ampicillin 250-mg capsules in stock. How many 250-mg capsules should you dispense?
    a. 40
    b. 60
    c. 80
    d. 160

14. A patient's total daily dose of diltiazem is 120 mg. The dose is to be divided q6h. How many milligrams of diltiazem should be given for each dose?
    a. 20 mg
    b. 30 mg
    c. 60 mg
    d. 480 mg

15. How many 30-mL individual prescriptions can you dispense from a 1-pt stock bottle?
    a. 16
    b. 32
    c. 50
    d. 100

16. Grains and drams are examples of measurements used in which system?
    a. Metric
    b. Apothecary
    c. Avoirdupois
    d. English

17. Express 25 as a Roman numeral.
    a. xxv
    b. vt
    c. xl
    d. vvvvv

18. The concentration of what type of product can be expressed in w/v percentage?
    a. Injectable solution
    b. Powder
    c. Topical ointment
    d. Tablets

19. How many milliliters are there in an 8-fl oz stock bottle of milk of magnesia?
    a. 120 mL
    b. 240 mL
    c. 360 mL
    d. 480 mL

20. What is the abbreviation for units (as in, insulin glargine 10 units qhs)?
    a. U
    b. u
    c. un
    d. Units should not be abbreviated

21. 23°C = _____°F
    a. −9
    b. −5
    c. 44.8
    d. 73.4

22. You receive a prescription for cephalexin 250 mg. The prescription states to dispense xiv. How many capsules should be dispensed?
    a. 7
    b. 14
    c. 28
    d. None

23. Tablespoon and teaspoon are examples of measurements used in which system?
    a. Metric
    b. Avoirdupois
    c. Intravenous
    d. Apothecary

24. Convert 560 µg to mg.
    a. 56,000 mg
    b. 5600 mg
    c. 5.6 mg
    d. 0.56 mg

25. How many milligrams of drug are in 20 mL of a 1:100 solution?
    a. 0.2 mg
    b. 2 mg
    c. 20 mg
    d. 200 mg

26. You receive a prescription written for phenobarbital gr 1/2. Which strength of phenobarbital tablets (in milligrams) should be dispensed?
    a. 15 mg
    b. 30 mg
    c. 60 mg
    d. 90 mg

27. The manufacturer produces dopamine intravenous solution in the concentration of 3200 µg/mL. How many milligrams of dopamine are in the 250-mL stock bag?
    a. 160 mg
    b. 400 mg
    c. 800 mg
    d. 1600 mg

28. What is the weight in pounds of a 12-kg child?
    a. 6.4 lb
    b. 12.6 lb
    c. 26.4 lb
    d. 30.8 lb

29. What number does the Roman numeral xl represent?
    a. 40
    b. 45
    c. 50
    d. 55

30. How many milliliters are in 3 tablespoons?
    a. 1.3 mL
    b. 3 mL
    c. 12 mL
    d. 15 mL

31. $\dfrac{10}{20} \times \dfrac{2}{3} =$
    a. 12/23
    b. 30/40
    c. 40/30
    d. 20/60

32. Express your answer to #31 as a decimal (round to 1 decimal place).
    a. 0.7
    b. 0.8
    c. 1.3
    d. 0.3

33. How many fluid ounces are in 480 mL?
    a. 8 fl oz
    b. 12 fl oz
    c. 16 fl oz
    d. 36 fl oz

34. A patient comes to your pharmacy needing help. She received a prescription from a pharmacy across town. Her prescription label says "Metoclopramide 5 mg/5 mL solution—take 10 mL every 8 hours." She does not know how to measure out 10 mL. How many teaspoons should you tell her to take per dose?
    a. 1.5
    b. 2
    c. 4
    d. This amount cannot be measured in teaspoons

35. How many milligrams of clindamycin are in a 60-g tube of 1% clindamycin topical gel?
    a. 0.6 mg
    b. 60 mg
    c. 600 mg
    d. 6000 mg

36. The concentration of what type of product is expressed in w/w percentage?
    a. Codeine sulfate oral solution
    b. Lidocaine topical ointment
    c. Digoxin injectable solution
    d. Amoxicillin oral suspension

37. How many milliliters does a 16-dram amber vial hold?
    a. 24 mL
    b. 32 mL
    c. 40 mL
    d. 80 mL

38. The strength of which of the following medications is expressed in milliequivalent?
    a. Insulin glargine
    b. Morphine sulfate
    c. Potassium chloride
    d. Tetracaine

39. You receive an order for fentanyl 12 µg/h transdermal patch: replace patch every 72 hours. The physician is concerned about the potential for abuse and only wants you to dispense enough for 1 week. How many patches should you dispense?
    a. 2 patches
    b. 3 patches
    c. 5 patches
    d. 7 patches

Use the following scenario for questions 40 to 44:

You are given a prescription for azithromycin 1% ophthalmic solution. The directions are to use a dose of 0.1 mL in the right eye twice daily for 2 days, then 0.1 mL in the right eye daily for an additional 7 days.

40. How many milligrams are in each dose of azithromycin 1% ophthalmic solution?
    a. 0.1 mg
    b. 1 mg
    c. 10 mg
    d. 100 mg

41. How many milligrams will the patient instill over the entire course of treatment?
    a. Not enough information
    b. 6 mg
    c. 9 mg
    d. 11 mg

42. Azithromycin 1% ophthalmic solution is available from the manufacturer in 2.5-mL bottles. How many doses will be in each bottle?
    a. 12 doses
    b. 13 doses
    c. 25 doses
    d. 30 doses

43. Will the 2.5-mL bottle be enough to last the entire course of treatment?
    a. Yes
    b. No
    c. Not enough information

44. The patient will not be able to measure out 0.1 mL to give himself each dose. How many drops should you tell the patient to instill in each eye in order to achieve the 0.1-mL dose?
    a. 1 drop
    b. 2 drops
    c. 3 drops
    d. 4 drops

45. $\dfrac{6}{7} \times \dfrac{3}{5} =$
    a. 30/21
    b. 9/12
    c. 35/18
    d. 18/35

46. Express your answer to #45 as a decimal (round to 2 decimal places).
    a. 1.43
    b. 0.75
    c. 1.94
    d. 0.51

47. You receive a prescription written as "ampicillin 0.5 g PO tid × 7 days." You only have ampicillin 250-mg capsules in stock. How many 250-mg capsules should you dispense?
    a. 24
    b. 42
    c. 84
    d. 168

48. In which unit of measure is a dose of insulin expressed?
    a. Milliequivalent
    b. Milligram
    c. Grains
    d. Units

49. A patient's total daily dose of diltiazem is 180 mg. The dose is to be divided q6h. How many milligrams of diltiazem should be given for each dose?
   a. 15 mg
   b. 45 mg
   c. 90 mg
   d. 180 mg

50. How many 60-mL individual prescriptions can you dispense from a 1-pt stock bottle?
   a. 8
   b. 16
   c. 32
   d. 60

Pharmacology for Technicians

CHAPTER
1

KNOWLEDGE AREAS

1.1 Generic and brand names of pharmaceuticals

1.2 Therapeutic equivalence

1.3 Drug interactions (ie, drug-disease, drug-drug, drug-dietary supplement, drug-OTC, drug-laboratory, drug-nutrient)

1.4 Strengths or dose, dosage forms, physical appearance, routes of administration, and duration of drug therapy

1.5 Common and severe side or adverse effects, allergies, and therapeutic contraindications associated with medications

1.6 Dosage and indication of legend, over-the-counter (OTC) medications, herbal and dietary supplements

KEY TERMS

Adverse drug reaction (ADR): Unintended effect of a medication

Anaphylaxis: Life-threatening allergic reaction

Angina: Chest pain

Antipyretic: Medications that decrease fever

Arrhythmia: Abnormal heart beat

Atrial fibrillation or flutter: Irregular, rapid heart beat

Candidiasis: Yeast infection

Conjunctivitis: Eye infection

Disulfiram reaction: Nausea, vomiting, headache

Diuresis: Urine production

Electrocardiogram: Monitors electrical activity of the heart

Epistaxis: Nose bleed

Extrapyramidal symptoms: Involuntary movements

Gastroparesis: Delayed gastric emptying

Gingival hypertrophy: Increased size of the gum encircling the teeth

Hemolytic anemia: Abnormal breakdown of red blood cells

Hepatotoxicity: Liver toxicity

Hypertrichosis: Abnormal amount of hair growth on the body

Malaise: Vague feeling of body discomfort

Mechanism of action (MOA): How a medication works in the body

Miosis: Pupil constriction

Myopathy: Muscular weakness

Narcolepsy: Excessive sleepiness and daytime sleep attacks

Otitis media: Ear infection

Paresthesia: Abnormal skin sensation (burning, pricking, numbness)

Periodontitis: Inflammation and infection of the ligaments and bones that support the teeth

Phototoxicity: Inflammatory skin reaction from exposure to sunlight

Prophylaxis: Prevention

Pulmonary embolism: Thrombosis (clot) in lung

Rosacea: Chronic skin condition causing facial redness and skin sores

Sleep apnea: Abnormal pauses in breathing during sleep

Somnolence: Drowsiness or sleepiness

Syncope: Fainting

Teratogen: Any substance causing fetal malformation

Trigeminal neuralgia: Intense pain on the face

Urticaria: Hives

CASE STUDY

You are assisting a pharmacist with a patient in the emergency room (ER). The patient's neighbor called 911 after finding her passed out in her kitchen. The patient is a 76-year-old woman with an unknown past medical history. The emergency medical service (EMS) first responders were able to bring the patient's medication bottles with her. The labels on the bottles include the following:

- Lisinopril 10 mg—Take 1 tablet by mouth daily—#30
- Alprazolam 1 mg—Take 1 tablet by mouth twice daily as needed—#60
- Levothyroxine 88 µg—Take 1 tablet by mouth daily—#30
- Oxycontin 10 mg—Take 1 tablet by mouth twice daily—#60

Self-Assessment Questions
- What are the indications for the medications taken by the patient?
- Could any of the medications taken cause her to be sedated?
- What are the brand and generic names for the medications taken by the patient?
- Are there any drug interactions between the patient's medications?

INTRODUCTION

In order to successfully practice as a pharmacy technician, it is important to understand pharmacology, or how medications work in the body. Included in this chapter are the brand and generic names of medications, indication, common adverse effects and drug interactions, as well as dosage forms and routes of administration. The chapter is broken down by drug category, the top 200 drugs are bolded throughout the chapter, and examples of other medications within each class.

PHARMACOLOGY

Pharmacology is the study of drugs, and is divided into 2 main subdivisions: pharmacokinetics and pharmacodynamics. Pharmacokinetics is the study of the 4 drug processes of absorption, distribution, metabolism, and excretion, which is commonly referred to as the ADME process. Pharmacodynamics involves the effect of the drug at the site of action within the body, based on the drug concentration.

DRUG CLASSIFICATION

Drugs are classified in different ways, based on the mechanism of action, receptor acted upon, body system affected, or by disorder. Drugs can also be classified based on Drug Enforcement Administration (DEA) schedule or pregnancy category. This chapter will review medications in classes based on the part of the body affected.

DRUG INTERACTIONS

A drug interaction occurs when a drug affects the activity of another drug when given together. There are multiple mechanisms for which this can occur, and it has the potential to increase or decrease the action of the drug. Examples of potential interactions include drug-disease, drug-dietary supplement, drug-OTC, drug-laboratory, and drug-nutrient interactions (Table 1-1).

The 3 primary mechanisms by which interactions occur include pharmaceutical, pharmacokinetic, and pharmacodynamic.

Pharmaceutical

Drug compatibility: Inactivation of medications when compounds are physically mixed together prior to administration.

Example: Ceftriaxone (Rocephin) and azithromycin (Zithromax) cannot be run through the same intravenous (IV) line as they are incompatible.

TABLE 1-1. **Drug Interactions**		
Interaction	*Description*	*Example*
Drug-disease	A medication interacts with a disease or condition	A patient with high blood pressure takes a decongestant (i.e. Pseudoephedrine) and it causes an additional increase in blood pressure
Drug-dietary supplement	An herbal or dietary supplement interacts with a prescription drug	St. John's wort can interact with oral contraceptives, making them less effective, causing breakthrough bleeding or unplanned pregnancy
Drug-OTC	An OTC medication can interact with a medication, increasing or decreasing its effects	Antacids can bind fluroquinolones and decrease their absorption and effectiveness.
Drug-laboratory	A drug may affect concentrations of specific laboratory values obtained, requiring additional testing	Metronidazole (Flagyl) can interfere with specific enzyme values, causing falsely low results
Drug-nutrient	A drug may affect the levels of certain nutrients in the body	Phenytoin (Dilantin), an anticonvulsive medication, can decrease vitamin D, vitamin K, and folic acid levels in the body after long-term use

Drug stability: Some medications are only stable in certain environmental situations.

Example: Insulin glargine (Lantus) is only stable for 28 days out of the refrigerator.

Pharmacokinetic

Absorption: Alteration in the amount of medication distributed through the stomach lining.

Example: Antacids (ie, calcium carbonate) decrease the absorption of quinolone (ie, levofloxacin, ciprofloxacin, etc) antibiotics, thus decreasing the effectiveness of the antibiotics.

Distribution: Alteration in the amount of medication flowing throughout the body.

Metabolism: Modification in the rate of metabolism throughout the body. This process usually occurs in the liver.

Example: Fluconazole decreases the metabolism of warfarin, which could lead to higher warfarin levels causing bleeding.

Elimination: Variation in the excretion of the drug from the body. This process usually occurs via the kidneys.

Example: Ibuprofen can decrease renal function, which could lead to increased lithium levels.

Pharmacodynamic

Antagonism: One medication works against another medication to prevent its action.

Example: β Blockers (ie, metoprolol) and β agonists (ie, albuterol) work at the same receptor site. Using them together may offset their action.

Potentiation: The combination of 2 medications increases the effect or length of effect.

Example: Opiates and benzodiazepines can both cause sedation. When given together, a patient may become comatose.

DRUG-FOOD INTERACTIONS

Foods can interact with medications at many stages. The most common effect is for food to interfere with drug absorption making it less effective. Food can also affect how a drug is utilized, as well as the excretion of medications. Depending on the drug, some should be taken with food and others without food.

Alcohol can also change the absorption and metabolism of medications. Additionally, alcohol itself can be altered by medications, leading to adverse effects for patients.

Grapefruit juice contains a compound not found in other citrus juices that increases the absorption of some medications. Several medications are metabolized in the small intestine by an enzyme, Cytochrome P450. Grape fruit juice inhibits the Cytochrome P450 enzyme, thus increasing the amount of medication absorbed. The increased absorption can enhance the effects and increase the risk of adverse effects of certain medications such as the statin drugs, calcium channel blockers, levothyroxine, and certain antiarrhythmic drugs.

PREGNANCY CATEGORY

The Food and Drug Administration (FDA) has developed 5 categories to indicate the potential of a drug to cause birth defects if taken during pregnancy (Table 1-2). These categories are based on risk to the fetus and available data.

DOSAGE FORMS

Medications are manufactured in many different dosage forms depending on the characteristics of the drug itself. There are many factors that go into deciding which dosage form should be chosen, such as route of administration, diagnosis of the patient, and availability of the medication desired.

Dosage forms can be divided into 3 different categories of liquids, semisolids, and solids.

★ *TECH ALERT: Category X medications are contraindicated in pregnancy. Examples of category X medications include: warfarin, statins, and isotretinoin.*

TABLE 1-2. **FDA Pregnancy Categories**	
Category	Definition
A	Adequate and well-controlled human studies have failed to demonstrate a risk to the fetus in the first trimester of pregnancy (and there is no evidence of risk in later trimesters).
B	Animal reproduction studies have failed to demonstrate a risk to the fetus and there are no adequate and well-controlled studies in pregnant women *or* animal studies have shown an adverse effect, but adequate and well-controlled studies in pregnant women have failed to demonstrate a risk to the fetus in any trimester.
C	Animal reproduction studies have shown an adverse effect on the fetus and there are no adequate and well-controlled studies in humans, but potential benefits may warrant use of the drug in pregnant women despite potential risks.
D	There is positive evidence of human fetal risk based on adverse reaction data from investigational or marketing experience or studies in humans, but potential benefits may warrant use of the drug in pregnant women despite potential risks.
X	Studies in animals or humans have demonstrated fetal abnormalities and/or there is positive evidence of human fetal risk based on adverse reaction data from investigational or marketing experience, and the risks involved in use of the drug in pregnant women clearly outweigh potential benefits. Category X medications are contraindicated in pregnancy.

Liquids

Elixir: Similar to a syrup, but also contains a high percentage of alcohol.

Emulsion: A mixture of 2 unblendable liquids (eg, water and oil). An emulsifying agent allows the 2 liquids to blend together.

Enema: A solution that is administered rectally.

Inhalant solution: A medication that is administered to the lungs via the mouth or nose. The solution can be delivered via a metered-dose inhaler (MDI) or nebulizer.

Lotion: Similar to a cream, however, it contains more water and is thinner.

Solution: Contains a drug that is completely dissolves into a liquid (eg, elixir, syrup).

Spray: A medication suspended in solution that is dispensed from a container into fine particles. It is usually applied locally (eg, nasal, topically).

Suspension: Solid particles dissolved into a liquid. It can be oral, injectable, or topical. Oral suspensions should be adequately mixed by being shaken well prior to administration.

Syrup: A sweetened liquid that contains the medication, sugar, and flavoring.

Semisolids

Cream: Contains medications in a base that is part oil and water. Creams may be applied topically or inserted rectally or vaginally.

Inhalant powder: Finely ground medication that is inhaled into the lungs.

Ointment: Contains medication in an oil base such as petroleum jelly. It is typically used topically and acts as water repellant.

Powder: Finely ground medication that can be administered internally or externally.

Suppository: Solid dosage form inserted into the rectum, vagina, or urethra.

Solids

Caplet: A tablet that is in the shape of an oval, similar to that of a capsule, to facilitate swallowing.

Capsule: A hard or soft gelatin container which holds active and inactive ingredients. Capsules are typically oval, but can vary in shape and color. The contents of the capsules can be powder, liquid, or granules.

Lozenge or Troche: A solid dosage form that contains an active ingredient in a flavored base. They are not meant to be swallowed, but to dissolve in the mouth slowly. The active ingredient in the lozenge or troche usually is indicated for a local infection in the mouth or throat.

Patch: A transdermal medication that is to be released over a specific period of time. The medication is absorbed through the skin and absorbed into the bloodstream.

Tablet: A molded or pressed powder of active and inactive ingredients. Tablets are manufactured in various sizes, shapes, and colors. They are most commonly administered orally, but can also be given rectally, vaginally, sublingually (under the tongue), or buccally (between the cheek and gum). Some medications are available in chewable tablets which may be the drug form of choice for who are unable to swallow tablets, such as children and elderly. Enteric-coated tablets have a hard-shell coating protect the drug from acid in the stomach. To preserve the integrity of the enteric-coated tablet, they should not be crushed or split.

ROUTES OF ADMINISTRATION

Drugs are administered to patients using the specific routes indicated on the drug label such as oral or intravenous. Some drugs are available in different forms. For example, an antibiotic may be available in both tablet and liquid forms. The various routes of administration are discussed below (Figure 1-1):

Inhalation (IH): Drugs are transformed into tiny droplets and inhaled through the mouth or nose so that they can be deposited into the lungs. The amount of absorption depends on where the drug deposits in the lungs.

Intramuscular (IM): A long needle is inserted into the muscle, which allows a large volume of drug to be administered. The absorption of the drug into the bloodstream is dependent on the drug properties and the muscle chosen for injection.

Intrathecal (IT): A needle is inserted into spinal canal in the lower spine. This route allows the drug to quickly produce effects on the spinal cord and brain. For example, morphine can be administered intrathecally to quickly alleviate pain during childbirth.

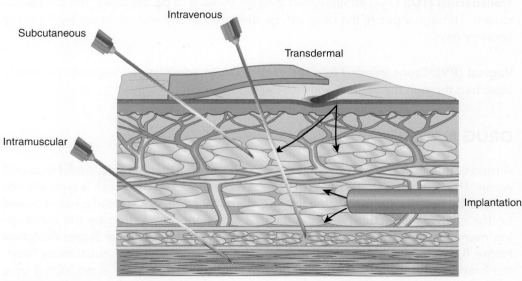

FIGURE 1-1 Routes of administration.

Intravenous (IV): A needle is directly inserted into a vein. A sterile solution is administered either as a single dose or continuous infusion. The drug is immediately carried to the bloodstream with a quick onset of action.

Nasal (Nsl): Drugs are transformed into tiny droplets and then administered into the nose. The drug is absorbed through the thin mucous membrane in the nose and quickly enters the bloodstream.

Ocular (OD, OS, OU): Drugs may be mixed with inactive substances to make a liquid, gel, or ointment, so that they can be applied to the eye. Most ophthalmic drugs are used for their local effects for eye disorders. (OD = right eye, OS = left eye, OU = both eyes)

★ TECH ALERT: Caution should be used if patients need to undergo an MRI while wearing a patch. There is potential for burns to occur.

Oral (PO): Most common route of administration. The medication is usually absorbed in the gastrointestinal (GI) tract and passes through the intestine wall and ultimately transported to the target site. Food and other drugs may affect the absorption, thus some drugs are taken with food, others on an empty stomach, and some drugs cannot be taken together. Oral administration also requires a person to be able to physically take the medication by mouth.

Rectal (PR): Drugs that are inserted into the rectum are readily absorbed. This is an alternate route for patients who are unable to swallow, nauseated, or have eating restrictions.

Subcutaneous (Sub-Q/SC): A short needle is inserted into the fatty tissue directly below the skin. Drugs are then slowly absorbed into the bloodstream. Common drugs administered subcutaneously include insulin and vaccines.

Sublingual (SL): Drugs placed under the tongue. This allows them to be rapidly absorbed to the bloodstream and bypass the gastrointestinal system. Only a few drugs are effective in this route, such as nitroglycerin.

Topical (Top): Drugs applied to the surface of the skin. The dosage form (ie, ointment, cream, lotion) determines the amount of drug that is absorbed and how quickly it is absorbed.

Transdermal (TD): Drug administered through the skin to be delivered into the bloodstream. Through a patch, the drug can be delivered slowly and continuously for many hours or days.

Vaginal (PV): Drugs inserted into the vagina. Drugs administered vaginally are slowly absorbed through the vaginal wall into the bloodstream.

DRUG NAMES

A medication may have up to 3 different names: chemical, generic, trade or brand name. The first name that a drug receives is its chemical name, which is typically not utilized by health care professionals. The chemical name is a scientific name based on the chemical structure. A generic name is assigned to a drug by the developing manufacturer. The generic name is also known as the United States Adopted Name (USAN), and helps to identify the active pharmaceutical substance. Next, the brand name is assigned by the manufacturer, and this name is protected by a patent, which means this company has exclusive rights to use it, and it is typically

TABLE 1-3. Examples of Chemical, Generic, and Brand Names	
Chemical name	(RS)-2-(4-(2-methylpropyl)phenyl)propanoic acid
Generic name	Ibuprofen
Brand or trade name	Advil, Motrin

designated with a registered trademark sign ®. A generic drug can have more than one brand name, as indicated in Table 1-3.

THERAPEUTIC EQUIVALENCE

The US FDA classifies drug products as therapeutically equivalent if the substituted product will have the same clinical and safety profile as the prescribed product. Therapeutically equivalent products must contain the same active ingredient, be the same dosage form, have the same route of administration, and be the same strength. Drugs are then assigned therapeutic equivalence codes which can be found in FDA, *The Orange Book*.

The Orange Book designates every drug with a 2-letter code, either A or B. The "A" code means that the drug is the therapeutic equivalent of the reference drug, for which it can be substituted. The "B" code means that drug is not therapeutically equivalent to the reference drug. The second letter (A, B, C, D, E, N, O, P, R, S, T, or X) provides information about the dosage form or potential bioequivalence problems. The "AB" code is the most commonly seen designation for equivalent drugs. Some "AB" products may have numbers behind them (1, 2, etc) which indicates that there is more than one product that is therapeutically equivalent (Table 1-4).

ANTIMICROBIALS

Microorganisms include bacteria, viruses, fungus, and protozoa. While most microorganisms are not harmful, some can lead to infection. Signs and symptoms of infection include increased heart rate (tachycardia), respiratory rate (tachypnea), temperature (fever), and white blood cells (leukocytosis).

There are many places in the body that bacteria can invade and cause infection. The location of the infection helps to guide antimicrobial therapy (Table 1-5).

Antimicrobials are any substance that kills or inhibits the growth of a microorganism, but causes little or no damage to the host. Antimicrobials include agents that act on all types of microorganisms, including bacteria (antibacterial/antibiotic), viruses (antiviral), fungus (antifungal), and protozoa (antiprotozoal).

★ *TECH ALERT: The term antibiotic is used interchangeably with antibacterial.*

ANTIBIOTICS

Antibiotics target bacteria in the body. Bacteria have only one cell and a cell wall which contains the proteins, DNA, and fluid needed for survival. The identification of bacteria via their bacterial shape (morphology) can help aid in the early diagnosis of the cause of infection. (Table 1-6) These bacteria can be found as single cells or grouped together. If several bacterial cells group together in a cluster, they are identified as *Staphylococcus*. Bacterial cells that form a chain are identified as *Streptococci*.

TABLE 1-4. Therapeutic Equivalence Codes and Their Descriptions

FDA Code	Description
A codes	**Drug product is therapeutically equivalent to the reference drug**
AA	Drugs in conventional dosage forms not presenting bioequivalence problems
AB	Drugs proven to meet the necessary bioequivalence requirement
AN	Solutions and powders for aerosolization that are therapeutically equivalent
AO	Injectable oil solutions that are therapeutically equivalent
AP	Injectable aqueous solutions that are therapeutically equivalent
AT	Topical products that are therapeutically equivalent
B codes	**Drug product is not therapeutically equivalent to the reference drug**
BC	Extended-release dosage form that is not therapeutically equivalent to the reference drug
BD	Active ingredients and dosage forms with documented bioequivalence problems
BE	Delayed-release oral dosage forms with documented bioequivalence problems
BN	Aerosol-nebulizer drug delivery systems with documented bioequivalence problems
BP	Active ingredients and dosage forms with potential bioequivalence problems
BR	Suppositories or enemas with bioequivalence problems
BS	Products having drug standard deficiencies
BT	Topical products with bioequivalence problems
BX	Drugs for which there is insufficient information to determine therapeutic equivalence

TABLE 1-5. Infection Location and Common Types

Location	Type	Treatment
Skin	**Cellulitis:** Bacterial skin infection with typical symptoms of redness, hot to touch, and painful. It may rapidly progress to serious infection.	Penicillin or cephalosporin antibiotics
Ear	**Otitis media:** Bacterial ear infection seen in young children. Typical symptoms are fever and ear pain.	Penicillin or cephalosporin antibiotics
Lung	**Pneumonia:** Bacterial or viral lung infection with typical symptoms of cough, chest pain, fever, and shortness of breath.	Varies from no antibiotics, penicillin, cephalosporin, macrolides, or fluoroquinolones
Kidney	**Urinary tract infection:** Bacterial infection of bladder or kidneys, occurring more commonly in women. Symptoms include painful urination, fever, and frequent urination.	Varies from no antibiotics, penicillin, cephalosporin, fluoroquinolones, sulfamethoxazole/trimethoprim, or nitrofurantoin
Nose and mouth	**Influenza:** Viral infection that presents with chills, fever, runny nose, and coughing. May be prevented with influenza vaccination.	Varies from symptomatic to antiviral. Antibiotics are not indicated.

TABLE 1-6. Morphology of Bacteria	
Shape	*Bacteria type*
Round	Cocci
Rod-like	Bacilli
Spiral	Spirochete

Antibiotics work by targeting the bacteria cell through different mechanism of actions (Figure 1-2). Some may break down the cell wall to destroy the bacteria, while others inhibit the cell from replicating. There are 2 basic type of antibiotics—those that work by killing the bacterial cell or bactericidal, and those that inhibit bacterial growth, or bacteriostatic.

Antibiotic resistance occurs when an antibiotic is no longer able to kill or stop the growth of bacteria. Overuse of antibiotics is one common reason antibiotic resistance is occurring more frequently. Due to bacterial resistance, patients often need more than one antibiotic is needed to kill the bacteria. Bacterial resistance can also occur when patients do not take their medications appropriately. Patients should be advised to finish their entire course of antibiotics. Even thought they may feel better, the antibiotic is still working against the bacteria.

Antibiotics have many drug interactions. Most antibiotics will decrease the effectiveness of oral contraceptives potentially leading to pregnancy. Patients should be advised to use an alternate form of birth control. Antibiotics can also increase the action of warfarin, thus international normalized ratios (INRs) will needs to be monitored closely. An INR is a laboratory test that measures the clotting time of the blood.

★ *TECH ALERT: Patients should be advised to finish their entire course of antibiotics. Even though they may feel better, the antibiotic is still working against the bacteria.*

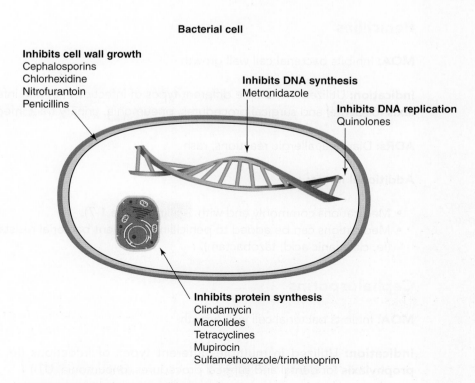

FIGURE 1-2 Antibiotic mechanism of action.

TABLE 1-7. Examples of Penicillins

Generic	Brand	Form	Strengths
Amoxicillin	**Amoxil, Moxatag**	**Capsule**	**250 mg, 500 mg**
		Suspension	**125 mg/5 mL, 200 mg/5 mL, 250 mg/5 mL, 400 mg/5 mL**
		Tablet	**500 mg, 875 mg**
		Chewable	**125 mg, 200 mg, 250 mg, 400 mg**
		Tablet, XR	**775 mg**
Amoxicillin/Clavulanate	**Augmentin**	**Suspension**	**125 mg/5 mL, 200 mg/5 mL, 250 mg/5 mL, 400 mg/5 mL, 600 mg/5 mL**
		Tablet	**250 mg, 500 mg, 875 mg**
		Chewable	**200 mg, 400 mg**
		Tablet, XR	**1000 mg**
Ampicillin	Principen	Capsule	250 mg, 500 mg
		Injection	125 mg, 250 mg, 500 mg, 1 g, 2 g, 10 g
		Suspension	125 mg/5 mL, 250 mg/5 mL
Penicillin V Potassium	**Pen VK**	**Suspension**	**125 mg/5 mL, 250 mg/5 mL**
		Tablet	**250 mg, 500 mg**
Piperacillin/Tazobactam	Zosyn	Injection	2.25 g, 3.375 g, 4.5 g, 40.5 g

Penicillins

MOA: Inhibits bacterial cell wall growth

Indication: Utilized in multiple different types of infections (ie, skin infections, **prophylaxis** for dental and surgical procedures, pneumonia, urinary tract infection [UTI])

ADRs: Diarrhea, allergic reactions, rash

Additional notes:

TECH ALERT: The top 200 drugs are listed in bold throughout the chapter.

- Medications commonly end with "-cillin" (Table 1-7).
- Medications can be added to penicillin to prevent bacterial resistance to penicillin (ie, clavulanic acid, tazobactam).

Cephalosporins

MOA: Inhibits bacterial cell wall growth

Indication: Utilized in multiple different types of infections (ie, skin infections, **prophylaxis** for dental and surgical procedures, pneumonia, UTI)

ADRs: Diarrhea, allergic reactions, rash

TABLE 1-8. Examples of Cephalosporins

Generic	Brand	Form	Strengths
Cefazolin	Ancef	Injection	500 mg, 1 g, 2 g, 10 g, 20 g, 300 g
Cefdinir	**Omnicef**	**Capsule**	**300 mg**
		Suspension	**125 mg/5 mL, 250 mg/5 mL**
Ceftriaxone	Rocephin	Injection	250 mg, 500 mg, 1 g, 2 g, 10 g
Cephalexin	**Keflex**	**Capsule**	**250 mg, 500 mg**
		Tablet	**250 mg, 500 mg**
		Suspension	**125 mg/5 mL, 250 mg/5 mL**

Additional notes:

- Medications commonly start with "ceph-" or "cef-" (Table 1-8).
- Cephalosporins are structurally similar to penicillins, thus an allergic reaction can occur if a patient is taking a cephalosporin and are allergic to penicillin.

*★ TECH ALERT: Patients with **anaphylaxis** to medications or food should wear a Medical-Alert Bracelet and carry an epinephrine Pen (Epi-Pen).*

Macrolides

MOA: Prevent bacteria growth by inhibiting protein synthesis

Indications: Otitis media, pneumonia, sexually transmitted disease

ADRs: Diarrhea, gastrointestinal upset, nausea

Additional notes:

- Medications have a common ending of "-mycin" (Table 1-9).
- Clarithromycin can leave a metallic taste in the mouth.
- Azithromycin is usually administered for 3 to 5 days, but lasts in the body twice as long.

TABLE 1-9. Examples of Macrolides

Generic	Brand	Form	Strengths
Azithromycin	**Zithromax, Zmax**	**Injection**	**500 mg**
		Suspension	**100 mg/5 mL, 200 mg/5 mL, 2 g/60 mL (XR)**
		Tablet	**250 mg, 500 mg, 600 mg**
Clarithromycin	**Biaxin**	**Suspension**	**125 mg/5 mL, 250 mg/5 mL**
		Tablet	**250 mg, 500 mg**
		Tablet, XR	**500 mg**
Erythromycin base	Ery-Tab, PCE	Coated tab	333 mg, 500 mg
		Tablet	250 mg, 500 mg
		Capsule, XR	250 mg
		Tablet, XR	250 mg, 333 mg, 500 mg
Erythromycin ethylsuccinate	EES, EryPed	Suspension	200 mg/5 mL, 400 mg/5 mL
		Tablet	400 mg
Erythromycin lactobionate	Erythrocin Lactobionate	Injection	500 mg

TABLE 1-10. Examples of Fluoroquinolones			
Generic	*Brand*	*Form*	*Strengths*
Ciprofloxacin	**Cipro**	**Injection**	**200 mg/100 mL, 400 mg/200 mL**
		Suspension	**250 mg/5 mL, 500 mg/5 mL**
		Tablet	**100 mg, 250 mg, 500 mg, 750 mg**
		Tablet, XR	**500 mg, 1000 mg**
Levofloxacin	**Levaquin**	**Injection**	**250 mg/50 mL, 500 mg/100 mL, 750 mg/150 mL**
		Solution	**25 mg/mL**
		Tablet	**250 mg, 500 mg, 750 mg**
Moxifloxacin	Avelox	Injection	400 mg/250 mL
		Tablet	400 mg

★ *TECH ALERT: The common cold is caused by a virus and should not be treated with antibiotics. Responsible antibiotic use helps prevent super-infections resistant to medications.*

Fluoroquinolones

MOA: Prevent bacteria growth by inhibiting protein replication

Indication: Utilized in multiple different types of infections (ie, abdominal infections, skin infections, pneumonia, sinusitis, UTI)

ADRs: Diarrhea, gastrointestinal upset, nausea, dizziness

Additional notes:

★ *TECH ALERT: A black box warning is the most serious warning from the FDA. It is a serious or life-threatening adverse effect.*

- Medications have a common ending of "-oxacin" (Table 1-10).
- Administer quinolones either 2 hours before or 6 hours after calcium (including dairy products), iron, or zinc.
- There have been reports of tendon inflammation or rupture with quinolones, thus they should not be used in children and have a black box warning for this use.

Tetracyclines

MOA: Inhibit protein synthesis within cell wall

Indications: Acne, bronchitis, malaria, **periodontitis**, pneumonia, **rosacea**, sexually transmitted diseases

ADRs: Gastrointestinal upset, **phototoxicity**

Additional notes:

- Medications have a common ending of "-cycline" (Table 1-11).
- Enters developing bone and teeth causing weakness, thus should be avoided in children and pregnant women.
- Tetracycline should be taken on an empty stomach and antacids should be avoided. Minocycline and doxycycline can be taken without regards to meals or antacids.

TABLE 1-11. Examples of Tetracyclines

Generic	Brand	Form	Strengths
Doxycycline	Adoxa, Doryx, Monodox, Vibramycin	Capsule	20 mg, 40 mg, 50 mg, 100 mg, 150mg
		Injection	100 mg
		Suspension	25 mg/5 mL
		Tablet	20 mg, 50 mg, 75 mg, 100 mg, 150 mg
		XR Tablet	75 mg, 100 mg, 150 mg, 200 mg
Minocycline	**Minocin, Dynacin, Solodyn**	**Capsule**	**50 mg, 75 mg, 100 mg**
		Injection	**100 mg**
		Tablet	**50 mg, 75 mg, 100 mg**
		Tablet, XR	**45 mg, 55 mg, 65 mg, 80 mg, 90 mg, 105 mg, 115 mg, 135 mg**
Tetracycline	Sumycin	Capsule	250 mg, 500 mg

Other Top 200 Antibiotics

CHLORHEXIDINE GLUCONATE

MOA: Interrupts bacterial cell wall production

Indications: Periodontitis (mouth infection), skin cleanser (Table 1-12)

TABLE 1-12. Other Top 200 Antibiotics

Generic	Brand	Form	Strengths
Chlorhexidine gluconate	**ChloraPrep, Chlorascrub, Hibiclens, Peridex, Periogard**	**Liquid, oral**	**0.12%**
			2%, 4%
		Liquid, topical	
Clindamycin	**Cleocin**	**Capsule**	**75 mg, 150 mg, 300 mg**
		Injection	**150 mg/1 mL**
		Suspension	**75 mg/5 mL**
Metronidazole	**Flagyl**	**Capsule**	**375 mg**
		Injection	**500 mg/100 mL**
		Tablet	**250 mg, 500 mg**
		Tablet, XR	**750 mg**
Mupirocin	**Bactroban, Centany**	**Cream**	**2%**
		Ointment	**2%**
Nitrofurantoin	**Macrodantin, Macrobid, Furadantin**	**Capsule**	**25 mg, 50 mg, 100 mg**
		Suspension	**25 mg/5 mL**
Sulfamethoxazole/ trimethoprim	**Bactrim, Septra**	**Injection**	**80-16 mg/1 mL**
		Suspension	**200-40 mg/5 mL**
		Tablet	**400-80 mg (SS), 800-160 mg (DS)**

DS, double strength; SS, single strength.

ADRs

- Oral: Increased tartar on teeth, staining of teeth, taste changes
- Topical: Dryness, skin irritation

Additional notes:

- Patients should use chlorhexidine after brushing teeth.
- Caution patient not to swallow chlorhexidine and not to eat for 2 to 3 hours after treatment.

CLINDAMYCIN

MOA: Inhibits bacterial growth by preventing formation

Indications: Pneumonia, skin infections, acne (topical), bacterial vaginosis (intravaginal)

ADRs: Nausea, vomiting, diarrhea

METRONIDAZOLE

MOA: Destroys bacterial and protozoa DNA

Indications: Intra-abdominal infections, *Clostridium difficile*, sexually transmitted diseases

ADRs: Nausea, metallic taste, urine discoloration (brown or black)

Additional note:

- Patients must avoid all alcohol when taking metronidazole. The combination can lead to a **disulfiram reaction** (flushing, headache, nausea, vomiting, sweating).

NITROFURANTOIN

MOA: Inhibits bacterial metabolism and cell wall synthesis

Indication: Treatment and prevention of UTIs

ADRs: Gastrointestinal upset, headache, urine discoloration (orange or brown)

Additional notes:

- Use should be avoided in pregnancy at term (38-42 weeks) due to possibility of **hemolytic anemia**.
- Therapeutic concentrations are not attained in patients with renal impairment.
- Macrobid is taken 2 times per day; Macrodantin is taken 4 times per day.

MUPIROCIN

MOA: Binds to bacterial inhibiting replication

Indication: Skin infections

ADRs: Rare

SULFAMETHOXAZOLE/TRIMETHOPRIM

MOA: Inhibits bacterial growth by preventing replication

Indications: Pneumonia, skin infections, UTIs

ADRs: Rash, **phototoxicity**, kidney failure

ANTIFUNGALS

Just like bacteria, most fungi are not harmful; although, some may be toxic. Typically, fungal infections are mild topical infections on the skin; however, patients with decreased immune systems (immunocompromised) may acquire a systemic fungal infection which is a severe illness. Common types of fungal infections are as follows:

- *Candida*: Type of yeast (fungi)
- Onychomycosis: Fungal infection of the nail
- Tinea capitis: Fungal infection of the neck and scalp
- Tinea corporis: Fungal infection of body—arms, legs, and shoulders
- Tinea cruris (jock itch): Fungal infection of the groin
- Tinea pedis (athlete's foot): Fungal infection of the foot

Antifungal Medications

MOA: Inhibit fungal formation

Indications: Candidiasis (esophageal, oral, systemic, urinary tract, vaginal), dermatitis

ADRs: Gastrointestinal upset, headache

Additional notes:

- Medications have a common ending of "-azole" (Table 1-13).
- High potential for drug interactions which could lead to **arrhythmias** and cardiac death.

TABLE 1-13. **Examples of Antifungals**			
Generic	*Brand*	*Form*	*Strengths*
Fluconazole	**Diflucan**	**Injection**	**100 mg, 200 mg, 400 mg**
		Suspension	**10 mg/mL, 40 mg/mL**
		Tablet	**50 mg, 100 mg, 150 mg, 200 mg**
Ketoconazole topical	**Extina, Nizoral, Xolegel**	**Foam**	**2%**
		Cream	**2%**
		Gel	**2%**
		Shampoo	**1%, 2%**

ANTIVIRALS

A virus is a simple cell that has only a protein coat and DNA or RNA. It is unable to replicate unless it is inside of another living cell, and can utilize this host cell's machinery for producing the viral DNA or RNA. Once inside of a cell, viruses multiply and kill the living cell. This makes it difficult to treat a viral infection because the virus is utilizing the body's own cells for replication.

Antibiotics do not work for viral infections, so it is important that they are not prescribed for illnesses of viral origin. Viruses can cause the common cold, influenza, herpes, and hepatitis.

Antiviral Medications

MOA: Inhibit viral replication

Indication: Herpes infection

ADRs: Gastrointestinal upset, injection site pain, **malaise**, renal failure

Additional notes:

- Medications have a common ending of "-cyclovir" (Table 1-14).
- These medications do not cure herpes, nor prevent transmission during sexual intercourse.

Antiviral, Neuraminidase Inhibitors

MOA: Inhibits release of viral particle from influenza

Indication: Prevention and treatment of influenza

ADRs: Nausea, vomiting, diarrhea

Additional notes:

- Medications have a common ending of "-amvir" (Table 1-15).
- Must be started within 2 days of contact with an infected patient or onset of flu symptoms.

TABLE 1-14. **Examples of Antivirals**			
Generic	*Brand*	*Form*	*Strengths*
Acyclovir	**Zovirax**	**Capsule**	**200 mg**
		Injection	**50 mg/mL**
		Suspension	**200 mg/5 mL**
		Tablet	**400 mg, 800 mg**
Valacyclovir	**Valtrex**	**Caplet**	**500 mg, 1 g**
		Tablet	**500 mg, 1 g**

TABLE 1-15. Examples of Antiviral, Neuraminidase Inhibitors

Generic	Brand	Form	Strengths
Oseltamivir	Tamiflu	Capsule	30 mg, 45 mg, 75 mg
		Suspension	6 mg/mL
Zanamivir	Relenza	Inhalation	5 mg/blister

ANTIRETROVIRALS

Human immunodeficiency virus (HIV) is a slow replicating virus that causes acquired immunodeficiency syndrome (AIDS). This condition is a progressive failure of the immune system leading to infection and possibly cancer (Tables 1-16 and 1-17).

MOA: Multiple options to block the virus

Indication: Treatment of HIV

ADRs: Nausea, vomiting, diarrhea—medication specific

Additional notes:

- Regimens typically require multiple pills at specific times throughout the day.
- Medications have many side effects and drug interactions.
- Patients must be monitored closely for response to treatment and side effects.

TABLE 1-16. Examples of Antiretrovirals

Generic	Brand	Form	Strengths
Atazanavir	Reyataz	Capsule	150 mg, 200 mg, 300 mg
Darunavir	Prezista	Suspension	100 mg/mL
		Tablet	75 mg, 150 mg, 400 mg, 600 mg, 800 mg
Efavirenz	Sustiva	Capsule	50 mg, 200 mg
		Tablet	600 mg
Emtricitabine	Emtriva	Capsule	200 mg
		Solution	10 mg/mL
Lamivudine	Epivir	Solution	10 mg/mL
		Tablet	150 mg, 300 mg
Rilpivirine	Edurant	Tablet	25 mg
Ritonavir	Norvir	Capsule	100 mg
		Solution	80 mg/mL
Tenofovir	Viread	Tablet	150 mg, 200 mg, 250 mg, 300 mg
Zidovudine	Retrovir	Capsule	100 mg
		Injection	10 mg/mL
		Syrup	50 mg/5 mL
		Tablet	300 mg

TABLE 1-17. **Example of Combination Antiretrovirals**			
Generic	*Brand*	*Form*	*Strengths*
Efavirenz/emtricitabine/tenofovir	Atripla	Tablet	600 mg/200 mg/300 mg
Emtricitabine/rilpivirine/tenofovir	Complera	Tablet	200 mg/25 mg/300 mg
Emtricitabine/tenofovir	Truvada	Tablet	200 mg/300 mg
Lamivudine/zidovudine	Combivir	Tablet	150 mg/300 mg

ANALGESIC MEDICATIONS

Pain is a perception that signals the patient that tissue damage is occurring or has occurred. This is a subjective feeling and can be difficult to control in some patients. Effective pain management often requires medications with different mechanisms of action and nonpharmacologic treatment (ie, physical therapy). The following are treatment types for pain.

Nonsteroidal Anti-Inflammatory Drugs

MOA: Reversibly inhibit cyclo-oxygenase-1 and -2 enzymes; has **antipyretic**, analgesic, and anti-inflammatory properties (Figure 1-3)

Indications: Arthritis, pain, reduction of fever

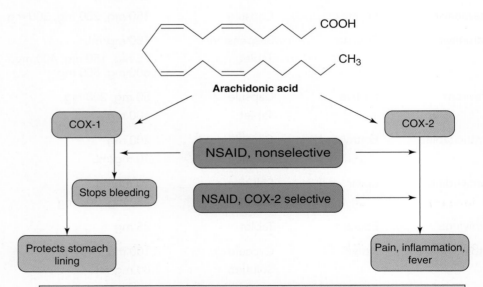

The COX-1 enzyme is responsible for protecting the stomach lining and assists in stopping the body from bleeding. The COX-2 enzyme is responsible for causing pain, inflammation, and fever. Nonselective NSAIDs block the COX-1 and COX-2 enzymes, which helps decreasing pain, inflammation, and fever; however, it can also cause gastrointestinal distress and increase the risk of bleeding. Since COX-2 selective NSAIDs only block the COX-2 enzyme, there is a decreased risk of side effects.

FIGURE 1-3 NSAID mechanism of action.

ADRs: Bleeding, dizziness, gastrointestinal upset

Additional notes:

- Increased risk of GI bleeding at any time during therapy and without warning.
- Use caution with concurrent therapy with aspirin, anticoagulants, smoking, alcohol, and with elderly patients.
- Lowest effective dose for shortest duration of time should be considered (Table 1-18).

★ *TECH ALERT: Patients should be cautioned not to take other OTC NSAIDs while taking prescription NSAIDs. Duplicate therapy can increase the risk of adverse events.*

TABLE 1-18. **Examples of Nonsteroidal Anti-inflammatory Drugs (NSAIDs)**			
Generic	*Brand*	*Form*	*Strengths*
Diclofenac	**Cambia, Cataflam, Voltaren**	**Capsule**	**25 mg**
		Powder	**50 mg/packet**
		Tablet	**50 mg**
		Tablet, EC, DR	**25,mg, 50,mg, 75,mg**
		Tablet, XR	**100 mg**
Etodolac	Lodine	Capsule	200 mg, 300 mg
		Tablet	400 mg, 500 mg
		Tablet, XR	400 mg, 500 mg, 600 mg
Ibuprofen	**Advil, Caldolor, Motrin**	**Caplet**	**100 mg, 200 mg**
		Capsule	**200 mg**
		Injection	**100 mg/mL**
		Suspension	**40 mg/mL, 100 mg/5 mL**
		Tablet, chewable	**200 mg, 400 mg, 600 mg, 800 mg**
		Tablet	**100 mg**
Indomethacin	Indocin	Capsule	25 mg, 50 mg
		Capsule, XR	75 mg
		Injection	1 mg
		Suppository	50 mg
		Suspension	25 mg/5 mL
Ketorolac	Toradol	Injection	15 mg/mL, 30 mg/mL
		Tablet	10 mg
Meloxicam	**Mobic**	**Suspension**	**7.5 mg/5 mL**
		Tablet	**7.5 mg, 15 mg**
Nabumetone	**Relafen**	**Tablet**	**500 mg, 750 mg**
Naproxen	Aleve, Anaprox, Naprelan, Naprosyn	Caplet	220 mg
		Suspension	125 mg/5 mL
		Tablet	220 mg, 250 mg, 275 mg, 375 mg, 500 mg, 550 mg
		Tablet, CR	412.5 mg, 550 mg, 825 mg
		Tablet, DR, EC	375 mg, 500 mg

Nonsteroidal Anti-inflammatory, COX-2 Inhibitors

MOA: Inhibits cyclo-oxygenase-2 enzymes, which result in decreased formation of prostaglandin precursors; has **antipyretic**, analgesic, and anti-inflammatory properties. It does not inhibit the cyclo-oxygenase-1 enzyme.

- Cyclo-oxygenase-1 plays a role in protecting the stomach.

Indications: Arthritis, fever, pain

ADRs: Bleeding, dizziness, gastrointestinal upset

★ TECH ALERT: *NSAIDs and opiates are often combined in order to minimize doses and side effects.*

Additional note:

- The advantage of COX-2 selective agents is that they cause less gastrointestinal upset (Table 1-19).

Narcotic (Opiate) Analgesics

MOA: Block the perception of pain in the brain

Indication: Relief of moderate-to-severe pain

ADRs: Constipation, hypotension, **miosis**, respiratory depression, sedation

Additional notes:

- Use caution in patients with drug abuse or alcoholism; potential for drug dependency
- Long-acting opiate analgesics should not be given to patients who have never taken an opiate. There is potential for increased risk of respiratory depression.
- When opiate analgesics are used in combination with other sedating medications (ie, benzodiazepines) the risk of sedation is increased significantly.
- Controlled-release opiates should not be used for "as needed" pain or mild pain. It should be reserved for patients who have received prior opiate prescriptions (Table 1-20).

Serotonin 5-HT (1b,1d) Receptor Agonist (Triptans)

MOA: Stimulates serotonin which causes vasoconstriction and decreases inflammation

Indication: Migraine

TABLE 1-19. Example Nonsteroidal Anti-inflammatory (NSAID), COX-2 Selective			
Generic	*Brand*	*Form*	*Strengths*
Celecoxib	**Celebrex**	**Capsule**	**50 mg, 100 mg, 200 mg, 400 mg**

TABLE 1-20. Examples of Narcotic (Opiate) Analgesics

Generic	Brand	Form	Strengths
Acetaminophen/codeine	**Tylenol #2, #3, #4**	**Solution**	**120/12 mg/5 mL**
		Tablet	**300/15 mg (#2), 300/30 mg (#3), 300/60 mg (#4)**
Fentanyl transdermal	**Duragesic**	**Patch**	**12 µg, 25 µg, 50 µg, 75 µg, 100 µg**
Hydrocodone	Zohydro ER	Capsule, 12 hour	10 mg, 15 mg, 20 mg, 30 mg, 40 mg, 50 mg
Hydrocodone/acetaminophen	**Lortab, Lorcet, Norco, Vicodin**	**Solution**	**7.5/325 mg/15 mL, 10/325 mg/15 mL**
		Tablet	**5/300 mg, 5/325 mg, 7.5/300 mg, 7.5/325 mg, 10/300 mg, 10/325 mg**
Oxycodone/acetaminophen	**Endocet, Percocet, Roxicet, Tylox**	**Solution**	**5/325 mg/5 mL**
		Tablet	**2.5/325 mg, 5/325 mg, 7.5/325 mg, 10/325 mg**
Hydromorphone	**Dilaudid, Exalgo**	**Injection**	**1 mg/mL, 2 mg/mL, 4 mg/mL, 10 mg/mL**
		Solution	**1 mg/mL**
		Suppository	**3 mg**
		Tablet	**2 mg, 4 mg, 8 mg**
		Tablet, XR	**8 mg, 12 mg, 16 mg, 32 mg**
Meperidine	**Demerol**	**Injection**	**25 mg/mL, 50 mg/mL, 75 mg/mL, 100 mg/mL**
		Solution	**50 mg/5 mL**
		Tablet	**50 mg, 100 mg**
Methadone	**Dolophine**	**Injection**	**10 mg/mL**
		Solution	**5 mg/5 mL, 10 mg/mL**
		Tablet	**5 mg, 10 mg**
		Tablet, dispersible	**40 mg**
Morphine	Avinza, Kadian, MS Contin, Oramorph SR	Capsule, XR	10 mg, 20 mg, 30 mg, 45 mg, 50 mg, 60 mg, 75 mg 80 mg, 90 mg, 100 mg, 120 mg, 130 mg, 150 mg, 200 mg
		Injection	1 mg/mL, 2 mg/mL, 4 mg/mL, 5 mg/mL, 8 mg/mL, 10 mg/mL, 15 mg/mL, 25 mg/mL,
		Solution	50 mg/mL, 10 mg/5 mL, 20 mg/5 mL,
		Suppository	100 mg/5 mL,
		Tablet	5 mg, 10 mg, 20 mg, 30 mg 15 mg, 30 mg
		Tablet, CR	15 mg, 30 mg, 60 mg, 100 mg, 200 mg
		Tablet, XR	15 mg, 30 mg, 60 mg, 100 mg, 200 mg
		Tablet, SR	15 mg, 30 mg, 60 mg, 100 mg

TABLE 1-20. **Examples of Narcotic (Opiate) Analgesics (*Continued*)**

Generic	Brand	Form	Strengths
Oxycodone	**Oxecta, Oxycontin, Roxicodone**	**Capsule**	**5 mg**
		Solution	**5 mg/5 mL, 20 mg/mL**
		Tablet	**5 mg, 7.5 mg 10 mg, 15 mg, 20 mg, 30 mg**
		Tablet, CR	**10 mg, 15 mg, 20 mg, 30 mg, 40 mg, 60 mg, 80 mg**
Oxymorphone	Opana	Injection	1 mg/mL
		Tablet	5 mg, 10 mg
		Tablet, XR	5 mg, 7.5 mg, 10 mg, 15 mg, 20 mg, 30 mg, 40 mg
Tramadol	**ConZip, Rybix, Ryzolt, Ultram**	**Capsule, VR**	**100 mg (25/75 mg), 150 mg (37.5/112 mg), 200 mg (50/150 mg), 300 mg (50/250 mg)**
		Tablet	**50 mg**
		Tablet, XR	**100 mg, 200 mg, 300 mg**
		Tablet, ODT	**50 mg**

ADRs: Chest pain, dizziness, nausea

- Note: When combined with other medications that increase serotonin levels, such as selective serotonin reuptake inhibitors (SSRIs), can cause a dangerous drug interaction known as "serotonin syndrome."

Additional notes:

- Medications have a common ending of "-triptan" (Table 1-21).
- Should be avoided in patients with cardiac disease.
- Indicated only for migraine treatment, not **prophylaxis**.

TABLE 1-21. **Example of Serotonin 5-HT (1b,1d) Receptor Agonist (Triptans)**

Generic	Brand	Form	Strengths
Almotriptan	Axert	Tablet	6.25 mg, 12.5 mg
Eletriptan	Relpax	Tablet	20 mg, 40 mg
Frovatriptan	Frova	Tablet	2.5 mg
Naratriptan	Amerge	Tablet	1 mg, 2.5 mg
Rizatriptan	Maxalt	Tablet	5 mg, 10 mg
		Tablet, ODT	5 mg, 10 mg
Sumatriptan	**Alsuma, Imitrex, Sumavel**	**Injection**	**4 mg, 6 mg**
		Intranasal	**5 mg**
		Tablet	**25 mg, 50 mg, 100 mg**
Zolmitriptan	Zomig	Intranasal	5 mg
		Tablet	2.5 mg, 5 mg
		Tablet, ODT	2.5 mg, 5 mg

TABLE 1-22. **Examples of Skeletal Muscle Relaxants**			
Generic	*Brand*	*Form*	*Strengths*
Baclofen	**Gablofen, Lioresal**	**Injection**	**500 µg/mL, 1000 µg/mL, 2000 µg/mL**
		Tablet	**10 mg, 20 mg**
Carisoprodol	**Soma**	**Tablet**	**250 mg, 350 mg**
Cyclobenzaprine	**Amrix, Fexmid, Flexeril**	**Capsule, ER**	**15 mg, 30 mg**
		Tablet	**5 mg, 7.5 mg, 10 mg**
Metaxalone	Skelaxin	Tablet	800 mg
Methocarbamol	**Robaxin**	**Injection**	**100 mg/mL**
		Tablet	**500 mg, 750 mg**
Orphenadrine	Norflex	Injection	30 mg/mL
		Tablet, ER	100 mg
Tizanidine	**Zanaflex**	**Capsule**	**2 mg, 4 mg, 6 mg**
		Tablet	**2 mg, 4 mg**

Skeletal Muscle Relaxant

MOA: Reduces motor tone and relaxes muscle

Indication: Muscle pain or spasms

ADRs: Gastrointestinal upset, headache, sedation

Additional notes:

- Cautious use in patients with history of alcohol or drug abuse.
- Tizanidine has many drug interactions; concurrent use with ciprofloxacin, fluvoxamine, and oral contraceptives is contraindicated (Table 1-22).

Other Top 200 Analgesic Medications

Butalbital/Acetaminophen/Caffeine

MOA

- Butalbital: Decreases motor activity and brain function and produces drowsiness
- Acetaminophen: Blocks pain impulse generation
- Caffeine: Improves skeletal muscle contraction

Indication: Headache

ADRs: Gastrointestinal upset, respiratory depression

Additional note:

- Not recommended for use in elderly; more sensitive to adverse drug reactions (Table 1-23).

★ *TECH ALERT: Fioricet may be confused with Fiorinal, Florinef, Lorcet, Percocet. Use caution with look-alike-sound-alike medications.*
How can you remember the difference between Fioricet and Fiorinal? FioriCET contains aCET-aminophen. FiorinAl contains Aspirin.

TABLE 1-23. Other Top 200 Analgesic Medications			
Generic	Brand	Form	Strengths
Butalbital/acetaminophen/ caffeine	Esgic, Fioricet	Capsule	50/300/40 mg, 50/325/40 mg
		Liquid	50/325/40 mg/15 mL
		Tablet	50/325/40 mg

QUICK QUIZ 1-1

1. Which class of antibiotics should be avoided in patients with an anaphylactic penicillin allergy?

2. List several examples of macrolide antibiotics.

3. Which antibiotic can cause a disulfiram reaction if taken with alcohol?

4. List the DEA classification for the following:
   a. Percocet
   b. Vicodin
   c. Dilaudid
   d. Duragesic

5. What are the most common side effects of meloxicam?

ANTICHOLESTEROL MEDICATIONS

Cholesterol is a lipid produced by the liver and also consumed through diet. Cholesterol has many functions throughout the body: maintaining cell membranes, production of hormones, metabolism of fat-soluble vitamins, and insulating nerve fibers. While cholesterol is necessary for the body to function, high levels of cholesterol (hypercholesterolemia) can cause the following:

- Atherosclerosis: Thickening and hardening of arteries
- Coronary heart disease: Heart receives inadequate oxygen due to atherosclerosis
- Myocardial infarction (heart attack): Blood flow to the heart is blocked due to a clogged artery
- Stroke: Inadequate oxygen to the brain

★ *TECH ALERT:*
A cholesterol screening measures your levels of low-density lipoprotein (LDL), high-density lipoprotein (HDL), and triglycerides.

LDL = bad cholesterol	LDL goal < 100 memory tip: LDL is Low
HDL = good cholesterol	HDL goal > 60 memory tip: HDL is High
Triglycerides	Triglyceride goal <150

HMG CoA Reductase Inhibitors (Statins)

MOA: Inhibit the first step in cholesterol synthesis (production of the enzyme HMG CoA reductase)

Indication: Hypercholesterolemia

TABLE 1-24. Examples of HMG CoA Reductase Inhibitor (Statins)

Generic	Brand	Form	Strengths
Atorvastatin	**Lipitor**	**Tablet**	**10 mg, 20 mg, 40 mg, 80 mg**
ªEzetimibe/simvastatin	**Vytorin**	**Tablet**	**10/10 mg, 10/20 mg, 10/40 mg, 10/80 mg**
Lovastatin	**Mevacor, Altoprev**	**Tablet** **Tablet, XR**	**10 mg, 20 mg, 40 mg** **20 mg, 40 mg, 60 mg**
Pitavastatin	Livalo	Tablet	1 mg, 2 mg, 4 mg
Pravastatin	**Pravachol**	**Tablet**	**10 mg, 20 mg, 40 mg, 80 mg**
Rosuvastatin	**Crestor**	**Tablet**	**5 mg, 10 mg, 20 mg, 40 mg**
Simvastatin	**Zocor**	**Tablet**	**5 mg, 10 mg, 20 mg, 40 mg, 80 mg**

ªEzetimibe is not a HMG CoA reductase inhibitor, but does reduce plasma cholesterol levels via a different mechanism.

ADRs: Hepatotoxicity, myopathy

Additional notes:

- Medications have a common ending of "-statin" (Table 1-24).
- Grapefruit juice (>1 quart/day) may increase levels of statins.
- Patients should report unusual muscle pain, weakness, or yellowing or skin or eyes.

> ⋆ *TECH ALERT: Statins should be taken at night, as more cholesterol is produced during the night than in the daytime.*

Cholestyramine Resins

MOA: Bind cholesterol in the stomach

Indication: Hypercholesterolemia

ADRs: Constipation, gastrointestinal upset

Additional notes:

- May lower absorption of many medications due to binding of medication, check proper administration times.
- Interferes with absorption of vitamins A, D, E, K, folic acid, and iron (Table 1-25).

Ezetimibe

MOA: Inhibits absorption of cholesterol in the stomach

Indication: Hypercholesterolemia

ADRs: Diarrhea, dizziness

Generic	Brand	Form	Strengths
TABLE 1-25. Examples of Medications for Hypercholesterolemia and Hypertriglyceridemia			
Cholestyramine resin	Prevalite, Questran	Powder for suspension	4 g
Ezetimibe	**Zetia**	**Tablet**	**10 mg**
Fenofibrate	**Antara, Fenoglide, Lipofen, Lofibra, TriCor, Triglide**	**Capsule** **Capsule, micronized** **Tablet**	**50 mg, 150 mg** **43 mg, 67 mg, 130 mg, 134 mg, 200 mg** **40 mg, 48 mg, 50 mg, 54 mg, 120 mg, 145 mg, 160 mg**
Fenofibric acid	**Fibricor, Trilipix**	**Capsule, DR** **Tablet**	**45 mg, 135 mg** **35 mg, 105 mg**
Gemfibrozil	**Lopid**	**Tablet**	**600 mg**
Niacin	**Niacor, Niaspan**	**Capsule** **Capsule, XR** **Tablet** **Tablet, CR** **Tablet, XR**	**50 mg, 250 mg** **250 mg, 500 mg** **50 mg, 100 mg, 250 mg, 500 mg** **250 mg, 500 mg, 750 mg** **500 mg, 750 mg 1000 mg**
Omega-3-acid ethyl esters	**Lovaza**	**Capsule**	**1 g**

Fenofibrate

MOA: Eliminates triglyceride particles from blood

Indication: Hypertriglyceridemia

ADRs: Hepatotoxicity, myopathy

Gemfibrozil

MOA: Unknown

Indication: Hypertriglyceridemia

ADRs: Gastrointestinal upset

Niacin

MOA: Inhibits the production of cholesterol

Indications: Hypercholesterolemia and hypertriglyceridemia

ADRs: Gastrointestinal upset, flushing, headache

Additional notes:

- Take an aspirin 30 to 60 minutes prior to decrease flushing and headache.
- Take at bedtime with a low-fat snack.

Omega-3-Acid Ethyl Esters

MOA: Unknown

Indication: Hypertriglyceridemia

ADRs: Gastrointestinal upset, prolongation of bleeding time

Additional notes:

- Derived from fish, thus use caution in patients with fish allergy.
- Many OTC products contain omega-3 fatty acids; however, these are not the same as the prescription products.

CARDIOVASCULAR MEDICATIONS

Arrhythmia

Arrhythmias are a heart rhythm, which is either too fast (tachycardia), too slow (bradycardia), or irregular (fibrillation). A common arrhythmia is atrial fibrillation, which occurs when the upper 2 chambers of the heart (atria) beat too fast and irregularly (Figures 1-4 and 1-5). Many different types of medications are used to treat atrial fibrillation including β-blockers, calcium channel blockers, and digoxin. Additionally, patients with atrial fibrillation often need anticoagulation with warfarin to prevent stroke.

Hypertension

Hypertension (HTN), also known as high blood pressure, occurs when an elevated force of blood pushes against the walls of the arteries, as the heart pumps the blood.

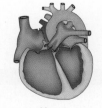

Heart
Beta Blockers
Calcium Channel Blockers

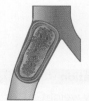

Blood Vessels
ACE inhibitors
ARBs
Calcium channel blockers
Nitrates

Kidneys
ACE inhibitors
ARBs
Diuretics

FIGURE 1-4 Antihypertensive medication mechanism of action.

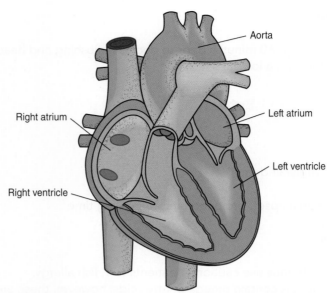

FIGURE 1-5 Schematic diagram of the structure of the heart.

Blood pressure readings are given as 2 numbers. The top number is called the systolic blood pressure (SBP) and the bottom number is called the diastolic blood pressure (DBP). Hypertension is defined as a blood pressure greater than 140/90 mm Hg.

There is a vast variety of treatment options for hypertension, although first-line treatment for this is lifestyle modification (Table 1-26). Initial pharmacologic therapy in most patients includes thiazide diuretics, angiotensin-converting enzyme (ACE) inhibitors, angiotensin receptor blockers (ARBs), or calcium channel blockers.

Congestive Heart Failure

Congestive heart failure (CHF) occurs when the heart is unable to sufficiently pump enough blood to meet the demands of the body. This in turn results in fatigue, shortness of breath, and leg swelling (edema). There are many causes of heart failure including hypertension, myocardial infarction, and heart disease. Nonpharmacologic treatment options include reduction of salt, smoking cessation, and weight loss. Pharmacologic treatment options include ACE inhibitors, ARBs, β-blockers, diuretics, and digoxin.

TABLE 1-26. **Lifestyle Modification**
• Weight loss to achieve healthy weight
• Dietary Approaches to Stop Hypertension (DASH) diet: fruits, vegetables, fat-free or low-fat milk, nuts, lean meats, fish, poultry, whole grains, heart healthy fats
• Limit alcohol
• Reduce sodium to 2.4 g/day
• Maintain adequate dietary potassium, calcium, and magnesium
• Stop smoking
• Aerobic exercise of at least 30 minutes per day for most days

Myocardial Infarction

A myocardial infarction (MI), or heart attack, is the irreversible damage to the heart due to lack of blood flow. Symptoms can include fatigue, chest pain, or indigestion. Myocardial infarctions require immediate care in the emergency room. Patients are treated in the hospital with various medications and nonpharmacologic treatment options. After a myocardial infarction, many medications are used to help prevent further infarction and to help preserve the remaining heart tissue. Treatment options include aspirin, clopidogrel, ACE inhibitors, ARBs, and β blockers.

Angina

Angina is chest pain due to a decrease in blood flow to the heart. It can vary in intensity and frequency. Severe angina can be a sign of a myocardial infarction. Angina is treated acutely with nitrates. Angina attacks may be prevented with long-acting nitrates, calcium channel blockers, and β blockers.

Angiotensin-Converting Enzyme Inhibitors

MOA: Inhibition of ACE

- ACE causes vasoconstriction and increased blood pressure.

Indications: Hypertension, heart failure, myocardial infarction

ADRs: Angioedema, cough, hyperkalemia, hypotension, renal failure

Additional notes:

- Medications have a common ending of "-pril" (Table 1-27).
- ACE inhibitors are contraindicated in pregnancy.
- The first dose should be taken at bedtime due to potential **syncope.**
- Electrolytes (ie, potassium) should be monitored on a regular basis.
- Angioedema is potentially life-threatening reaction. It involves the swelling of the tongue which could block a patient's airway. The most common antihypertensive to cause angioedema is ACE inhibitors and ARBs.

TABLE 1-27. Examples of Angiotensin-Converting Enzyme Inhibitors			
Generic	*Brand*	*Form*	*Strengths*
Benazepril	**Lotensin**	**Tablet**	**5 mg, 10 mg, 20 mg, 40 mg**
Captopril	Capoten	Tablet	12.5 mg, 25 mg, 50 mg, 100 mg
Enalapril	**Vasotec**	**Tablet**	**2.5 mg, 5 mg, 10 mg, 20 mg**
Lisinopril	**Prinivil, Zestril**	**Tablet**	**2.5 mg, 5 mg, 10 mg, 20 mg, 30 mg,40 mg**
Lisinopril/hydrochlorothiazide	**Prinzide, Zestoretic**	**Tablet**	**10/12.5 mg, 20/12.5 mg, 20/25 mg**
Quinapril	**Accupril**	**Tablet**	**5 mg, 10 mg, 20 mg, 40 mg**
Ramipril	**Altace**	**Capsule**	**1.25 mg, 2.5 mg, 5 mg, 10 mg**

Angiotensin II Receptor Blockers

MOA: Inhibit angiotensin II

- Angiotensin II acts as a vasoconstrictor and increases blood pressure.

Indications: Hypertension, heart failure, myocardial infarction

ADRs: Angioedema, hyperkalemia, hypotension, renal failure

Additional notes:

- Medications have a common ending of "-sartan" (Table 1-28)
- ARBs are very similar to ACE inhibitors.
- An ARB is an alternative medication for patients who experience a cough from an ACE inhibitor.

β Blockers

MOA: Decrease rate and force of heart contractions

Indications: Angina, atrial fibrillation or flutter, heart failure, hypertension, migraine headache **prophylaxis**, myocardial infarction

ADRs: Hypotension, bradycardia, dizziness, fatigue

TABLE 1-28. Examples of Angiotensin II Receptor Blockers

Generic	Brand	Form	Strengths
Azilsartan	Edarbi	Tablet	40 mg, 80 mg
Candesartan	Atacand	Tablet	4 mg, 8 mg, 16 mg, 32 mg
Eprosartan	Teventen	Tablet	400 mg, 600 mg
Irbesartan	**Avapro**	**Tablet**	**75 mg, 150 mg, 300 mg**
Losartan	**Cozaar**	**Tablet**	**25 mg, 50 mg, 100 mg**
Losartan/hydrochlorothiazide	**Hyzaar**	**Tablet**	**50/12.5 mg, 100/12.5 mg, 100/25 mg**
Olmesartan	**Benicar**	**Tablet**	**5 mg, 20 mg, 40 mg**
Olmesartan/hydrochlorothiazide	**Benicar HCT**	**Tablet**	**20/12.5 mg, 40/12.5 mg, 40/25 mg**
Olmesartan/amlodipine/hydrochlorothiazide	Tribenzor	Tablet	20/5/12.5 mg, 40/5/12.5 mg, 40/5/25 mg, 40/10/12.5 mg, 40/10/25 mg
Telmisartan	Micardis	Tablet	20 mg, 40 mg, 80 mg
Valsartan	**Diovan**	**Tablet**	**40 mg, 80 mg, 160 mg, 320 mg**
Valsartan/hydrochlorothiazide	**Diovan HCT**	**Tablet**	**80/12.5 mg, 160/12.5 mg, 160/25 mg, 320/12.5 mg, 320/25 mg**

TABLE 1-29. Examples of β Blockers

Generic	Brand	Form	Strengths
Atenolol	**Tenormin**	**Tablet**	**25 mg, 50 mg, 100 mg**
Bisoprolol	Zebeta	Tablet	5 mg, 10 mg
Bisoprolol/ hydrochlorothiazide	**Ziac**	**Tablet**	**2.5/6.25 mg, 5/6.25 mg, 10/6.25 mg**
Carvedilol	**Coreg**	**Capsule, ER**	**10 mg, 20 mg, 40 mg, 80 mg**
		Tablet	**3.125 mg, 6.25 mg, 12.5 mg, 25 mg**
Esmolol	Brevibloc	Injection	10 mg/mL
Metoprolol succinate	**Toprol XL**	**Tablet, ER**	**25 mg, 50 mg, 100 mg, 200 mg**
Metoprolol tartrate	**Lopressor**	**Injection**	**1 mg/mL**
		Tablet	**25 mg, 50 mg, 100 mg**
Nebivolol	**Bystolic**	**Tablet**	**2.5 mg, 5 mg, 10 mg, 20 mg**
Propranolol	**InnoPran, Inderal**	**Capsule, ER**	**60 mg, 80 mg, 120 mg, 160 mg**
		Capsule, SR	**60 mg, 80 mg, 120 mg, 160 mg**
		Injection	**1 mg/mL**
		Solution	**4 mg/mL, 8 mg/mL**
		Tablet	**10 mg, 20 mg, 40 mg, 60 mg, 80 mg**
Sotalol	Betapace, Sorine	Injection	15 mg/mL
		Tablet	80 mg, 120 mg, 160 mg, 240 mg

Additional notes:

- Medications have a common ending of "-lol" (Table 1-29).
- Caution diabetics that β blockers may mask the signs of hypoglycemia.
- Abrupt withdrawal may lead to tachycardia, hypertension, or myocardial infarction.
- May exacerbate asthma.

Calcium Channel Blockers

MOA: Vasodilation of arteries and decrease heart rate

Indications: Angina, atrial fibrillation or flutter, hypertension (Table 1-30)

ADRs: Syncope, headache, constipation

DIURETICS

Loop Diuretics

MOA: Increased urinary excretion of sodium, potassium, and water

Indications: Edema, hypertension, heart failure

★ *TECH ALERT: Metoprolol succinate (Toprol XL) and metoprolol tartrate (Lopressor) are not interchangeable. Metoprolol succinate is an extended-release product and metoprolol tartrate is an immediate-release product. Use caution when filling these products.*

TABLE 1-30. Examples of Calcium Channel Blockers

Generic	Brand	Form	Strengths
Amlodipine	**Norvasc**	**Tablet**	**2.5 mg, 5 mg, 10 mg**
Diltiazem	**Cardizem, Cartia, Dilacor, Diltia, Diltzac, Matzim, Taztia, Tiazac**	**Capsule, XR**	**120 mg, 180 mg, 240 mg, 300 mg, 360 mg, 420 mg**
		Injection	**5 mg/mL**
		Tablet	**30 mg, 60 mg, 90 mg, 120 mg**
		Tablet, XR	**120 mg, 180 mg, 240 mg, 300 mg, 360 mg, 420 mg**
Felodipine	Plendil	Tablet, XR	2.5 mg, 5 mg, 10 mg
Nicardipine	Cardene	Capsule	20 mg, 30 mg
		Capsule, SR	30 mg, 45 mg, 60 mg
		Injection	2.5 mg/mL, 20 mg/200 mL, 40 mg/200 mL
Nifedipine	**Adalat, Nifedical, Procardia**	**Capsule**	**10 mg, 20 mg**
		Tablet, XR	**30 mg, 60 mg, 90 mg**
Verapamil	**Calan, Covera, Isoptin, Verelan**	**Caplet, SR**	**120 mg, 180 mg, 240 mg**
		Capsule, ER	**120 mg, 180 mg, 240 mg**
		Capsule, SR	**120 mg, 180 mg, 240 mg, 360 mg**
		Injection	**2.5 mg/mL**
		Tablet	**40 mg, 80 mg, 120 mg**
		Tablet, XR	**120 mg, 180 mg, 240 mg**
		Tablet, SR	**120 mg, 180 mg, 240 mg**

ADRs: Electrolyte disturbances, dizziness, gastrointestinal upset, hypotension

Additional notes:

⋆ TECH ALERT: *A patient in the hospital is receiving Lasix 100mg/10mL IVPB at 10mg/hour. How fast should the nurse run the drip (mL/hour).*

- Medications have a common ending of "-mide" (Table 1-31).
- Take early in day to avoid nighttime **diuresis.**
- Take with food or milk to avoid GI distress.
- Monitor electrolytes regularly. Patients commonly need to take potassium supplements.

Thiazide Diuretics

MOA: Increased urinary excretion of sodium, potassium, and water

Indications: Edema, hypertension, heart failure

TABLE 1-31. Examples of Loop Diuretics

Generic	Brand	Form	Strengths
Bumetanide	Bumex	Injection	0.25 mg/mL
		Tablet	0.5 mg, 1 mg, 2 mg
Furosemide	**Lasix**	**Injection**	**10 mg/mL**
		Solution	**40 mg/5 mL, 10 mg/mL**
		Tablet	**20 mg, 40 mg, 80 mg**
Torsemide	Demadex	Injection	10 mg/mL
		Tablet	5 mg, 10 mg, 20 mg, 100 mg

TABLE 1-32. Examples of Thiazide Diuretics			
Generic	*Brand*	*Form*	*Strengths*
Chlorothiazide	Diuril	Injection	500 mg
		Suspension	250 mg/5 mL
		Tablet	250 mg, 500 mg
Hydrochlorothiazide	**Microzide**	**Capsule**	**12.5 mg**
		Tablet	**12.5 mg, 25 mg, 50 mg**

ADRs: Electrolyte disturbances, dizziness, hypotension

Additional notes:

- Medications have a common ending of "-thiazide" (Table 1-32).
- Take early in day to avoid nighttime **diuresis.**
- Combined with multiple medications to enhance antihypertensive action.

Potassium-Sparing Diuretics

MOA: Increased urinary excretion of sodium and water, increased retention of potassium

Indications: Edema, heart failure, hypertension, hypokalemia

ADRs: Electrolyte disturbances, dizziness, GI distress, hypotension

Additional notes:

- Avoid potassium supplements, salt substitutes, and natural licorice.
- Men may develop breast tissue (gynecomastia) when taking spironolactone.
- May be combined with other diuretics to offset electrolyte disturbances.(Table 1-33).

Nitrates

MOA: Vasodilator which decreases heart filling thus increasing its efficacy and increases cardiac blood flow

Indications: Angina, heart failure, hypertension, anal fissure (rectal ointment)

ADRs: Dizziness, headache, hypotension

★ *TECH ALERT: The abbreviation "HCTZ" should be avoided for hydrochlorothiazide as it is error prone.*

TABLE 1-33. Examples of Potassium-Sparing Diuretics			
Generic	*Brand*	*Form*	*Strengths*
Amiloride	Midamor	Tablet	5 mg
Eplerenone	Inspra	Tablet	25 mg, 50 mg
Hydrochlorothiazide/ triamterene	**Dyazide, Maxzide**	**Capsule**	**25/37.5 mg**
		Tablet	**25/37.5 mg, 50/75 mg**
Spironolactone	**Aldactone**	**Tablet**	**25 mg, 50 mg, 100 mg**
Triamterene	Dyrenium	Capsule	50 mg, 100 mg

TABLE 1-34. Examples of Nitrates

Generic	Brand	Form	Strengths
Isosorbide dinitrate	Dilatrate, IsoDitrate, Isordil	Capsule, SR	40 mg
		Tablet	5 mg, 10 mg, 20 mg, 30 mg
		Tablet, SL	2.5 mg, 5 mg
		Tablet, ER	40 mg
Isosorbide Mononitrate	**Imdur, Monoket**	**Tablet**	**10 mg, 20 mg**
		Tablet, ER	**30 mg, 60 mg, 120 mg**
Nitroglycerin	**Minitran, Nitro-Bid, Nitro-Dur, NitroMist, Rectiv**	**Capsule, ER**	**2.5 mg, 6.5 mg, 9 mg**
		Injection	**100 µg/mL, 200 µg/mL, 400 mg/mL**
		Ointment, rectal	**0.4%**
		Ointment, topical	**2%**
		Patch	**0.1 mg/hr, 0.2 mg/hr, 0.3 mg/hr, 0.4 mg/hr, 0.6 mg/hr, 0.8 mg/hr**
		Spray, SL	**0.4 mg/spray**
		Tablet, SL	**0.3 mg, 0.4 mg, 0.6 mg**

★ TECH ALERT: Patients should be advised to sit down when using nitroglycerin sublingual or spray as it can cause dizziness. If chest pain is unresolved for more than 15 minutes, they should call 911.

★ TECH ALERT: Patients may take an antiplatelet and anticoagulant together depending on the indication. However, they are at a higher risk for serious bleeding.

Additional note:

- Avoid use with PDE-5 inhibitors (sildenafil, tadalafil, vardenafil) as concurrent administration can lead to extreme hypotension (Table 1-34).

ANTIPLATELET AND ANTICOAGULANT MEDICATIONS

Thrombosis is a stationary blood clot that forms when blood thickens and clumps together. Usually thrombosis occurs in the legs, but can occur in other parts of the body. This thrombosis is called a deep vein thrombosis (DVT). If a thrombosis becomes loose and moves throughout the body, it is then called an embolism. The clot typically moves to the lungs, which is called a pulmonary emboism (PE). A thrombosis can also move to the brain and cause a stroke. These conditions are treated with anticoagulant medications.

Blood flow can also be decreased by a plaque that blocks an artery. A plaque consists of fatty material and platelets. When a plaque blocks an artery in the heart it causes a myocardial infarction (MI), this is also known as a heart attack. A plaque can also occur in the brain and cause a stroke.

Antiplatelet Agents

MOA: Inhibit platelet clumping

Indications: Angina, myocardial infarction, stroke

ADRs: Bleeding, bruising

Additional notes:

- Aspirin may also be used for pain, inflammation, and fever.

TABLE 1-35. Examples of Antiplatelet Agents

Generic	Brand	Form	Strengths
Aspirin	Ascriptin, Bayer, Bufferin, Ecotrin	Caplet	81 mg, 325 mg, 500 mg
		Caplet, EC	325 mg
		Suppository	300 mg, 600 mg
		Tablet	325 mg
		Tablet, chewable	81 mg
		Tablet, EC	81 mg, 162 mg, 325 mg, 650 mg
Cilostazol	Pletal	Tablet	50 mg, 100 mg
Clopidogrel	**Plavix**	**Tablet**	**75 mg, 300 mg**
Prasugrel	Effient	Tablet	5 mg, 10 mg
Ticagrelor	Brilinta	Tablet	90 mg

- When antiplatelet agents are used in combination with warfarin, there is an increased risk of bleeding (Table 1-35).

★ TECH ALERT: An INR is used to tell if the blood is too thick (low INR, <2) or too thin (high INR, >3).

Anticoagulants

MOA: prevent the coagulation or clotting of blood

Indications: Atrial fibrillation, cardiac valve replacement, clotting disorders, myocardial infarction, stroke

ADRs: Bleeding

Additional notes:

- Indications vary depending on agent.
- Warfarin.
  ○ Has many drug interactions including OTC medications. Patients should be counseled to notify their physician of any medication changes.
  ○ Can be affected by food such as green leafy vegetables, which can decrease a patient's INR. Patients should be advised to eat a consistent diet (Table 1-36).
  ○ Requires frequent laboratory monitoring.

Other Top 200 Cardiovascular Drugs

CLONIDINE

MOA: Stimulates α_2 receptor in the brain stem which decreases blood pressure and heart rate

Indications: Attention deficit hyperactivity disorder (ADHD), hypertension, pain (epidural)

ADRs: Bradycardia, central nervous system (CNS) depression, hypotension

TABLE 1-36. Examples of Anticoagulants

Generic	Brand	Form	Strengths
Dabigatran	Pradaxa	Capsule	75 mg, 150 mg
Enoxaparin	Lovenox	Injection	30 mg, 40 mg, 60 mg, 80 mg, 100 mg, 120 mg, 150 mg
Dalteparin	Fragmin	Injection	2500 units, 5000 units, 7500 units, 12,500 units, 15,000 units, 18,000 units
Heparin		Injection	1 Units/mL, 2 Units/mL, 10 Units/mL, 100 Units/mL, 1000 Units/mL, 5000 Units/mL, 10,000 Units/mL, 20,000 Units/mL
Rivaroxaban	Xarelto	Tablet	10 mg, 15 mg, 20 mg
Warfarin	**Coumadin, Jantoven**	**Injection**	**5 mg**
		Tablet	**1 mg, 2 mg, 2.5 mg, 3 mg, 4 mg, 5 mg, 6 mg, 7.5 mg, 10 mg**

Additional notes:

- Has many off-label uses—alcohol and drug abuse, migraine **prophylaxis**, insomnia, and menopause.
- Abrupt withdrawal may lead to tachycardia, hypertension, or myocardial infarction.

★ *TECH ALERT: The term "off-label" is used when a medication is used outside of the FDA-approved indication, dose, or age group. This is a common practice as it is difficult to get funding for research for generic medications.*

Digoxin

MOA: Prevents **arrhythmias** and increases heart contraction

Indications: Atrial fibrillation, heart failure

ADRs: Dizziness, gastrointestinal upset

Hydralazine

MOA: Vasodilation of arteries which decreases blood pressure

Indications: Heart failure, hypertension

ADRs: Hypotension, tachycardia

Additional note:

- Rarely, can cause a drug-induced rash; advise patient to contact physician with new-onset rash (Table 1-37).

ENDOCRINE MEDICATIONS

Insulin is the hormone responsible for the uptake of glucose (sugar) from the blood into cells where it is utilized for energy or stored as glycogen for future use. When there is a lack of insulin, the body is unable to process the glucose, which leads to excessive sugar in the blood (hyperglycemia) in addition to symptoms such as increased urine production, dehydration, and other metabolic derangements.

TABLE 1-37. Examples of Other Top 200 Cardiovascular Drugs

Generic	Brand	Form	Strengths
Clonidine	Catapres, Duraclon, Kapvay	Injection	100 µg/mL
		Patch	0.1 mg, 0.2 mg, 0.3 mg
		Tablet	0.1 mg, 0.2 mg, 0.3 mg
		Tablet, XR	0.1 mg, 0.2 mg
Digoxin	Lanoxin	Injection	250 µg/mL
		Solution	50 µg/mL
		Tablet	125 µg, 250 mg
Hydralazine	Apresoline	Injection	20 mg/mL
		Tablet	10 mg, 25 mg, 50 mg, 100 mg

Diabetes mellitus is the term used to refer to the lack of insulin, or lack of response to insulin. There are 3 main types of diabetes:

1. Type 1 diabetics make no insulin, thus can only be treated with exogenous insulin not oral medication. They are usually diagnosed as children or young adults.
2. Type 2 diabetics make limited insulin; however, they have become insulin resistant. Type 2 diabetic patients are usually obese adults. However, there has been an increase of type 2 diabetes in children due to the increasing incidence of childhood obesity. Depending on the severity of illness, they can be treated with lifestyle changes, oral medication, or insulin.
3. Gestational diabetes occurs in women who are pregnant. The increased blood sugar typically only lasts through pregnancy; however, the patient is at a higher risk of developing type 2 diabetes later in life. Patients can be treated with lifestyle medications or insulin.

Normal blood sugar readings are between 70 and 140 mg/dL. When blood glucose levels drop below 70, patients become hypoglycemic; symptoms include sweating, shaking, and clamminess. Patient should be treated immediately with oral glucose tablets, juice, or something sugary to instantly increase the sugar present in the blood.

Diabetics should be counseled on lifestyle medications such as healthy diet, weight loss, smoking cessation, and exercise. Diabetes puts patients at a higher risk of developing many complications such as cardiac disease, renal failure, infection, and peripheral neuropathy. Patients should frequently monitor their blood sugar and follow up with their physician for regular monitoring.

⋆ *TECH ALERT:*
Hemoglobin A_{1c} is a laboratory test that averages the blood sugar over a prolonged period of time. The hemoglobin A_{1c} goal for most diabetic patients should be less than 7%.

TYPE 2 DIABETIC MEDICATIONS

Biguanide

MOA: Decreases glucose production and absorption; improves insulin sensitivity

Indications: Type 2 diabetes mellitus

ADRs: Gastrointestinal upset, diarrhea, headache, hypoglycemia

Additional notes:

- Should not be used in patients with renal insufficiency
- Drug should be temporarily stopped in patients undergoing a radiology exam that uses contrast dye
- The extended release tablet shell may remain intact and be visible in the stool

Dipeptidyl Peptidase IV (DDP-IV) Inhibitor

MOA: Increase release of insulin; decrease release of glucose

Indication: Type 2 diabetes mellitus

ADRs: Gastrointestinal upset

Additional note:

- Medications have a common ending of "-gliptin"

Meglitinide

MOA: Increases release of insulin

Indication: Type 2 diabetes mellitus

ADRs: Hypogylcemia, gastrointestinal upset

Additional notes:

- Medications have a common ending of "-glinide"
- Drug should be taken 15-30 minutes prior to a meal; it should not be taken if meal is skipped

Sulfonylurea

MOA: Stimulates release of insulin

Indications: Type 2 diabetes mellitus

ADRs: Hypoglycemia, GI upset

Additional notes:

- Take 30 minutes before meals (immediate release); extended release products should be taken with breakfast
- Patients with decreased caloric intake may need to hold doses to avoid hypoglycemia

★ *TECH ALERT: Micronized glyburide (Glynase) and conventional glyburide (DiaBeta) are NOT bioequivalent. Use caution when filling prescriptions for these medications.*

Thiazolidinedione

MOA: Improves cell response to insulin

Indications: Type 2 diabetes mellitus

ADRs: Edema, hypoglycemia, headache

Additional notes:

- Medications have a common ending of "-glitazone"
- May cause or exacerbate heart failure; patients should notify physician if they experience rapid weight gain, edema, or shortness of breath (Table 1-38)

★ *TECH ALERT: Insulin is a high-alert medication. Due to the number of insulin preparations, it is essential to identify/clarify the type of insulin to be used.*

TYPE 1 AND 2 DIABETES MELLITUS MEDICATIONS

Insulin

MOA: Replaces or supplements insulin normally secreted by the pancreas

Indication: Type 1 diabetes mellitus, type 2 diabetes mellitus

ADRs: Hypoglycemia, pain at injection site

Additional notes:

- Available as pen formulations and in vials.
- Should be stored in a refrigerator (not frozen); may be kept out of the refrigerator for 28 days
- Regular insulin may be given IV in emergency situations (Table 1-39)

★ *TECH ALERT: Tech Alert: Insulin Regular, Insulin NPH, and the combination do not require a prescription. They are considered nonprescription medications; however, must be kept behind the pharmacy counter.*

THYROID DRUGS

The thyroid is a butterfly shaped gland located in the neck above the collarbone. Thyroid hormones regulate the body's metabolism and affect every organ system in the body. Signs of an overactive thyroid (hyperthyroid) include tachycardia, weight loss, anxiety, and exopthalmia, or protruding eyeballs. An underactive thyroid (hypothyroid) manifests as bradycardia, weight gain, and fatigue.

Treatment for Hypothyroidism

Levothyroxine

MOA: Synthetic thyroid hormone replacement (T4).

TABLE 1-38. Examples of Oral Hypoglycemic Agents

Generic	Brand	Form	Strengths
Biguanides			
Metformin	**Fortamet, Glucophage, Glumetza, Riomet**	**Solution** **Tablet** **Tablet, XR**	**100 mg/mL** **500 mg, 850 mg, 1000 mg** **500 mg, 750 mg, 1000 mg**
Dipeptidyl Peptidase IV (DDP-IV) Inhibitors			
Linagliptin	Tradjenta	Tablet	5 mg
Saxagliptin	Onglyza	Tablet	2.5 mg, 5 mg
Sitagliptin	Januvia	Tablet	25 mg, 50 mg, 100 mg
Meglitinides			
Nateglinide	Starlix	Tablet	60 mg, 120 mg
Repaglinide	Prandin	Tablet	0.5 mg, 1 mg, 2 mg
Sulfonylureas			
Glimepiride	**Amaryl**	**Tablet**	**1 mg, 2 mg, 4 mg**
Glipizide	**Glucotrol**	**Tablet** **Tablet, XR**	**5 mg, 10 mg** **2.5 mg, 5 mg, 10 mg**
Glyburide	**DiaBeta, Glynase**	**Tablet** **Tablet, micronized**	**1.25 mg, 2.5 mg. 5 mg** **1.5 mg, 3 mg, 5 mg, 6 mg**
Thiazolidinediones			
Pioglitazone	**Actos**	**Tablet**	**15 mg, 30 mg, 45 mg**
Rosiglitazone	**Avandia**	**Tablet**	**2 mg, 4 mg, 8 mg**
Combination Hypoglycemics			
Glipizide/metformin	Metaglip	Tablet	2.5/500 mg, 2.5/500 mg, 5/500 mg
Glyburide/metformin	**Glucovance**	**Tablet**	**1.25/250 mg, 2.5/500 mg, 5/500 mg**
Linagliptin/metformin	Jentadueto	Tablet	2.5/500 mg, 2.5/850 mg, 2.5/1000 mg
Pioglitazone/glimepiride	Duetact	Tablet	30/2 mg, 30/4 mg
Repaglinide/metformin	PrandiMet	Tablet	1/500 mg, 2/500 mg
Rosiglitazone/glimepiride	Avandaryl	Tablet	4/1 mg, 4/2 mg, 4/4 mg, 8/2 mg, 8/4 mg
Saxagliptin/metformin	Kombiglyze XR	Tablet, XR	2.5/1000 mg, 5/500 mg, 5/1000 mg
Sitagliptin/metformin	Janumet, Janumet XR	Tablet Tablet, XR	50/500 mg, 50/1000 mg 50/500 mg, 50/1000 mg, 100/1000 mg

TABLE 1-39. Examples of Insulin		
Generic	*Brand*	*Length of Action*
Insulin aspart	**Novolog**	**Rapid**
Insulin glulisine	Apidra	Rapid
Insulin lispro	Humalog	Rapid
Insulin regular	Humulin R, Novolin R	Short
Insulin NPH	Humulin N, Novolin N	Intermediate
Insulin detemir	Levemir	Intermediate, long
Insulin glargine	**Lantus**	**Long**
Insulin Combination Products		
Insulin aspart protamine/ insulin aspart	Novolog 70/30	Intermediate (70%)/rapid (30%)
Insulin lispro protamine/ insulin lispro	Humalog 50/50	Intermediate (50%)/rapid (50%)
	Humalog 75/25	Intermediate (75%)/rapid (25%)
Insulin NPH/insulin regular	Humulin 70/30	Intermediate (70%)/short (30%)
	Novolin 70/30	Intermediate (70%)/short (30%)

Thyroid, Desiccated

MOA: Porcine thyroid hormone replacement (T4 and T3)

ADRs: Based on thyroid levels

Additional notes:

- Thyroid products should not be used as weight loss agents.
- Should be taken on an empty stomach with a full glass of water, 30 minutes before breakfast.
- Do not take antacids or iron preparations within 4 hours of thyroid medications.

Treatment for Hyperthyroidism

Methimazole

MOA: Blocks the production of thyroid hormones

Propylthiouracil

MOA: Blocks the production of thyroid hormones

ADRs: Based on thyroid levels

Additional note:

- Propylthiouracil can cause bone marrow suppression, which may be fatal (Table 1-40).

★ TECH ALERT: Hyperthyroid symptoms include tachycardia, anxiety, weight loss, and insomnia. Hypothyroid symptoms include somnolence and weight gain.

TABLE 1-40. **Examples of Thyroid Products**			
Generic	*Brand*	*Form*	*Strengths*
Levothyroxine	**Levothroid, Levoxyl, Synthroid, Tirosint, Unithroid**	**Capsule**	**13 mcg, 25 mcg, 50 mcg, 75 mcg, 88 mg, 100 mcg, 112 mcg 125 mcg, 137 mcg, 150 mcg**
		Injection	**100 mcg, 500 mcg**
		Tablet	**25 mcg, 50 mcg, 75 mcg, 88 mcg, 100 mcg, 112 mcg, 125 mcg, 137 mcg, 150 mcg, 175 mcg, 200 mcg, 300 mcg**
Thyroid, Desiccated	**Armour Thyroid, Nature-Thyroid, Westhroid**	**Tablet**	**15 mg, 16.25 mg, 30 mg, 32.5 mg, 60 mg, 65 mg, 90 mg, 120 mg, 130 mg, 180 mg, 195 mg, 240 mg, 300 mg**
Methimazole	Tapazole	Tablet	5 mg, 10 mg
Propylthiouracil	PTU	Tablet	50 mg

QUICK QUIZ 1-2

1. What electrolyte replacement medication is commonly taken with diuretics?

2. What are the most common adverse drug reactions of statins?

3. Nitrates should not be taken with which class of medications?

4. Can a type 1 diabetic be treated with oral antidiabetic medications?

5. What is the generic name of Plavix?

CENTRAL NERVOUS SYSTEM MEDICATIONS

Many Central Nervous System (CNS) medications work by modifying neurotransmitters within the brain. Neurotransmitters are the chemical messengers which transmit signals or messages to targets within the brain. Many neurological disorders are thought to stem from disrupted levels of neurotransmitters. Therefore, by manipulating the levels of these neurotransmitters a desired response can be obtained to help patients. Neurotransmitters involved in the CNS include serotonin, dopamine, acetylcholine, epinephrine, norepinephrine, gama-aminobutyric acid (GABA) and glutamate.

Diabetic neuropathy is a nerve disorder caused by diabetes. Symptoms include **parasthesias**, pain, numbness, and loss of feeling. The neuropathy typically occurs in the legs, feet, toes, arms, and hands. Treatment options include anticonvulsants and antidepressants.

Fibromyalgia is widespread musculoskeletal pain with fatigue, sleep disturbances, and joint stiffness. There are no specific diagnostic criteria or cure. It can be treated with exercise and stress reduction. Medications used to treat fibromyalgia include anticonvulsants and antidepressants.

Restless leg syndrome (RLS) is a neurological disorder that affects the legs. Patients experience pain, pulling, **parasthesias**, and a uncontrollable urge to move their legs.

Symptoms typically occur at night when relaxing and they can interfere with sleeping. Treatment options vary from anticonvulsants and dopaminergic agents.

Seizures are the result of abnormal electrical activity in the brain. Some seizures present with convulsions. Convulsions are the uncontrollable shaking of the body. However, some seizures may cause a patient to blankly stare off. Seizures can last from seconds to minutes, and rarely last longer. There are many different types of anticonvulsants that are used for seizures. Therapy depends on the type and severity of the seizure.

ANTICONVULSANTS

Carbamazepine

MOA: Multiple mechanisms; depresses activity in brain

Indications: Bipolar disease, post-traumatic stress disorders, restless leg syndrome, seizures

ADRs: Dizziness, headache, nausea

Additional notes:

- A wide variety of blood disorders have been reported; patients should notify their physician of easy bruising
- Severe dermatologic disorders have been reported; patients should notify their physician of any rashes
- Patients of Asian descent should be screened prior to use because of significant increase in dermatologic disorders.

Divalproex

MOA: Increased concentration of GABA

- GABA is an inhibitory neurotransmitter in the brain.

Indications: Diabetic neuropathy, migraine **prophylaxis**, seizures

ADRs: Gastrointestinal upset, headaches, tremor, vision changes

* TECH ALERT: *Valproic acid delayed-release and extended-release products are **not** interchangeable. Use caution when dispensing these products.*

Gabapentin

MOA: Interacts with GABA neurotransmitters in brain which may cause seizures

Indications: Fibromyalgia, neuropathic pain, restless legs syndrome, seizures

ADRs: CNS depression, dizziness

Additional note:

- Extended-release gabapentin has not indicated for seizures.

* TECH ALERT: *Gabapentin immediate release and extended release are not interchangeable with each other or with gabapentin enacarbil.*

Pregabalin

MOA: Inhibits excitatory transmitter release in the brain

Indications: Fibromyalgia, neuropathic pain, seizures

ADRs: CNS depression, dizziness, weight gain

Lacosamide

MOA: Stabilizes neuron membranes in the brain

Indication: Seizures

ADRs: Dizziness, headache, nausea

Additional note:

- Patients with cardiac disease should have an **electrocardiogram** (ECG/EKG) prior to therapy.

Lamotrigine

MOA: Stabilizes neuron membranes in the brain

Indications: Bipolar disease, seizures

ADRs: GI distress

Additional notes:

- Severe and life-threatening skin rashes have been reported.
- Hormonal contraceptives decrease lamotrigine concentrations requiring a dose increase.

Levetiracetam

MOA: Unknown

Indication: Seizures

ADRs: Agitation, headache, sedation, weakness

Oxcarbazepine

MOA: Unknown

Indications: Bipolar disorder, neuropathic pain, seizures

ADRs: Dizziness, nausea, sedation

Additional note:

- May decrease the effectiveness of oral contraceptives; alternate methods are suggested.

Phenytoin

MOA: Stabilizes neuron membranes in the brain

Indication: Seizures

ADRs: Cardiac **arrhythmia** (IV formulation), dizziness, **gingival hypertrophy**, **hypertrichosis**

Additional notes:

- A wide variety of blood disorders have been reported; patients should notify their physician of easy bruising.
- IV phenytoin must be administered slowly to avoid hypotension and cardiac **arrhythmias**; cardiac monitoring is advised.
- Severe dermatologic disorders have been reported; patients should notify their physician of any rashes.
- Sedation, confusion, and loss of motor coordination may occur at higher drug levels; patients should have their phenytoin levels monitored.

Topiramate

MOA: Stabilizes neuron membranes in the brain

Indications: Diabetic neuropathy, migraine **prophylaxis**, neuropathic pain, seizures

ADRs: Anorexia, **paresthesia**, **somnolence**, weight loss

Additional notes:

- Cognitive dysfunction and sedation may occur with use; patients should be cautioned about performing tasks that require mental alertness (ie, driving).
- Off-label use for alcoholism and cocaine addiction (Table 1-41).

ANTIDEPRESSANT MEDICATIONS

Depression

Depression is a persistent feeling of sadness and loss of interest. The exact cause is not known but a variety of risk factors are there including decreased levels of serotonin and norepinephrine, hormones, life events, and childhood trauma. It may be treated with therapy, dopamine reuptake inhibitors, selective serotonin reuptake inhibitors, and various other medications.

Seasonal Affective Disorders

Seasonal affective disorder (SAD) is depression that occurs at the same time each year (ie, winter). Treatment includes light therapy, therapy, and antidepressant medications.

TABLE 1-41. Examples of Anticonvulsants

Generic	Brand	Form	Strengths
Carbamazepine	Carbatrol	Capsule, ER	100 mg, 200 mg, 300 mg
	Epitol	Suspension	100 mg/5 mL
	Equetro	Tablet	200 mg
	Tegretol	Tablet, chewable	100 mg
		Tablet, ER	100 mg, 200 mg, 400 mg
Divalproex	**Depakote**	**Capsule**	**125 mg**
		Tablet, DR	**125 mg, 250 mg, 500 mg**
		Tablet, ER	**250 mg, 500 mg**
Gabapentin	**Gralise, Neurontin**	**Capsule**	**100 mg, 300 mg, 400 mg**
		Solution	**250 mg/5 mL**
		Tablet	**600 mg, 800 mg**
Gabapentin enacarbil	Horizant	Tablet, ER	600 mg
Lacosamide	Vimpat	Injection	10 mg/mL
		Solution	10 mg/mL
		Tablet	50 mg, 100 mg, 150 mg, 200 mg
Lamotrigine	**Lamictal**	**Tablet**	**25 mg, 100 mg, 150 mg, 200 mg**
		Tablet, chewable	**2 mg, 5 mg, 25 mg**
		Tablet, ER	**25 mg, 50 mg, 100 mg, 200 mg, 250 mg, 300 mg**
		Tablet, ODT	**25 mg, 50 mg, 100 mg, 200 mg**
Levetiracetam	**Keppra**	**Infusion**	**500 mg, 1000 mg, 150 mg**
		Solution	**100 mg/mL**
		Tablet	**250 mg, 500 mg, 750 mg, 1000 mg**
		Tablet, ER	**500 mg, 750 mg**
Oxcarbazepine	Trileptal	Suspension	300 mg/5 mL
		Tablet	150 mg, 300 mg, 600 mg
Phenytoin	**Dilantin, Phenytek**	**Capsule, ER**	**30 mg, 100 mg, 200 mg, 300 mg**
		Injection	**50 mg/mL**
		Suspension	**100 mg/4 mL, 125 mg/5 mL**
		Tablet, chewable	**50 mg**
Pregabalin	**Lyrica**	**Capsule**	**25 mg, 50 mg 75 mg, 100 mg, 150 mg, 200 mg, 225 mg, 300 mg**
		Solution	**20 mg/mL**
Topiramate	**Topamax**	**Capsule**	**15 mg, 25 mg**
		Tablet	**25 mg, 50 mg, 100 mg, 200 mg**

Dopamine Reuptake Inhibitor

MOA: Blocks norepinephrine and dopamine reuptake allowing for more activity

- Low levels of norepinephrine and dopamine are associated with depression

Indications: Depression, SAD, smoking cessation

TABLE 1-42. **Example of Dopamine Reuptake Inhibitor**			
Generic	*Brand*	*Form*	*Strengths*
Bupropion	**Aplenzin, Budeprion, Buproban, Forfivo, Wellbutrin, Zyban**	**Tablet**	**75 mg, 100 mg**
		Tablet, ER	**174 mg, 348 mg, 522 mg**
		Tablet, ER	**100 mg, 150 mg, 200 mg, 300 mg, 450 mg**
		Tablet, SR	**100 mg, 150 mg, 200 mg**

ADRs: Headache, insomnia, weight loss

Additional note:

- Risk of seizures, higher incidence with high-dose, binge drinking (Table 1-42).

Selective Serotonin Reuptake Inhibitor (SSRI)

MOA: Blocks serotonin reuptake allowing for more serotonin availability

- Low levels of serotonin are associated with depression

Indications: Bulimia nervosa, depression, obsessive-compulsive disorder, panic disorder, posttraumatic stress disorder, premenstrual dysphoric disorder, social anxiety disorder

ADRs: Dizziness, fatigue, GI upset, headache

Additional notes:

- Increased risk of suicide in children and young adults (age 18-24 years)
- Gradually taper drug upon discontinuation due to withdrawal syndrome (irritability, agitation, dizziness) (Table 1-43)

TABLE 1-43. **Examples of Selective Serotonin Reuptake Inhibitor**			
Generic	*Brand*	*Form*	*Strengths*
Citalopram	**Celexa**	**Solution**	**10 mg/5 mL**
		Tablet	**10 mg, 20 mg, 40 mg**
Escitalopram	**Lexapro**	**Solution**	**1 mg/mL**
		Tablet	**5 mg, 10 mg, 20 mg**
Fluoxetine	**Prozac, Sarafem**	**Capsule**	**10 mg, 20 mg, 40 mg**
		Capsule, DR	**90 mg**
		Solution	**20 mg/5 mL**
		Tablet	**10 mg, 20 mg, 60 mg**
Paroxetine	**Paxil, Pexeva**	**Solution**	**10 mg/5 mL**
		Tablet	**10 mg, 20 mg, 30 mg, 40 mg**
		Tablet, CR	**12.5 mg, 25 mg, 37.5 mg**
Sertraline	**Zoloft**	**Solution**	**20 mg/mL**
		Tablet	**25 mg, 50 mg, 100 mg**
Vilazodone	Viibryd	Tablet	10 mg, 20 mg, 40 mg

TABLE 1-44. Example of Serotonin Reuptake Inhibitor/Antagonist			
Generic	*Brand*	*Form*	*Strengths*
Trazodone	**Desyrel, Oleptro**	**Tablet**	**50 mg, 100 mg, 150 mg, 300 mg**
		Tablet, ER	**150 mg, 300 mg**

Serotonin Reuptake Inhibitor/Antagonist

MOA: Blocks serotonin reuptake allowing for more serotonin availability

- Low levels of serotonin are associated with depression

Indications: Depression, insomnia

ADRs: Headache, hypotension, sedation

Additional note:

- Take immediate-release tablet after meals and extended release on an empty stomach (Table 1-44).

Serotonin/Norepinephrine Reuptake Inhibitor (SNRI)

MOA: Blocks norepinephrine and serotonin reuptake allowing for more activity

- Low levels of norepinephrine and serotonin are associated with depression

Indications: Depression, fibromyalgia, generalized anxiety disorders, musculoskeletal pain, peripheral neuropathic pain

ADRs: Fatigue, headache, nausea

Additional notes:

- Increased risk of suicide in children and young adults (age 18-24 years).
- Gradually taper drug upon discontinuation due to withdrawal syndrome (irritability, agitation, dizziness) (Table 1-45).

TABLE 1-45. Examples of Serotonin/Norepinephrine Reuptake Inhibitor			
Generic	*Brand*	*Form*	*Strengths*
Desvenlafaxine	Pristiq	Tablet, ER	50 mg, 100 mg
Duloxetine	**Cymbalta**	**Capsule, DR**	**20 mg, 30 mg, 60 mg**
Milnacipran	Savella	Tablet	12.5 mg, 25 mg, 50 mg, 100 mg
Venlafaxine	**Effexor**	**Capsule, ER**	**37.5 mg, 75 mg, 150 mg**
		Tablet	**25 mg, 3.5 mg 50 mg, 75 mg, 100 mg**
		Tablet, ER	**37.5 mg, 75 mg, 150 mg, 225 mg**

TABLE 1-46. **Examples Tricyclic Antidepressants**			
Generic	*Brand*	*Form*	*Strengths*
Amitriptyline	**Elavil**	**Tablet**	**10 mg, 25 mg, 50 mg, 75 mg, 100 mg, 150 mg**
Imipramine	Tofranil	Capsule	75 mg, 100 mg, 125 mg, 150 mg
		Tablet	10 mg, 25 mg, 50 mg
Nortriptyline	**Pamelor**	**Capsule**	**10 mg, 25 mg, 50 mg, 75 mg**
		Solution	**10 mg/5 mL**

Tricyclic Antidepressants (TCA)

MOA: Increase concentration of serotonin and norepinephrine

- Low levels of norepinephrine and serotonin are associated with depression.

Indications: Depression, migraine **prophylaxis**, neuropathic pain

ADRs: Hypotension, sedation (Table 1-46)

> **★ *TECH ALERT:*** *Overdoses of tricycle antidepressants (TCAs) can be fatal; large quantities should not be dispensed.*

ANTI-PARKINSON AGENT

Parkinson disease is a chronic and progressive movement disorder. It is characterized by tremor, slowness of movement (bradykinesia), rigidity, and instability. Parkinson disease is associated with low levels of dopamine. Dopamine helps muscle control, thus decreased levels lead to movement dysfunction. Thus, the mechanism of most anti-Parkinson agents is to increase dopamine levels in the brain.

MOA: Increased levels of dopamine

Indications: Parkinson disease, restless leg syndrome

ADRs: Dizziness, **somnolence**, nausea

Additional note:

- Associated with compulsive behaviors and loss of impulse control (ie, gambling) (Table 1-47).

TABLE 1-47. **Examples of Anti-Parkinson Agents**			
Generic	*Brand*	*Form*	*Strengths*
Carbidopa/levodopa	Parcopa, Sinemet	Tablet	10/100 mg, 25/100 mg, 25/250 mg
		Tablet, ER	25/100 mg, 50/200 mg
		Tablet, ODT	10/100 mg, 25/100 mg, 25/250 mg
		Tablet, SR	25/100 mg, 50/200 mg
Pramipexole	Mirapex	Tablet	0.125 mg, 0.25 mg, 0.5 mg, 0.75 mg, 1 mg, 1.5 mg
		Tablet, ER	0.375 mg, 0.75 mg, 1.5 mg, 2.25 mg, 3 mg, 3.75 mg, 4.5 mg
Ropinirole	**Requip**	**Tablet**	**0.25 mg, 0.5 mg, 1 mg, 2 mg, 3 mg, 4 mg, 5 mg**
		Tablet, ER	**2 mg, 4 mg, 6 mg, 8 mg, 12 mg**

DEMENTIA MEDICATIONS

Dementia is the loss of brain function that leads to a decline in memory. Symptoms usually develop slowly and worsen over time, eventually interfering with activities of daily life. Alzheimer disease is the most common form of dementia.

Acetylcholinesterase Inhibitors

MOA: Increase acetylcholine in brain

- Low levels of acetylcholine are associated with cognitive deficits. Acetylcholinesterase is the enzyme which destroys acetylcholine and prevents it from be absorbed into the neuron. Preventing the destruction of acetylcholine increases levels in the brain and decreases symptoms.

Indication: Dementia

ADRs: GI distress, insomnia

Additional note:

- These drugs do not cure the disease, but help decrease symptoms (Table 1-48).

N-Methyl-D-Aspartate Receptor Antagonist

MOA: Blocks overstimulation of glutamate receptor

- Excess glutamate may contribute to brain cell death

Indication: Dementia

ADRs: Confusion, cough, constipation, dizziness

Additional note:

- Donepezil and memantine may be used alone or in combination to decrease the progression of dementia (Table 1-49).

TABLE 1-48. Examples of Acetylcholinesterase Inhibitors			
Generic	*Brand*	*Form*	*Strengths*
Donepezil	**Aricept**	**Tablet**	**5 mg, 10 mg, 23 mg**
		Tablet, ODT	**5 mg, 10 mg**
Galantamine	Razadyne	Capsule, ER	8 mg, 16 mg, 24 mg
		Solution	4 mg/mL
		Tablet	4 mg, 8 mg, 12 mg
Rivastigmine	Exelon	Capsule	1.5 mg, 3 mg, 4.5 mg, 6 mg
		Patch	4.6 mg, 9.5 mg, 13.3 mg
		Solution	2 mg/mL

TABLE 1-49. **Example of *N*-Methyl-ᴅ-Aspartate Receptor Antagonist**			
Generic	*Brand*	*Form*	*Strengths*
Memantine	**Namenda**	**Solution**	**2 mg/mL**
		Tablet	**5 mg, 10 mg**

PSYCHIATRIC DISORDERS

Attention Deficit Hyperactivity Disorder

Attention deficit hyperactivity disorder (ADHD) is characterized by inattention, hyperactivity, and impulsivity. ADHD is commonly diagnosed in childhood. The drug of choice for treatment is stimulant medications, such as amphetamines.

Bipolar Disorder

Bipolar disorder is a mood disorder that is characterized by alternating periods of depression and mania (elevated or agitated mood). Treatment can include therapy or medications such as lithium, anticonvulsants, and antipsychotics.

Insomnia

Insomnia is a sleep disorder in which there is an inability to fall asleep and/or stay asleep throughout the night. Nonpharmacologic treatment options for insomnia include limiting electronics, exercise, caffeine, and alcohol before bed, keeping a consistent sleep schedule, relaxation techniques, and limiting daytime napping. Pharmacologic treatment choices include hypnotics and benzodiazepines.

Schizophrenia

Schizophrenia is a mental disorder in which patients interpret reality as an abnormal perception. They may have visual or auditory hallucinations, delusions, and disordered thinking and behavior. Patients may be treated with therapy and antipsychotic medications.

Atypical Antipsychotics

MOA: Inhibition of dopamine and serotonin receptors

- Excessive levels of dopamine and serotonin can lead to psychiatric disorders

Indications: Bipolar disorder, delirium, schizophrenia, adjunct treatment for depression

ADRs: Hypotension, hypercholesterolemia, sedation, weight gain

Additional notes:

- Patients with diabetes may experience increased blood sugars.
- Elderly patients with dementia treated with antipsychotics are at an increased risk of death.
- Tend to have less side effects than typical antipsychotics (Table 1-50).

Typical Antipyschotics

MOA: Inhibition of dopamine receptors

- Typical antipyschotics block dopamine receptors more strongly than atypical antipyschotics

Indications: Schizophrenia, delirium, pyschosis

ADRs: Sedation, extrapyramidal symptoms (movement disorder), tardive dyskinesia (involuntary movement)

Additional note:

- Side effects are more severe than atypical antipsychotics, thus reserved for more severe cases. (Table 1-51)

TABLE 1-50. Examples of Atypical Antipsychotics			
Generic	*Brand*	*Form*	*Strengths*
Aripiprazole	**Abilify**	**Injection**	**7.5 mg/mL**
		Solution	**1 mg/mL**
		Tablet	**2 mg, 5 mg, 10 mg, 15 mg, 20 mg, 30 mg**
		Tablet, ODT	**10 mg, 15 mg**
Asenapine	Saphris	Tablet, SL	5 mg, 10 mg
Lurasidone	Latuda	Tablet	20 mg, 40 mg, 80 mg
Olanzapine	**Zyprexa**	**Injection**	**10 mg**
		Injection, ER	**210 mg, 300 mg, 405 mg**
		Tablet	**2.5 mg, 5 mg, 7.5 mg, 10 mg, 15 mg, 20 mg**
		Tablet, ODT	**5 mg, 10 mg, 15 mg, 20 mg**
Quetiapine	**Seroquel**	**Tablet**	**25 mg, 50 mg, 100 mg, 250 mg, 200 mg, 300 mg, 400 mg**
		Tablet, ER	**50 mg, 150 mg, 200 mg, 300 mg, 400 mg**
Risperidone	**Risperdal**	**Injection, ER**	**12.5 mg, 25 mg, 37.5 mg, 50 mg**
		Solution	**1 mg/mL**
		Tablet	**0.25 mg, 0.5 mg, 1 mg, 2 mg, 3 mg, 4 mg**
		Tablet, ODT	**0.25 mg, 0.5 mg, 1 mg, 2 mg, 3 mg, 4 mg**
Ziprasidone	**Geodon**	**Capsule**	**20 mg, 40 mg, 60 mg, 80 mg**
		Injection	**20 mg**

TABLE 1-51. Examples of Typical Antipsychotics			
Generic	*Brand*	*Form*	*Strengths*
Fluphenazine	Prolixin	Injection	2.5 mg/mL
		Solution	2.5 mg/5 mL
		Tablet	1 mg, 2.5 mg, 5 mg, 10 mg
Haloperidol	Haldol	Injection	5 mg/mL
		Solution	2 mg/mL
		Tablet	0.5 mg,1 mg, 2 mg, 5 mg, 10 mg, 20 mg
Thioridazine		Tablet	10 mg, 25 mg, 50 mg, 100 mg
Thiothixene	Navane	Capsules	1 mg, 2 mg, 5 mg, 10 mg

SEDATING MEDICATIONS

Benzodiazepines

MOA: Inhibition of GABA neurons in the brain, which decreases rate of neuron firing causing relaxation

Indications: Anxiety, ethanol withdrawal, insomnia, sedation, seizures

ADRs: CNS depression, memory impairment, sedation

Additional notes:

- Medications have a common ending of "-am" (Table 1-52).
- Paradoxical (hyperactivity) reactions have been reported, mainly in children and elderly.
- Use caution in patients with drug abuse or alcoholism, potential for drug dependency.
- Withdrawal symptoms such as seizures may occur with abrupt discontinuation.

Hypnotics

MOA: Inhibition of GABA neurons in the brain, which decreases rate of neuron firing causing relaxation

TABLE 1-52. Examples of Benzodiazepines

Generic	Brand	Form	Strengths
Alprazolam	**Niravam, Xanax**	**Solution**	**1 mg/mL**
		Tablet	**0.25 mg, 0.5 mg, 1 mg, 2 mg**
		Tablet, ER	**0.5 mg, 1 mg, 2 mg, 3 mg**
		Tablet, ODT	**0.25 mg, 0.5 mg, 1 mg, 2 mg**
Clorazepate	Tranxene	Tablet	3.75 mg, 7.5 mg, 15 mg
Clonazepam	**Klonopin**	**Tablet**	**0.5 mg, 1 mg, 2 mg**
		Tablet, ODT	**0.125 mg, 0.25 mg, 0.5 mg, 1 mg, 2 mg**
Diazepam	**Diastat, Valium**	**Rectal gel**	**5 mg, 10 mg, 20 mg**
		Injection	**5 mg/mL**
		Solution	**5 mg/mL, 5mg/5 mL**
		Tablet	**2 mg, 5 mg, 10 mg**
Lorazepam	**Ativan**	**Injection**	**2 mg/mL, 4 mg/mL**
		Solution	**2 mg/mL**
		Tablet	**0.5 mg, 1 mg, 2 mg**
Midazolam	Versed	Injection	1 mg/mL, 5 mg/mL
		Solution	2 mg/mL
Temazepam	**Restoril**	**Capsule**	**7.5 mg, 15 mg, 22.5 mg, 30 mg**
Triazolam	Halcion	Tablet	0.125 mg, 0.25 mg

TABLE 1-53. Examples of Hypnotics			
Generic	*Brand*	*Form*	*Strengths*
Eszopiclone	**Lunesta**	**Tablet**	**1 mg, 2 mg, 3 mg**
Ramelteon	Rozerem	Tablet	8 mg
Zaleplon	Sonata	Capsule	5 mg, 10 mg
Zolpidem	**Ambien, Edluar, Intermezzo, Zolpimist**	**Oral spray** **Tablet** **Tablet, SL** **Tablet, ER**	**5 mg/actuation** **5 mg, 10 mg** **1.75 mg, 3.5 mg, 5 mg, 10 mg** **6.25 mg, 12.5 mg**

Indication: Insomnia

ADRs: Amnesia, headache

Additional notes:

- There is an increased risk of sleep-related activities such as sleep-driving, eating, phone calls.
- Use caution in patients with lung disorders or **sleep apnea** (Table 1-53).

Stimulants

MOA: Amphetamine that releases dopamine and norepinephrine

- Increased levels of dopamine and norepinephrine increase concentration and mood

Indications: ADHD, **narcolepsy**

ADRs: Decreased appetite, headache, insomnia

Additional note:

- Modafinil should not be used in pediatrics for any indication due to serious skin reactions and psychiatric events (Table 1-54).

Other Top 200 Central Nervous System Drugs

BUPRENORPHINE/NALOXONE

MOA

- Buprenorphine: Binds to opiate receptors in CNS
- Naloxone: Displaces narcotics from opiate receptors

Indications: Maintenance treatment for opioid dependence

ADRs: Headache, pain, withdrawal syndrome

TABLE 1-54. Examples of Stimulants

Generic	Brand	Form	Strengths
Dextroamphetamine/ amphetamine	Adderall	Capsule, ER	5 mg, 10 mg, 15 mg, 20 mg, 25 mg, 30 mg
		Tablet	5 mg, 7.5 mg, 10 mg, 12.5 mg, 15 mg, 20 mg, 30 mg
Lisdexamfetamine	Vyvanse	Capsule	20 mg, 30 mg, 40 mg, 50 mg, 60 mg, 70 mg
Methylphenidate	Concerta, Daytrana, Metadate, Methylin, Ritalin	Capsule, ER	10 mg, 20 mg, 30 mg, 40 mg, 50 mg, 60 mg
		Patch	10 mg, 15 mg, 20 mg, 30 mg
		Solution	5 mg/5 mL, 10 mg/mL
		Tablet	5 mg, 10 mg, 20 mg
		Tablet, chewable	2.5 mg, 5 mg 10 mg
		Tablet, ER	10 mg, 20 mg
		Tablet, ER	18 mg, 27 mg, 36 mg, 54 mg
		Tablet, SR	20 mg
Modafinil	Provigil	Tablet	100 mg, 200 mg

Additional note:

- The addition of naloxone to buprenorphine deters the injection of the tablet.

BUSPIRONE

MOA: Unknown

Indications: Generalized anxiety

ADRs: Dizziness, drowsiness

MIRTAZAPINE

MOA: α_2 antagonist that increase concentration of serotonin and norepinephrine

- Low levels of norepinephrine and serotonin are associated with depression.

Indications: Depression, posttraumatic stress disorder

ADRs: Somnolence, weight gain (Table 1-55)

TABLE 1-55. Examples of Other Top 200 Central Nervous System Drugs

Generic	Brand	Form	Strengths
Buprenorphine/ naloxone	Suboxone	Film	2 mg/0.5 mg, 8 mg/2 mg
		Tablet	2 mg/0.5 mg, 8 mg/2 mg
Buspirone	Buspar	Tablet	5 mg, 7.5 mg, 10 mg, 15 mg, 30 mg
Mirtazapine	Remeron	Tablet	7.5 mg, 15 mg, 30 mg, 45 mg
		Tablet, ODT	15 mg, 30 mg, 45 mg

PULMONARY MEDICATIONS

Allergic Rhinitis

Allergic rhinitis is inflammation of the nasal airways from an allergen (ie, dust, pollen, animal dander). Symptoms include runny nose, itching, eye redness, and swelling. Treatment of allergic rhinitis includes nasal corticosteroids.

Asthma

Asthma is an inflammation of the airways in the lungs, which causes the lungs to swell and narrow. Common symptoms include wheezing, shortness of breath, and coughing. Asthma can be exacerbated by smoking, allergens (ie, smoke, dust, animals), and infection. Acute asthma exacerbations are treated with short-acting β_2 agonists. Long-term control of asthma is achieved with long-acting β_2 agonists, inhaled corticosteroids, and oral corticosteroids.

Bronchospasm

Bronchospasm is the sudden constriction of the bronchioles in the lungs. It can occur in patients with asthma, bronchitis, and anaphylaxis. Bronchospasm is treated with short-acting β_2 agonists.

Chronic Obstructive Pulmonary Disease

Chronic obstructive pulmonary disease (COPD) consists of 2 main forms:

- Chronic bronchitis: Long-term cough with mucus
- Emphysema: Destruction of lungs over time

Patients with COPD usually have a combination of the 2 forms. The most common cause of COPD is smoking. COPD is a progressive disorder without a cure. Patients should be encouraged to stop smoking. Treatment options include β_2 agonists, inhaled corticosteroids, inhaled anticholinergics, and oral corticosteroids.

β_2 Agonists

MOA: Open up lungs by relaxing bronchial muscles

Indications: Asthma, bronchospasm, chronic obstructive pulmonary disease

ADRs: Dizziness, nervousness, tachycardia

Additional note:

- Long-acting β_2 agonists (formoterol, salmeterol) should not be used for acute exacerbations. They are indicated for the prevention of exacerbations (Table 1-56).

TABLE 1-56. Examples of β₂ Agonists

Generic	Brand	Form	Strengths
Albuterol	**AccuNeb, ProAir, Proventil, Ventolin, VoSpire**	**Inhaler**	**90 μg/inhalation**
		Nebulization	**0.063 mg/3 mL (0.021%), 1.25 mg/3 mL (0.042%), 2.5 mg/3 mL (0.83%), 2.5 mg/5 mL (0.5%)**
		Solution	**2 mg/5 mL**
		Tablet	**2 mg, 4 mg**
		Tablet, ER	**4 mg, 8 mg**
Formoterol	Foradil, Perforomist	Inhaler	12 μg/inhalation
		Nebulization	20 μg/2 mL
Levalbuterol	Xopenex	Inhaler	45 μg/inhalation
		Nebulization	0.31 mg/3 mL, 0.63 mg/3 mL, 1.25 mg/mL
Salmeterol	Serevent	Inhaler	50 μg/inhalation

Corticosteroid, Inhaled

MOA: Decrease inflammation in lungs

Indications: Asthma, COPD

ADRs: Oral **candidiasis**, respiratory infection

Additional notes:

- Medications have a common ending of "-asone" (Table 1-57).
- Full benefit of medication not seen for days, thus not used for acute exacerbations.
- May cause a reduction in growth in pediatric patients, lowest effective dose should be used.

★ *TECH ALERT: Patients should be instructed to rinse mouth and throat after use of inhaled corticosteroids to decrease the risk of oral* ***candidiasis***.

Anticholinergic, Inhaled

MOA: Bronchodilation and decreased secretion production

Indications: Bronchitis, bronchospasm, COPD, emphysema

ADRs: Cough, paradoxical bronchospasm

TABLE 1-57. Examples of Inhaled Corticosteroids

Generic	Brand	Form	Strengths
Beclomethasone	QVAR	Inhaler	40 μg, 80 μg
Fluticasone	**Flovent**	**Inhaler**	**44 μg, 110 mg, 220 μg**
		Disk Inhaler	**50 μg, 100 μg, 250 mg**
Mometasone	Asmanex	Twisthaler	110 μg, 220 μg

TABLE 1-58. Examples of Inhaled Anticholinergic Agents

Generic	Brand	Form	Strengths
Aclidinium	Tudorza	Inhaler	400 µg/inhalation
Ipratropium	Atrovent	Inhaler	17 µg/actuation
		Nebulizer	500 µg/2.5 mL (0.02%)
Tiotropium	**Spiriva**	**HandiHaler**	**18 µg/inhalation**

Additional notes:

- Close the eyes when administering—blurred vision can occur if sprayed in eyes.
- Should only be used for acute attacks when used in combination with short-acting β_2 agonists (albuterol).
- The contents of Spiriva capsules are for inhalation only via the HandiHaler. The HandiHaler pierces the capsule to allow for inhalation of the contents. Capsules should never be swallowed (Tables 1-58 and 1-59).

Corticosteroid, Nasal

MOA: Decreases inflammation in nose

Indication: Allergic rhinitis

ADRs: Dizziness, **epistaxis**, gastrointestinal upset

Additional note:

- Maximal benefit may take 2 weeks (Table 1-60).

Corticosteroids, Systemic

MOA: Decreases inflammation and immune system

Indication: Anti-inflammatory or immunosuppressant in a variety of diseases

- Examples: Allergic reactions, arthritis, asthma, Chron's disease, dermatitis, organ transplant

TABLE 1-59. Examples of Combination Inhaled Products

Generic	Brand	Form	Strengths
Budesonide/formoterol	**Symbicort**	**Inhaler**	**80 µg/4.5 µg, 160 µg/4.5 g**
Fluticasone/salmeterol	**Advair**	**Inhaler**	**45 µg/21 µg, 115 µg/21 µg, 230 µg/21 µg**
		Disk inhaler	**100 µg/50 µg, 250 µg/50 µg, 500 µg/50 µg**
Ipratropium/albuterol	**Combivent, DuoNeb**	**Inhaler**	**18 µg/90 µg/inhalation**
		Nebulizer	**0.5 mg/2.5 mg/3 mL**
Mometasone/formoterol	Dulera	Inhaler	100/5 µg, 200/5 µg

TABLE 1-60. Examples of Corticosteroid, Nasal

Generic	Brand	Form	Strengths
Beclomethasone nasal	Beconase AQ, Qnasl	Aerosol	80 µg/inhalation
		Suspension	42 µg/inhalation
Budesonide nasal	Rhinocort AQ	Suspension	32 µg/inhalation
Ciclesonide nasal	Omnaris, Zetonna	Aerosol	37 µg/inhalation
		Suspension	50 µg/inhalation
Fluticasone nasal	**Flonase, Veramyst**	**Suspension**	**27.5 µg/inhalation, 50 µg/inhalation**
Mometasone nasal	**Nasonex**	**Suspension**	**50 µg/spray**
Triamcinolone nasal	Nasacort AQ	Suspension	55 µg/inhalation

ADRs: Adrenal suppression, hyperglycemia, infection, nausea, osteoporosis, psychiatric disorders, weight gain

Additional notes:

- Medications have a common ending of "-sone" (Table 1-61).
- Lowest dose for the shortest period of time is based on disease state.
- A gradual tapering of dose may be needed prior to stopping the therapy.

TABLE 1-61. Examples of Systemic Corticosteroids

Generic	Brand	Form	Strengths
Dexamethasone	Baycadron, Decadron	Injection	4 mg, 10 mg
		Solution	0.5 mg/5 mL, 1 mg/mL
		Tablet	0.5 mg, 0.75 mg, 1 mg, 1.5 mg, 2 mg, 4 mg, 6 mg
Hydrocortisone	Cortef, Solu-Cortef	Injection	100 mg, 250 mg, 500 mg, 1 g
		Tablet	5 mg, 10 mg, 20 mg
Methylprednisolone	**Depo-Medrol, Medrol, Solu-Medrol**	**Injection**	**40 mg, 125 mg, 500 mg, 1 g, 2 g**
		Tablet	**4 mg, 8 mg, 16 mg, 32 mg**
Prednisolone	**Flo-Pred, Millipred, Orapred, Pediapred, Veripred**	**Solution**	**5 mg/5 mL, 10 mg/5 mL, 15 mg/5 mL, 20 mg/5 mL, 25 mg/5 mL**
		Suspension	**15 mg/5 mL**
		Tablet	**5 mg**
		Tablet, ODT	**10 mg, 15 mg, 30 mg**
Prednisone	**Deltasone, Rayos**	**Solution**	**1 mg/mL, 5 mg/mL**
		Tablet	**1 mg, 2.5 mg, 5 mg, 10 mg, 20 mg, 50 mg**
		Tablet, DR	**1 mg, 2 mg, 5 mg**

TABLE 1-62. Examples of Antitussives

Generic	Brand	Form	Strengths
Benzonatate	**Tessalon Perles, Zonatuss**	**Capsule**	**100 mg, 150 mg, 200 mg**
Codeine		Solution	30 mg/5 mL
		Tablet	15 mg, 30 mg, 60 mg
Dextromethorphan	Delsym, Robafen, Robitussin, Triaminic, Vicks	Capsule	15 mg
		Liquid	7.5 mg/5 mL, 10 mg/5 mL, 10 mg/15 mL, 15 mg/5 mL, 15 mg/15 mL, 20 mg/15 mL 30 mg/5 mL, 30 mg/30 mL
		Lozenge	5 mg
		Strip, ODT	7.5 mg
		Tablet	15 mg

COUGH/COLD MEDICATIONS

Antitussives

MOA: Suppress cough

Indication: Symptomatic relief of cough

ADRs: Confusion, sedation

Additional notes:

★ *TECH ALERT: Benzonatate must be swallowed whole; it exerts its action topically on respiratory receptors.*

- Dextromethorphan has potential to be abused.
- Codeine is a C-II when prescribed as a stand-alone product.
- Other agents that can be used in combination as antitussive agents include hydro-codone and homatropine (Table 1-62).

Decongestants

MOA: Decrease inflammation, swelling, and mucus in nose and lungs

Indication: Relief of nasal congestion

★ *TECH ALERT: Pseudoephedrine is used to make crystal meth-amphetamine. In order to deter illegal manu-facturing, many states have restricted sales of pseudoephedrine.*

ADRs: Dizziness, nervousness, tachycardia

Additional note:

- Use caution in patients with hypertension and heart disease (Table 1-63).

TABLE 1-63. Examples of Decongestants

Generic	Brand	Form	Strengths
Pseudoephedrine	Sudafed, SudoGest, Sudo-Tab	Caplet, ER	120 mg
		Liquid	15 mg/5 mL, 30 mg/5mL
		Tablet	30 mg, 60 mg
		Tablet, ER	120 mg, 240 mg

TABLE 1-64. Example of Expectorant

Generic	Brand	Form	Strengths
Guaifenesin	Humibid, Mucinex, Q-Tussin	Caplet	400 mg
		Granules	50 mg, 100 mg
		Liquid	100 mg/5 mL, 200 mg/5 mL
		Tablet	200 mg, 400 mg
		Tablet, ER	600 mg, 1200 mg

Expectorant

MOA: Decreases thickness of and break up of mucous and stimulates coughing

Indication: Loosen phlegm and thin bronchial secretions to make coughs more productive

ADRs: Minimal—Dizziness, headache (Tables 1-64 and 1-65)

Leukotriene Receptor Antagonists

MOA: Inhibit the leukotriene receptor

- Leukotriene receptors are associated with inflammation and contraction of the lungs

Indications: Allergic rhinitis, asthma

ADRs: Headache, dizziness

Additional note:

- Should not be used for acute exacerbations of asthma (Table 1-66).

★ *TECH ALERT: Montelukast granules may be mixed with applesauce, carrots, rice, ice cream, baby formula, or breast milk.*

TABLE 1-65. Examples of Combination Products

Generic	Brand	Form	Strengths
Guaifenesin/codeine	**Cheratussin AC, Guaiatussin AC, Robafen AC**	**Capsule**	**200 mg/9 mg**
		Liquid	**100 mg/10 mg/5 mL, 300 mg/10 mg/5 mL**
		Tablet	**400 mg/10 mg, 400 mg/20 mg**
Guaifenesin/ dextromethorphan	Cheracol, Mucinex DM, Q-Tussin DM, Robitussin DM	Caplet	400 mg/15 mg, 400 mg/20 mg
		Capsule	200 mg/10 mg
		Granules	100 mg/5 mg
		Liquid	100 mg/10 mg/5 mL, 200 mg/10 mg/5 mL, 200 mg/20 mg/5 mL
		Tablet	1000 mg/60 mg, 1200 mg/60 mg, 100 mg/10 mg
		Tablet, ER	600 mg/30 mg, 1200 mg/60 mg
Promethazine/ codeine	**Phenergan/Codeine**	**Syrup**	**6.25/10 mg/5 mL**

TABLE 1-66. **Examples of Leukotriene Receptor Antagonists**			
Generic	*Brand*	*Form*	*Strengths*
Montelukast	**Singulair**	**Granules**	**4 mg/packet**
		Tablet	**10 mg**
		Tablet, chewable	**4 mg, 5 mg**
Zafirlukast	Accolate	Tablet	10 mg, 20 mg

Histamine-1 Antagonist (Antihistamines)

First generation: Diphenhydramine, hydroxyzine

Second generation: Cetirizine, desloratadine, fexofenadine, levocetirizine, loratadine

MOA: Inhibits histamine-1 receptors

- Histamine-1 receptors cause bronchoconstriction, hives, itching.

Indications

- First generation: Allergic rhinitis, anxiety, insomnia, sedation, **urticaria**
- Second generation: Allergic rhinitis, **urticaria**

ADRs: Headache, gastrointestinal upset, sedation (first generation)

Additional note:

- First-generation agents have more sedating effects (Table 1-67).

★ *TECH ALERT: Medications are sometimes separated into "generations." First generations are the first version of the medication that was discovered. Second generations are the next, and so on with additional generations created. Each generation has a similar mechanism of action, but different side effects which tend to get better as the generation increases.*

ELECTROLYTE SUPPLEMENTS

Calcium

MOA: Prevents rate of bone loss, neutralizes gastric acid

Indications: Antacid, hypocalcemia, osteoporosis

ADRs: Constipation

Additional note:

- Should be given with meals to increase absorption.

Potassium

MOA: Major electrolyte in the body that involves with heart, brain, and skeletal muscles

Indication: Hypokalemia (low potassium)

ADRs: Gastrointestinal upset, hyperkalemia (high potassium)

TABLE 1-67. **Examples of Histamine-1 Antagonists**			
Generic	*Brand*	*Form*	*Strengths*
Cetirizine	Zyrtec	Capsule	10 mg
		Syrup	5 mg/5 mL
		Tablet	5 mg, 10 mg
		Tablet, chewable	5 mg, 10 mg
Desloratadine	Clarinex	Syrup	0.5 mg/mL
		Tablet	5 mg
		Tablet, ODT	2.5 mg, 5 mg
Diphenhydramine	Benadryl, Q-Dryl, Unisom	Caplet	25 mg, 50 mg
		Capsule	25 mg, 50 mg
		Injection	50 mg/mL
		Syrup	12.5 mg/5 mL
		Tablet	25 mg, 50 mg
		Tablet, ODT	12.5 mg, 25 mg
Fexofenadine	**Allegra**	**Suspension**	**6 mg/mL**
		Tablet	**30 mg, 60 mg, 180 mg**
		Tablet, ODT	**30 mg**
Hydroxyzine	**Atarax, Vistaril**	**Capsule**	**25 mg, 50 mg, 100 mg**
		Injection	**25 mg/mL, 50 mg/mL**
		Syrup	**10 mg/5 mL**
		Tablet	**10 mg, 25 mg, 50 mg**
Levocetirizine	Xyzal	Solution	0.5 mg/mL
		Tablet	5 mg
Loratadine	Alavert, Claritin	Capsule	10 mg
		Syrup	5 mg/5 mL
		Tablet	10 mg
		Tablet, chewable	5 mg
		Tablet, ODT	10 mg
Meclizine	Antivert, Bonine, Dramamine, VertiCalm	Caplet	12.5 mg
		Tablet	12.5 mg, 25 mg, 50 mg
		Tablet, chewable	25 mg

Additional notes:

- Oral formulations should be taken with food to prevent GI upset.
- IV formulations should *not* be administered undiluted or IV push; inappropriate administration could be fatal.

Magnesium

MOA: Cofactor in many enzyme processes in the body

Indications: Constipation, hypomagnesemia, indigestion

ADRs: Diarrhea (Table 1-68)

TABLE 1-68. Examples of Electrolyte Supplements

Generic	Brand	Form	Strengths
Calcium carbonate	Caltrate, Maalox, Rolaids, Tums	Capsule	1250 mg, 364 mg
		Suspension	1250 mg/5 mL
		Tablet	650 mg, 1250 mg, 1500 mg
		Tablet, chewable	500 mg, 650 mg, 750 mg, 1250 mg
Potassium chloride	**Epiklor, K-Tab, Kaon-CL, Klor-Con, microK**	**Capsule, ER**	**8 mEq, 10 mEq**
		Injection	**2 mEq/mL**
		Powder	**20 mEq/packet, 25 mEq/packet**
		Solution	**20 mEq/15 mL, 40 mEq/15 mL**
		Tablet, ER	**8 mEq, 10 mEq, 20 mEq**
Magnesium oxide	Mag-Ox, Phillips' Laxative, Uro-Mag	Caplet	250 mg, 500 mg
		Capsule	140 mg
		Tablet	400 mg, 500 mg

GASTROINTESTINAL

Gastroesophageal Reflux Disease

TECH ALERT:
Gastroesophageal reflux disease is commonly abbreviated as GERD.

Gastroesophageal reflux disease (GERD) is a chronic condition of stomach contents flowing back into the esophagus. Refluxed stomach acid that reaches the esophagus can cause heartburn. Other symptoms include coughing, wheezing, or a sore throat. If GERD continues over time it can lead to an irritation of the esophagus (esophagitis) causing ulcers or bleeding. GERD can be treated with lifestyle modifications (Table 1-69) or medications such as antacids, histamine-2 blockers, and proton pump inhibitors (PPIs). Severe GERD may require surgical intervention.

Helicobacter pylori

Helicobacter pylori (*H pylori*) is a bacterium in the stomach that can lead to development of stomach ulcers. As it is a bacterium it can be treated with antibiotics.

Antidiarrheal

MOA: Works via the opioid receptor to prolong transit time (time from beginning to end of the GI tract) (Table 1-70)

TABLE 1-69. Lifestyle Modifications for GERD

- Maintain a healthy weight
- Wear loose-fitting clothing around the stomach area
- Remain upright 3 hours after meals
- Raise the head of the bed 6 to 8 in
- Avoid smoking
- Avoid exacerbating foods and drinks like chocolate, coffee, peppermint, greasy and spicy foods, tomato-based products, and alcohol

TABLE 1-70. **Examples of Antidiarrheal**			
Generic	*Brand*	*Form*	*Strengths*
Diphenoxylate and atropine	Lomotil	Tablet	2.5 mg/0.025 mg
		Solution	2.5 mg/0.025 mg/5 mL
Loperamide	Imodium	Caplet	2 mg
		Liquid	1 mg/7.5 mL

Indication: Controlling symptoms of diarrhea, including traveler's diarrhea

ADRs: Constipation

ANTIEMETICS

Metoclopramide

MOA: Decreases dopamine and serotonin activity which are responsible for nausea

Indications: Gastroparesis, gastroesophageal reflux, nausea

ADRs: Drowsiness, movement disorders (tremor, rigidity)

Additional notes:

- Pediatric and elderly patients at risk for movement disorders.
- Should be taken 30 minutes prior to a meal.

Ondansetron

MOA: Decreases serotonin activity which is responsible for nausea

Indications: Nausea, vomiting

ADRs: Constipation, headache

Promethazine

MOA: Decreases activity at chemoreceptor trigger zone (CTZ) which is responsible for nausea

Indications: Nausea, vomiting

ADRs: Constipation, dizziness, drowsiness

Additional note:

- Injection can lead to serious tissue injury (Table 1-71).

★ *TECH ALERT: Atropine is added to diphenoxylate to decrease abuse potential. Observe for atropine side effects (ie, dryness, tachycardia, thirst, flushing).*

TABLE 1-71. Examples of Antiemetics

Generic	Brand	Form	Strengths
Metoclopramide	Metozolv, Reglan	Injection	5 mg/mL
		Solution	5 mg/5 mL
		Tablet	5 mg, 10 mg
		Tablet, ODT	5 mg, 10 mg
Ondansetron	Zofran, Zuplenz	Film	4 mg, 8 mg
		Injection	2 mg/mL
		Solution	4 mg/5 mL
		Tablet	4 mg, 8 mg
		Tablet, ODT	4 mg, 8 mg
Promethazine	Phenadoz, Phenergan, Promethegan	Injection	25 mg/mL, 50 mg/mL
		Suppository	12.5 mg, 25 mg, 50 mg
		Syrup	6.25 mg/mL
		Tablet	12.5 mg, 25 mg, 50 mg

Antacids

MOA: Neutralize acid formation in stomach (Figure 1-6)

Indications: Hyperacidity, dyspepsia

ADRs: Constipation (aluminum), diarrhea (magnesium)

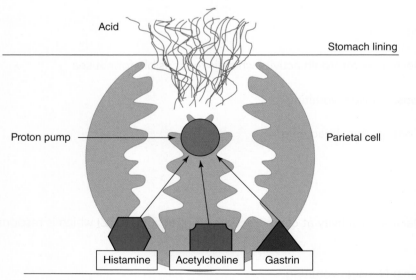

Histamine, acetylcholine, and gastrin stimulate the proton pump to release acid into the stomach. Antacids work by neutralizing the acid in the stomach. Proton pump inhibitors block the final step of acid release by inactivating the proton pump. H_2 blockers inhibit histamine stimulation of the proton pump.

FIGURE 1-6 Antacid medication mechanism of action.

TABLE 1-72. Examples of Antacids

Generic	Brand	Form	Strengths
Aluminum hydroxide	AlternaGel	Suspension	320 mg/5 mL, 600 mg/5 mL
Calcium carbonate	Maalox, Rolaids, Tums	Tablet, chewable	400 mg, 600 mg, 750 mg, 1177 mg
Magnesium hydroxide	Milk of Magnesia	Tablet	311 mg
		Suspension	400 mg/5 mL, 800 mg/5 mL

Additional notes:

- All antacids may decrease the absorption of iron, fluoroquinolone, and tetracycline antibiotics.
- Multiple combination products are available (Table 1-72).

Histamine-2 Blockers

MOA: Inhibit histamine production at the Histamine-2 receptor of the gastric parietal cell, which decreases gastric acid secretion and volume

Indications: Treatment of GERD, erosive esophagitis, ulcers, heartburn, *H. pylori* eradication (in combination with antibiotics)

ADRs: Headache, diarrhea, dizziness, constipation

Additional notes:

- Medications have a common ending of "-tidine" (Table 1-73).
- All medications have at least one strength which are available OTC.
- May be taken without regards to meals.
- Confusion may occur in elderly and patients with renal or hepatic impairment.

★ *TECH ALERT: H. pylori is a bacterium found in the stomach. It is linked to an increased risk of gastrointestinal ulcers. It can be eradicated with a course of antibiotics and PPIs.*

TABLE 1-73. Examples of Histamine-2 Blockers

Generic	Brand	Form	Strengths
Ranitidine	**Zantac**	**Capsule**	**150 mg, 300 mg**
		Tablet	**75 mg, 150 mg, 300 mg**
		Syrup	**15 mg/mL**
		IV	**25 mg/mL**
Famotidine	**Pepcid**	**Tablet**	**10 mg, 20 mg, 40 mg**
		Suspension	**40 mg/mL**
		IV	**10 mg/mL**
Cimetidine	Tagamet	Tablet	200 mg, 300 mg, 400 mg, 800 mg
		Suspension	300 mg/mL
Nizatidine	Axid	Capsule	150 mg
		Suspension	15 mg/mL

TABLE 1-74. Examples of Laxatives

Generic	Type	Brand	Form	Strengths
Bisacodyl	Stimulant	Biscolax, Dulcolax	Suppository	10 mg
			Tablet	5 mg, 10 mg
			Tablet, DR	5 mg
			Tablet, EC	5 mg
Docusate	Softener	Colace, DSS, Kaopectate, Phillips	Capsule	50 mg, 100 mg, 240 mg, 250 mg
			Liquid	50 mg/5 mL
			Tablet	100 mg
Polyethylene glycol	**Osmotic**	**Colyte, GaviLyte, Miralax, MoviPrep, NuLytely, TriLyte**	**Powder**	**17 gm (Miralax) 227-420 gm**
Senna	Stimulant	Little Tummys Laxative, Senna-Lax, Senokot	Liquid	8.8 mg/5 mL, 8.8 mg/mL, 33.3 mg/mL
			Strip	8.6 mg
			Tablet	8.6 mg, 15 mg, 25 mg
			Tablet, chewable	10 mg, 15 mg

Laxative

MOA

- Osmotic: Increases water retention in stool
- Softener: Increases water and fat in stool
- Stimulant: Increases movement of intestine

Indication: Constipation

ADRs: Diarrhea, stomach cramping

Additional note:

- Polyethylene glycol may be used for bowel cleansing prior to a colonoscopy (Table 1-74).

Proton Pump Inhibitors

MOA: Suppress gastric acid secretion by inhibiting the parietal cell hydrogen-potassium adenosine triphosphate pump

Indications: Treatment of GERD, erosive esophagitis, ulcers, heartburn, *H. pylori* eradication (in combination with antibiotics)

ADRs: Headache, abdominal pain, diarrhea

Additional notes:

- Medications have a common ending of "-prazole" (Table 1-75).
- PPIs may increase the risk of *C. difficile*, bone fractures, and hypomagnesemia.

TABLE 1-75. Examples of Proton Pump Inhibitors

Generic	Brand	Form	Strengths
Dexlansoprazole	Dexilant	Capsule	30 mg, 60 mg
Esomeprazole	**Nexium**	**Capsule**	**20 mg, 40 mg**
		Granules	**10 mg, 20 mg, 40 mg**
		IV	**20 mg, 40 mg**
Lansoprazole	**Prevacid**	**Capsule**	**15 mg, 30 mg**
		Suspension	**3 mg/mL**
Omeprazole	**Prilosec, Zegerid**	**Capsule**	**10 mg, 20 mg, 40 mg**
		Tablet	**20 mg**
		Granules	**2.5 mg, 10 mg**
		Suspension	**2 mg/mL**
Pantoprazole	**Protonix**	**Tablet**	**20 mg, 40 mg**
		Granules	**40 mg**
		IV	**40 mg**
Rabeprazole	Aciphex	Tablet	20 mg

- Should be taken on an empty stomach.
- Do not crush capsule and tablets; granules may be mixed with applesauce for administration.

★ *TECH ALERT: C. difficile is a bacterium in the GI tract that causes severe diarrhea. Typically, it occurs after the normal flora of the stomach is destroyed by antibiotics. The incidence can be increased if a patient is also taking a PPI.*

QUICK QUIZ 1-3

1. List the DEA category for the following:
   a. Methylphenidate
   b. Alprazolam

2. What is the indication of memantine?

3. What are the common side effects of Topamax?

4. List common adverse drug reactions for methylprednisolone.

5. Montelukast is indicated for the acute treatment of asthma.
   a. True
   b. False

REPRODUCTIVE AND URINARY MEDICATIONS

Benign Prostatic Hyperplasia

Benign prostatic hyperplasia (BPH) is enlargement of the prostate gland. It can lead to the block of flow of urine out of the bladder and cause bladder, kidney, or urinary tract complications. Patients with BPH experience symptoms of urinary hesitancy, frequency, and retention. BPH can be treated with α blockers or α-reductase inhibitors.

Overactive Bladder

Overactive bladder (OAB) is the requirement of frequent urination and may lead to involuntary loss of urine (incontinence). Nonpharmacologic management of OAB includes limiting fluids, avoiding caffeine, and bladder retraining. Medications for OAB include anticholinergic agents.

α Blockers

MOA: Inhibition of α receptors which cause relaxation of smooth muscle in prostate and bladder

Indications: BPH, hypertension

ADRs: Dizziness, headache, hypotension

Additional notes:

- Medications have a common ending of "-osin" (Table 1-76).
- Only doxazosin and terazosin are indicated for hypertension as they are nonspecific α blockers; they also cause vasodilation in the peripheral smooth muscles causing hypotension.

α-Reductase Inhibitor

MOA: Decreases testosterone levels

Indications: BPH, baldness

ADRs: Impotence

Additional notes:

- Medications have a common ending of "-teride" (Table 1-77).
- Should not be handled by pregnant women because it is absorbed through the skin and is a **teratogen**.

TABLE 1-76. Examples of α Blockers

Generic	Brand	Form	Strengths
Alfuzosin	Uroxatral	Tablet, ER	10 mg
Doxazosin	**Cardura**	**Tablet**	**1 mg, 2 mg, 4 mg, 8 mg**
		Tablet, ER	**4 mg, 8 mg**
Silodosin	Rapaflo	Capsule	4 mg, 8 mg
Tamsulosin	**Flomax**	**Capsule**	**0.4 mg**
Terazosin	**Hytrin**	**Capsule**	**1 mg, 2 mg, 5 mg, 10 mg**

TABLE 1-77. Examples of 5-α-Reductase Inhibitor

Generic	Brand	Form	Strengths
Dutasteride	**Avodart**	**Capsule**	**0.5 mg**
Finasteride	Propecia, Proscar	Tablet	1 mg, 5 mg

Anticholinergic Agent

MOA: Urinary bladder contraction

Indication: OAB

ADRs: Dry mouth, headache, constipation (Table 1-78)

Contraceptives

MOA: Inhibition of ovulation

Indications: Acne, dysfunctional uterine bleeding, pregnancy prevention

ADRs: Edema, nausea

Additional notes:

- Increased risk of cardiovascular side effects (myocardial infarction, thromboembolism) in women who smoke and who are greater than 35 years of age.
- Patients who are noncompliant have a risk of becoming pregnant.
- Do not protect against HIV or other sexually transmitted diseases.
- Emergency contraception is approved by the FDA as an OTC. Pharmacies are required to keep the product behind the counter (Table 1-79).

Hormone Replacement Products

MOA: Replace estrogen that has decreased during menopause

Indications: Symptoms of menopause (bone loss, hot flashes, vaginal symptoms), cancer (high dose)

ADRs: Abdominal pain, headache

TABLE 1-78. Examples of Anticholinergic Agents

Generic	Brand	Form	Strengths
Darifenacin	Enablex	Tablet, ER	7.5 mg, 15 mg
Fesoterodine	Toviaz	Tablet, ER	4 mg, 8 mg
Tolterodine	**Detrol**	**Capsule, ER** **Tablet**	**2 mg, 4 mg** **1 mg, 2 mg**
Trospium	Sanctura	Capsule, ER Tablet	60 mg 20 mg

TABLE 1-79. Examples of Contraceptives

Generic	Brand	Form
Estradiol/dienogest	Natazia	Tablet
Ethinyl estradiol/desogestrel	Apri, Azurette, Caziant, Cyclessa, Desogen, Emoquette, Kariva, Mircette, Ortho-Cept	Tablet
Ethinyl estradiol/drospirenone	**Gianvi, Loryna, Ocella, Syeda, Vestura, Yasmin, Yaz, Zarah**	**Tablet**
Ethinyl estradiol/ethynodiol diacetate	Kelnor, Zovia	Tablet
Ethinyl estradiol/etonogestrel	**NuvaRing**	**Ring, vaginal**
Ethinyl estradiol/levonorgestrel	Aviane, Enpresse, Jolessa, Lessina, Levora, Nordette, Portia, Seasonique, Trivora	Tablet
Ethinyl estradiol/norelgestromin	Ortho Evra	Patch
Ethinyl estradiol/norethindrone	**Estrostep, Loestrin, Microgestin, Neocon, Ortho-Novum, Ovcon**	**Tablet**
Ethinyl estradiol/norgestimate	**MonoNessa, Ortho-Tri-Cyclen, Previfem, Sprintec, Tri-Previfem, Tri-Sprintec, TriNessa**	**Tablet**

Additional notes:

- May increase risk of breast and endometrial cancer.
- Increased risk of cardiovascular disease (heart attack), stroke, and blood clots.
- Lowest dose for shortest period of time recommended (Table 1-80).

TABLE 1-80. Example of Hormone Replacement Products

Generic	Brand	Form	Strengths
Estradiol	**Alora, Climara, Delestrogen, Depo-Estradiol, Estrace, EstroGel, FemRing, Femtrace, Vivelle-Dot**	**Gel**	**0.06%, 1%**
		Injection	**5 mg, 10 mg, 20 mg, 40 mg**
		Patch	**0.014 mg, 0.025 mg, 0.375 mg, 0.05 mg, 0.06 mg, 0.075 mg, 0.1 mg**
		Ring	**0.05 mg, 0.1 mg**
		Spray	**1.53 mg**
		Tablet	**0.5 mg, 1 mg, 2 mg**
Estrogens (conjugated A/synthetic)	**Cenestin**	**Tablet**	**0.3 mg, 0.45 mg, 0.625 mg, 0.9 mg, 1.25 mg**
Estrogens (conjugated B/synthetic)	**Enjuvia**	**Tablet**	**0.3 mg, 0.45 mg, 0.625 mg, 0.9 mg, 1.25 mg**
Estrogens (conjugated/equine)	**Premarin**	**Cream**	**0.625 mg/g**
		Injection	**25 mg**
		Tablet	**0.3 mg, 0.45 mg, 0.625 mg, 0.9 mg, 1.25 mg**
Estrogens (esterified)	Menest	Tablet	0.3 mg, 0.625 mg, 1.25 mg, 2.5 mg
Estropipate	Ogen	Tablet	0.75 mg, 1.5 mg, 3 mg

TABLE 1-81. Examples of Phosphodiesterase-5 Enzyme (PDE) Inhibitor			
Generic	*Brand*	*Form*	*Strengths*
Avanafil	Stendra	Tablet	50 mg, 100 mg, 200 mg
Sildenafil	**Revatio, Viagra**	**Injection**	**0.8 mg/mL**
		Tablet	**20 mg, 25 mg, 50 mg, 100 mg**
Tadalafil	**Adcirca, Cialis**	**Tablet**	**2.5 mg, 5 mg, 10 mg, 20 mg**
Vardenafil	Levitra, Staxyn	Tablet	2.5 mg, 5 mg, 10 mg, 20 mg
		Tablet, ODT	10 mg

Phosphodiesterase-5 Enzyme Inhibitor

MOA: Increase flow of blood into the penis during sexual stimulation; vasodilation in the lungs

Indications: Erectile dysfunction, pulmonary artery hypertension

ADRs: Headache, gastrointestinal upset, rhinitis

Additional notes:

- Medications have a common ending of "-afil" (Table 1-81).
- Avoid use with nitrates, concurrent administration can lead to extreme hypotension.

Selective Estrogen Receptor Modulator

MOA: Acts on estrogen receptor to prevent bone loss (Table 1-82)

Indications: Osteoporosis, risk reduction for breast cancer

ADRs: Edema, hot flashes, muscle pain

Urinary Analgesic

MOA: Unknown mechanism

Indications: Symptomatic relief of burning, itching, frequency, urgency associated with urinary tract infections

ADRs: Dizziness, headache, urinary discoloration

TABLE 1-82. Example of Selective Estrogen Receptor Modulator			
Generic	*Brand*	*Form*	*Strength*
Raloxifene	**Evista**	**Tablet**	**60 mg**

TABLE 1-83. Example of Urinary Analgesic

Generic	Brand	Form	Strengths
Phenazopyridine	AZO, Baridium, Phenazo, Pyridium	Tablet	95 mg, 100 mg, 200 mg

Additional note:

- Phenazopyridine will not treat urinary tract infections, only the associated symptoms. Patients should be advised to follow up with a physician for treatment of a urinary tract infection (Table 1-83).

OPHTHALMIC AGENTS

Glaucoma

Glaucoma is caused by an increase in intraocular pressure that can damage the optic nerve, ultimately resulting in loss of vision. Treatment includes the use of ophthalmic agents that decrease intraocular pressure.

Antiglaucoma Ophthalmic Agents

MOA: Decrease intraocular pressure

Indication: Glaucoma

ADRs: Blurred vision, burning, stinging

Additional note:

- Medications ending in -prost may permanently change eye color to brown; also increases eyelash length and number (Table 1-84).

TABLE 1-84. Examples of Antiglaucoma Ophthalmic Agents

Generic	Brand	Form	Strengths
Bimatoprost	Latisse, Lumigan	Solution	0.01%, 0.03%
Brimonidine	Alphagan P	Solution	0.1%, 0.15%
Latanoprost	**Xalatan**	**Solution**	**0.005%**
Tafluprost	Zioptan	Solution	0.0015%
Timolol	Betimol, Timolol, Timoptic	Gel Solution	0.25%, 0.5% 0.25%, 0.5%
Travoprost	Travatan Z	Solution	0.004%

TABLE 1-85. Examples of Antibiotic Ophthalmic Agents

Generic	Brand	Form	Strengths
Ciprofloxacin Ophthalmic	Ciloxan	Ointment	0.3%
		Solution	0.3%
Moxifloxacin Ophthalmic	**Moxeza, Vigamox**	**Solution**	**0.5%**
Tobramycin	AK-Tob, Tobrex	Ointment	0.3%
		Solution	0.3%

Antibiotic Ophthalmic Agents

MOA: Inhibition of bacteria locally in eye (Table 1-85)

Indication: Bacterial **conjunctivitis**

ADRs: Dry eye, eye irritation

TOPICAL MEDICATIONS

Antifungals

MOA: Inhibit fungal formation (Table 1-86)

Indications: Tinea, dermatitis

ADRs: Burning, irritation, itching

Corticosteroids

MOA: Decrease inflammation

Indications: Dermatitis, eczema, psoriasis, rashes

ADRs: Burning, irritation, itching

★ *TECH ALERT: Creams, lotions, and ointments are not interchangeable. Use caution with dispensing.*

★ *TECH ALERT: Lidocaine patches may be cut to appropriate size. The patch should be applied to the most painful site and up to 3 patches at a time may be used. Patches should only remain on for 12 hours during a 24-hour period.*

VITAMINS

Vitamins are classified as either water or fat soluble. Fat-soluble vitamins (Table 1-87) are dissolved in the lipids or fat of the body, and therefore can remain stored in the body. Water-soluble vitamins (Table 1-88) dissolve in water, so they are excreted in the urine and not stored within the body. The

TABLE 1-86. Examples of Topical Medications

Generic	Category	Brand	Form	Strengths
Triamcinolone	**Corticosteroid**	**Kenalog, Oralone, Pediaderm, Trianex, Triderm, Zytopic**	**Aerosol** **Cream** **Lotion** **Ointment** **Paste**	**0.2 mg** **0.025%, 0.1%, 0.5%** **0.025%, 0.1%** **0.025%, 0.05%, 0.1%, 0.5%** **0.1%**
Betamethasone/ clotrimazole	**Corticosteroid/ antifungal**	**Lotrisone**	**Cream** **Lotion**	**0.05%/1%** **0.05%/1%**
Ciclopirox	Antifungal	Ciclodan, Loprox, Penlac	Cream Gel Shampoo Nail polish Suspension	0.77% 0.77% 1% 8% 0.77%
Clobetasol	**Corticosteroid**	**Clobex, Cormax, Olux, Temovate**	**Foam** **Cream** **Gel** **Lotion** **Ointment** **Shampoo** **Solution**	**0.05%** **0.05%** **0.05%** **0.05%** **0.05%** **0.05%** **0.05%**
Ketoconazole	Antifungal	Extina, Nizoral, Xolegel	Foam Cream Gel Shampoo	2% 2% 2% 1%, 2%
Lidocaine Patch	**Analgesic**	**Lidoderm**	**Patch**	**5%**
Nystatin	Antifungal	Nystop, Pedi-Dri	Cream Ointment Powder	100,000 units/g 100,000 units/g 100,000 units/g

TABLE 1-87. Fat-Soluble Vitamins

Vitamin	Name	Use
A	Retinol	Vision, immune system, reproduction
D_2	Ergocalciferol	Absorption of calcium, osteoporosis prevention
D_3	Cholecalciferol	Absorption of calcium, osteoporosis prevention
E	α-Tocopherol	Antioxidant, immune system
K	Phytonadione	Blood clotting

TABLE 1-88. Water-Soluble Vitamins		
Vitamin	Name	Use
B₁	Thiamine	Energy generation from carbohydrates
B₂	Riboflavin	Energy production
B₃	Niacin	Energy transfer and metabolism of glucose, fat, and alcohol
B₅	Pantothenic acid	Oxidation of fatty acids and carbohydrates
B₆	Pyridoxine	Metabolism of amino acids and lipids
B₇	Biotin	Metabolism of lipids, proteins, and carbohydrates
B₉	Folic acid	Formation of coenzymes
B₁₂	Cyanocobalamin	Production of red blood cells
C	Ascorbic acid	Cofactor in enzyme reactions

fat-soluble vitamins include A, D, E, and K, and the water-soluble vitamins are the B-complexes and vitamin C.

Folic Acid

MOA: Formation of many coenzymes in the body

Indications: Anemia, prevents neural tube defects during pregnancy

ADRs: Minimal

Iron Salts

MOA: Allows transport of oxygen via red blood cells

Indication: Anemia

ADRs: Constipation, dark stools, nausea

Additional note:

- Multiple salt forms and doses; caution should be used in dispensing (Table 1-89).

WEIGHT LOSS AGENTS

Obesity

Obesity is an excessive amount of body fat. It can increase the risk of heart disease, diabetes, and high blood pressure. Medications for weight loss are usually recommended for patients with a body mass index (BMI) of greater than 30 or greater than 27 with medical complications of obesity.

★ *TECH ALERT:*
*BMI = weight (kg)/height(m²)
A patient who is 64 in and weighs 240 lb would have a BMI of 41.2.*

TABLE 1-89. Examples of Vitamins			
Generic	*Brand*	*Form*	*Strengths*
Folic acid	**Folvite, Folacin**	**Injection**	**5 mg/mL**
		Tablet	**0.4 mg, 0.8 mg, 1 mg**
Ferrous fumarate	Femiron, Ferrets, Ferrocite, Hemocyte	Tablet	63 mg, 200 mg, 324 mg, 325 mg
		Tablet, TR	150 mg
Ferrous gluconate	Ferate, Fergon	Tablet	240 mg, 246 mg, 324 mg, 325 mg
Ferrous sulfate	**Feosol, Fer-In-Sol, Fer-iron, SlowFE**	**Liquid**	**75 mg/mL, 220 mg/5 mL, 300 mg/5 mL**
		Tablet	**324 mg, 325 mg**
		Tablet, EC	**324 mg, 325 mg**
		Tablet, ER	**140 mg**
		Tablet, SR	**140 mg, 142 mg, 160 mg**

Anorexiant

MOA: Appetite suppressant

Indication: Obesity

ADRs: Dizziness, dry mouth, euphoria, overstimulation

Additional note:

- Phentermine is a DEA schedule class IV. It is only indicated for short-term weight loss. States vary in prescribing laws.

Lipase Inhibitor

MOA: Inhibition of enzyme for fat digestion in the stomach

Indication: Obesity

ADRs: Abdominal pain, diarrhea, headache

Additional note:

- If dietary fats are greater than 30% of calories, gastrointestinal events increase (Table 1-90).

Other Top 200 Medications

Crohn disease is an inflammatory bowel disease that can cause abdominal pain, diarrhea, and malnutrition. It can affect different areas of the digestive tract.

Ectopic pregnancy is a complication of pregnancy when the embryo implants outside the uterus. This is a nonviable pregnancy that is life threatening to the mother.

TABLE 1-90. Examples of Anorexiants

Generic	Category	Brand	Form	Strengths
Lorcaserin	Anorexiant	Belviq	Tablet	10 mg
Orlistat	Lipase inhibitor	Alli, Xenical	Capsule	60 mg, 120 mg
Phentermine	**Anorexiant**	**Adipex-P, Suprenza**	**Capsule** **Tablet** **Tablet, ODT**	**15 mg, 30 mg, 37.5 mg** **37.5 mg** **15 mg, 30 mg**
Phentermine/ topiramate	Anorexiant	Qsymia	Capsule	3.75/23 mg, 7.5/46 mg, 11.25/69 mg, 15/92 mg

Gout is a type of arthritis that occurs with a buildup of uric acid in the body. It often leads to inflammation and pain, usually only in one joint.

Malaria is a mosquito-born infectious disease that causes fevers and flu-like symptoms. It is usually acquired in a subtropical or tropical country.

Osteoporosis is the loss of bone density due to a decrease in calcium and minerals. The bones then become more fragile and have an increased risk of fracture.

Psoriasis is an immune condition that causes skin cells to grow quickly leading to redness and irritation.

Rheumatoid arthritis (RA) is an autoimmune disease that causes chronic inflammation. It typically affects the joints and surrounding tissues causing pain and swelling.

Systemic lupus erythematosus (SLE) is a chronic autoimmune disease in which the body mistakenly attacks healthy tissue. It can affect every organ system leading to failure.

Aminoquinoline

MOA: Inhibits malaria parasite function; decreases inflammation

Indications: Malaria, SLE, rheumatoid arthritis

ADRs: Dizziness, headache, nausea, ophthalmic effects, sunlight sensitivity

Additional note:

- Patients should have eye examinations every 3 months while on this medication (Table 1-91).

TABLE 1-91. Example of Aminoquinoline

Generic	Brand	Form	Strengths
Hydroxychloroquine	**Plaquenil**	**Tablet**	**200 mg**

TABLE 1-92. **Examples of Anticholinergics**			
Generic	*Brand*	*Form*	*Strengths*
Benztropine	**Cogentin**	**Injection**	**1 mg/mL**
		Tablet	**0.5 mg, 1 mg, 2 mg**
Dicyclomine	**Bentyl**	**Capsule**	**10 mg**
		Injection	**10 mg/mL**
		Syrup	**10 mg/5 mL**
		Tablet	**20 mg**

ANTICHOLINERGIC AGENTS

MOA: Decrease involuntary movements in stomach, bladder, lungs

Indications

- Dicyclomine: Irritable bowel, urinary incontinence
- Benztropine: Parkinson disease, drug-induced **extrapyramidal symptoms**

ADRs: Dizziness, drowsiness, dry mouth, vision changes (Table 1-92)

ANTIGOUT MEDICATIONS

Allopurinol and Febuxostat

MOA: Decrease uric acid

- High concentrations of uric acid lead to gout

Indication: Gout

ADRs: Liver function abnormalities, nausea, rash

Colchicine

MOA: Anti-inflammatory

Indication: Acute gout flare

ADRs: Diarrhea, gastrointestinal upset, nausea

Additional note:

- It has no analgesic activity throughout the rest of the body, thus should only be used to treat pain from gout. (Table 1-93)

Bisphosphonate

MOA: Increase in bone density

TABLE 1-93. **Examples of Antigout Agents**			
Generic	*Brand*	*Form*	*Strengths*
Allopurinol	**Aloprim, Zyloprim**	**Injection**	**500 mg**
		Tablet	**100 mg, 300 mg**
Colchicine	**Colcrys**	**Tablet**	**0.6 mg**
Febuxostat	Uloric	Tablet	40 mg, 80 mg

Indications: Osteoporosis

ADRs: Gastrointestinal upset, hypocalcemia

Additional notes:

- Medications have a common ending of "-dronate" (Table 1-94).
- Ensure adequate calcium and vitamin D intake.
- Must be taken first thing in the morning on an empty stomach, and patient must remain upright for at least 30 minutes after taking.
- The required administration frequency of bisphosphonates varies based on the dose. It ranges from daily, weekly, monthly, to yearly depending on the product formulation.

Methotrexate

MOA: Inhibits DNA synthesis, repair, replication allowing it to be used in oncology; anti-inflammatory activity

Indications: Chron's disease, ectopic pregnancy, oncology, psoriasis, rheumatoid arthritis

ADRs: Dizziness, immunosuppression, reddening of skin

Additional note:

- Severe reactions include renal failure, bone marrow suppression, dermatologic toxicity, liver failure, cancer, neurotoxicity, infection (Table 1-95).

TABLE 1-94. **Examples of Bisphosphonates**			
Generic	*Brand*	*Form*	*Strengths*
Alendronate	**Binosto, Fosamax**	**Tablet**	**5 mg, 10 mg, 35 mg, 40 mg, 70 mg**
		Tablet, effervescent	**70 mg**
Ibandronate	**Boniva**	**Injection**	**1 mg/mL**
		Tablet	**150 mg**
Risedronate	Actonel, Atelvia	Tablet	5 mg, 30 mg, 35 mg, 150 mg
		Tablet, DR	35 mg

TABLE 1-95. **Methotrexate**			
Generic	*Brand*	*Form*	*Strengths*
Methotrexate	**Rheumatrex, Trexall**	**Injection**	**25 mg/mL**
		Tablet	**2.5 mg, 5 mg, 7.5 mg, 10 mg, 15 mg**

QUICK QUIZ 1-4

1. Why should dutasteride not be touched by a pregnant woman?

2. What is the indication of latanoprost?

3. Ferrous sulfate causes diarrhea.

   a. True

   b. False

4. What are the side effects of dicyclomine?

5. Phentermine is a DEA schedule class IV.

   a. True

   b. False

CASE STUDY REVIEW

You are assisting a pharmacist with a patient in the emergency room. The patient's neighbor called 911 after finding her passed out in her kitchen. The patient is a 76-year-old woman with an unknown past medical history. The EMS first responders were able to bring the patient's medication bottles with her. The labels on the bottles include the following:
- Lisinopril 10 mg—Take 1 tablet by mouth daily—#30
- Alprazolam 1 mg—Take 1 tablet by mouth twice daily as needed—#60
- Levothyroxine 88 µg—Take 1 tablet by mouth daily—#30
- Oxycontin 10 mg—Take 1 tablet by mouth twice daily—#60

Self-Assessment Questions
- What are the indications for the medications taken by the patient?
  - Lisinopril: Hypertension, heart failure, or myocardial infarction
- Could any of the medications taken cause her to be sedated?
  - Alprazolam and Oxycontin can both cause sedation.
- What are the brand and generic names for the medications taken by the patient?
  - Lisinopril: Prinivil, Zestril
  - Alprazolam: Xanax
  - Levothyroxine: Levothroid, Levoxyl, Synthroid
  - Oxycodone CR: Oxycontin
- Are there any drug interactions between the patient's medications?
  - Alprazolam and Oxycontin combined can increase the risk of sedation.

CHAPTER SUMMARY

- Know the generic and brand name of the top 200 pharmaceuticals.
- Understand the definition of therapeutic equivalence and the difference between the categories.
- Identify common drug interactions (ie, drug-disease, drug-drug, drug-dietary supplement, drug-OTC, drug-laboratory, drug-nutrient).
- Recognize the strengths or dose, dosage forms, physical appearance, routes of administration, and duration of drug therapy.
- Name common and severe side or adverse effects, allergies, and therapeutic contraindications associated with medications.
- List dosage and indication of legend, OTC medications, herbal and dietary supplement.

ANSWERS TO QUICK QUIZZES

Quick Quiz 1-1

1. Cephalosporins
2. Azithromycin, clarithromycin, erythromycin
3. Metronidazole
4. Percocet: C-II; Vicodin: C-III; Dilaudid: C-II; Duragesic: C-II
5. Bleeding, dizziness, gastrointestinal upset

Quick Quiz 1-2

1. Potassium chloride
2. Hepatotoxicity, myopathy
3. PDE-5 inhibitors
4. No
5. Clopidogrel

Quick Quiz 1-3

1. Methylphenidate: C-II; alprazolam: C-IV
2. Dementia
3. Anorexia, paresthesia, somnolence, weight loss
4. Adrenal suppression, hyperglycemia, infection, nausea, osteoporosis, psychiatric disorders, weight gain
5. False

Quick Quiz 1-4

1. Teratogen

2. Glaucoma

3. False

4. Dizziness, drowsiness, dry mouth, vision changes

5. True

CHAPTER QUESTIONS

1. Which of the following antifungals is not a topical agent?
   a. Diflucan
   b. Extina
   c. Nizoral
   d. Xolegel

2. A 55-year-old female patient brings in a prescription for Mobic. His current prescription list includes aspirin 81 mg daily, Coumadin 5 mg daily, Zocor 40 mg daily, and fentanyl transdermal patch every 72 hours. What should you alert the pharmacist about?
   a. Mobic is contraindicated in females.
   b. A potential drug interaction between Mobic and Zocor.
   c. Mobic can increase the sedation caused by fentanyl transdermal.
   d. The drug interaction between Mobic, aspirin, and Coumadin.

3. What is the generic name of Voltaren?
   a. Diclofenac
   b. Ibuprofen
   c. Meloxicam
   d. Nabumetone

4. NSAID medications can increase the risk of which serious side effect?
   a. Gastrointestinal bleeding
   b. Seizures
   c. Respiratory depression
   d. Arrhythmias

5. Which of the following is *not* a side effect of opioids?
   a. Diarrhea
   b. Constipation
   c. Sedation
   d. Respiratory depression

6. Fentanyl transdermal is in which DEA class?
   a. I
   b. II
   c. III
   d. IV

7. Sumatriptan is indicated for which of the following?
   a. Hypertension
   b. Back pain
   c. Migraine
   d. Parkinson disease

8. Which beverage should not be consumed with a HMG CoA reductase inhibitor?
   a. Water
   b. Grapefruit juice
   c. Wine
   d. Orange juice

9. What is the generic name of Crestor?
   a. Atorvastatin
   b. Lovastatin
   c. Pravastatin
   d. Rosuvastatin

CHAPTER 1: Pharmacology for Technicians

10. Which of the following patients should not be prescribed Lotensin?
   a. A 34 year-old pregnant woman
   b. A 7 year-old girl
   c. A 65 year-old man
   d. A 95 year-old man

11. What is the generic name of Altace?
   a. Benazepril
   b. Lisinopril
   c. Quinapril
   d. Ramipril

12. Which of the following is available in an injection formulation?
   a. Levothyroxine
   b. Thyroid, desiccated
   c. Methimazole
   d. Propylthiouracil

13. Which of the following is not a side effect of Augmentin?
   a. Diarrhea
   b. Allergic reaction
   c. Constipation
   d. Rash

14. Lisinopril is in which class of medication?
   a. Angiotensin-converting enzyme inhibitor
   b. Angiotensin II receptor blocker
   c. β Blocker
   d. Calcium channel blocker

15. Which of the following disease states may be exacerbated by Inderal?
   a. Hypercholesterolemia
   b. Diabetes
   c. Asthma
   d. Anxiety

16. Which of the following medications should not be crushed?
   a. Tenormin
   b. Ziac
   c. Coreg
   d. Toprol XL

17. Which of the following is not used to treat hypertension?
   a. ACEIs
   b. ARBs
   c. β Blockers
   d. Statins

18. You receive a prescription for atenolol 25 mg #30—1 tab PO qd. What is the likely indication?
   a. Diabetes
   b. Hypercholesterolemia
   c. Hypertension
   d. Depression

19. When should Lasix 20 mg daily be taken?
   a. With breakfast
   b. With lunch
   c. Before dinner
   d. At bedtime

20. Which of the following is not an indication for nitroglycerin?
   a. Anal fissure
   b. Angina
   c. Heart failure
   d. Hyperlipidemia

21. What is the generic name of Plavix?
   a. Cilostazol
   b. Clopidogrel
   c. Prasugrel
   d. Ticagrelor

22. Which patient should not be taking metformin?
   a. A 24 year-old woman with seizures
   b. A 56 year-old man with renal failure
   c. A 55 year-old woman with hypertension
   d. A 78 year-old man with heart failure

23. If a patient has a severe allergic reaction to amoxicillin, which antibiotic they should not take?
   a. Levofloxacin
   b. Azithromycin
   c. Cefdinir
   d. Minocycline

24. What time of the day should Amaryl be taken?
    a. Before meals
    b. At bedtime
    c. After meals
    d. Immediately upon rising

25. Which of the following routes has the fastest onset of action?
    a. Oral
    b. Intravenous injection
    c. Transdermal
    d. Intramuscular

26. What is the primary indication of trazodone?
    a. Seizures
    b. Anxiety
    c. Attention deficit hyperactivity disorder
    d. Depression

27. What does the abbreviation OD mean?
    a. Right eye
    b. Left eye
    c. Right ear
    d. Left ear

28. Pioglitazone may exacerbate which of the following disease states?
    a. Heart failure
    b. Migraines
    c. Seizures
    d. Hypothyroidism

29. What is the brand name of rosiglitazone?
    a. Actos
    b. Avandia
    c. Glucophage
    d. Glynase

30. What is methimazole is indicated for?
    a. Hypothyroidism
    b. Hypoglycemia
    c. Hyperthyroidism
    d. Hyperglycemia

31. What is a common side effect of ACEIs?
    a. Sore throat
    b. Cough
    c. Anxiety
    d. Sedation

32. How many milligrams of codeine are in Tylenol #4?
    a. 15 mg
    b. 30 mg
    c. 45 mg
    d. 60 mg

33. A patient brings in a prescription for Zyban. What is the patient trying to stop?
    a. Smoking cigarettes
    b. Drinking alcohol
    c. Eating fatty foods
    d. Texting while driving

34. Which of the following medication cannot be crushed?
    a. Celexa
    b. Prozac
    c. Effexor XR
    d. Keppra

35. What is the main indication of ketoconazole?
    a. Antifungal
    b. Antibacterial
    c. Antiviral
    d. Antianxiety

36. A patient brings in a prescription for Ativan. How many months can this prescription be refilled?
    a. 0
    b. 1
    c. 6
    d. 12

37. What is the indication of zolpidem?
    a. Insomnia
    b. Bipolar
    c. Depression
    d. Anxiety

38. What is a side effect of Spiriva?
    a. Blurred vision
    b. Dry mouth
    c. Thrush
    d. Tachycardia

39. Diuretics can cause a decrease in which of the following?
    a. Electrolytes
    b. Cholesterol
    c. Blood sugar
    d. Serotonin

40. Which of the following is an expectorant?
    a. Dextromethorphan
    b. Pseudoephedrine
    c. Guaifenesin
    d. Codeine

41. Which of the following patients is at a high risk of cardiovascular side effects while taking Ovcon?
    a. A 40-year-old woman, nonsmoker
    b. A 25-year-old woman, smoker
    c. A 36-year-old woman, smoker
    d. All of the above

42. Which pharmacy reference book contains therapeutic equivalence?
    a. *The Red Book*
    b. *The Blue Book*
    c. *The Orange Book*
    d. *The Purple Book*

43. Lyrica is in which DEA class?
    a. II
    b. III
    c. IV
    d. V

44. Which of the following brand/generic pair is not correct?
    a. Lipitor/atorvastatin
    b. Zocor/simvastatin
    c. Crestor/lovastatin
    d. Pravachol/pravastatin

45. Which medication cannot treat seizures?
    a. Neurontin
    b. Keppra
    c. Wellbutrin
    d. Topamax

46. Sinemet increases the concentration of which of the following?
    a. Norepinephrine
    b. Epinephrine
    c. Dopamine
    d. Serotonin

47. Atypical antipsychotics can increase which of the following?
    a. Electrolytes
    b. Cholesterol
    c. Blood sugar
    d. Blood pressure

48. What is a common side effect of Zyprexa?
    a. Weight loss
    b. Depression
    c. Weight gain
    d. Constipation

49. Which of the following is a side effect of Ritalin?
    a. Insomnia
    b. Sedation
    c. Gastrointestinal upset
    d. Rash

50. Antacids should not be taken simultaneously with which of the following?
    a. Ferrous sulfate
    b. Ciprofloxacin
    c. Doxycycline
    d. All of the above

Pharmacy Law and Regulations for the Pharmacy Technician

CHAPTER 2

PTCB KNOWLEDGE AREAS

2.1. Storage, handling, and disposal of hazardous substances and wastes (eg, material safety data sheet [MSDS])

2.2. Hazardous substance exposure, prevention, and treatment (eg., eyewash, spill kit, MSDS)

2.3. Controlled substance transfer regulations (DEA)

2.4. Controlled substance documentation requirements for receiving, ordering, returning, loss or theft, destruction

2.5. Formula to verify the validity of a prescriber's DEA number (DEA)

2.6. Record keeping, documentation, and record retention (eg, length of time prescriptions are maintained on file)

2.7. Restricted drug programs and related prescription-processing requirements (eg, thalidomide, isotretinoin, clozapine)

2.8. Professional standards related to data integrity, security, and confidentiality (eg, HIPAA, backing up and archiving)

2.9. Requirement for consultation (eg, OBRA '90)

2.10. Food and Drug Administration's (FDA's) recall classification

2.11. Infection control standards (eg, laminar air flow, clean room, hand washing, cleaning counting trays, countertop, and equipment) (OSHA, USP <795> and <797>)

2.12. Record keeping for repackaged and recalled products and supplies (TJC, BOP)

2.13. Professional standards regarding the roles and responsibilities of pharmacists, pharmacy technicians, and other pharmacy employees (TJC, BOP)

2.14. Reconciliation between state and federal laws and regulations

2.15. Facility, equipment, and supply requirements (eg, space requirements, prescription file storage, cleanliness, reference materials) (TJC, USP, BOP)

KEY TERMS

Controlled substance: Any drug that is in schedule I through V and regulated by the Drug Enforcement Administration (DEA)

Cross contamination: The unintentional transfer of one drug onto another through powder residue or insufficient cleaning practices

Drug Enforcement Administration (DEA): The federal agency that enforces controlled substance laws and regulations of the United States

Food and Drug Administration (FDA): An agency within the US Department of Health and Human Services responsible for protecting the public health, regulating tobacco products, assuring safe cosmetics and dietary supplements, and also promoting advancements in public health

Health Insurance Portability and Accountability Act (HIPAA): A federal act which protects the privacy of individually identifiable health information and sets standards for the security and sharing of this information

Monograph: Detailed information about a drug, including indication, dosage, description, side effect information, pharmacologic properties, and warnings

National Association of the Boards of Pharmacy (NABP): Comprised of all the State Boards of Pharmacy, has no regulatory authority

National Formulary (NF): Standards for excipients, botanicals, and other similar products

Over-the-counter (OTC): Medication that can be purchased without a prescription

Protected health information (PHI): Information that is related to the health of a patient (eg diagnosis, current treatments, surgeries, etc)

State Boards of Pharmacy (BOP): Specific to each state, can discipline pharmacy personnel, and has regulatory authority to develop new standards

United States Pharmacopeia (USP): A scientific nonprofit organization that sets standards for the identity, strength, quality, and purity of medicines, food ingredients, and dietary supplements manufactured, distributed, and consumed worldwide.

CASE STUDY

A customer, John Smith, enters your pharmacy and presents a prescription to you. You recognize the customer but the name on the prescription is for Ted Turner. He tells you that Ted is his neighbor. The prescription is written for alprazolam tablets to be used as needed for restlessness. The prescription is from Paige Turner, DDS. You see that the DEA number on the prescription is BT1578395. The prescription was written 3 weeks ago.

John really wants to get this script filled and give it back to his neighbor. You take the prescription back to the pharmacist for some clarification prior to entering the information into the computer. After reviewing the prescription, the pharmacist decides to ask Mr. Smith a few more questions and then makes a phone call to Dr. Paige Turner's office.

The pharmacist has decided not to fill the prescription and informs Mr. Smith that a full explanation of the reason for not filling the script will be reviewed with Mr. Turner over the phone. Take a look at the example of a typical prescription shown in Figure 2-1.

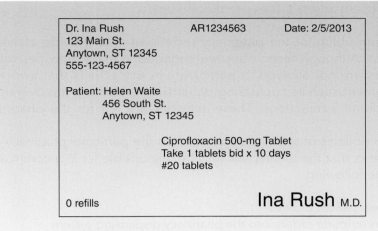

Dr. Ina Rush	AR1234563	Date: 2/5/2013
123 Main St.		
Anytown, ST 12345		
555-123-4567		

Patient: Helen Waite
456 South St.
Anytown, ST 12345

Ciprofloxacin 500-mg Tablet
Take 1 tablets bid x 10 days
#20 tablets

0 refills   **Ina Rush** M.D.

FIGURE 2-1 Sample prescription.

INTRODUCTION

This chapter will describe significant pharmacy laws and the importance of regulations in pharmacy practice. Pharmacy technicians are in the privileged position to assist the pharmacist in caring for the public. Because of this tremendous responsibility, it is necessary to govern the profession with rules and regulations. These laws help protect the patient and standardize the process of dispensing medications.

In this chapter, the laws which have shaped the practice of pharmacy over the last century will be introduced. Additionally, there will be an overview of the governing bodies that are responsible for protecting the public and the practice of pharmacy. There will also be a discussion on the specific laws and regulations that apply to every pharmacy technician and pharmacy to describe how to practice carefully and safely.

PHARMACY PERSONNEL

The pharmacy must have an adequate number of licensed pharmacists in order to meet the needs of the patients. The pharmacist may also fulfill the role of a manager or director depending on the overall business unit and structure of the organization. Pharmacists are in the position to oversee the daily workflow of the pharmacy and to ensure effective communication between pharmacy support personnel, pharmacy technicians, and patients.

Pharmacy technicians will have a job description outlining the responsibilities of the role as well as the level of competency required to perform all of the functions to support the pharmacist and the organization. State Boards of Pharmacy may have specific rules and laws associated with the scope of technician responsibilities within the pharmacy. Pharmacy technicians should be familiar with State Board of Pharmacy requirements for the state in which they practice. Employers that place technicians into roles requiring advanced skill sets should have additional training available with a mechanism to evaluate competency as required by regulatory bodies.

Pharmacy Technician's Responsibilities

The main responsibility of the pharmacy technician is to provide assistance to the pharmacist. Although technicians are engaged in many activities within the pharmacy, they are not allowed to participate in any activity that involves professional judgment such as counseling patients or evaluating the overall potential for medication interactions. These activities are left for the pharmacist to complete.

The responsibilities of technicians depend on the particular pharmacy setting. Some of the tasks that the technicians may be responsible for in a community setting include the following:

- Creating new patient profiles
- Entering prescription orders into the pharmacy dispensing system
- Communicating with insurance carriers to obtain proper billing information and troubleshoot claims
- Assisting with all filling and labeling requirements
- Compounding nonsterile prescriptions, such as creams or ointments
- Reconstituting oral suspensions
- Assisting with training and educating other technicians
- Greeting customers, answering telephone calls, and ensuring the patient receives the correct prescription
- Obtaining refill authorizations from prescribers
- Putting away drug orders and assisting in drug inventory

Some tasks that the technician may be responsible for in a hospital or institutional setting include the following:

- Delivering medications to nursing units
- Filling automated dispensing cabinets or medication carts
- Compounding both sterile and nonsterile products, including chemotherapy
- Repacking bulk medications into unit doses
- Performing monthly unit inspections and checking for outdated medications
- Purchasing drugs and managing drug inventory
- Assisting with training and educating other technicians

★ TECH ALERT: The American Association of Pharmacy Technicians (AAPT) has a pharmacy technician code of ethics that can be viewed at www.pharmacytechnician. com.

Pharmacist's Responsibilities

Whether practicing in a retail setting, a health care system, or even a more nontraditional environment, the pharmacist will always be responsible for overseeing the work of the technician. Following are some other tasks a pharmacist may be responsible for:

- Enter and fill orders and verify instructions for each prescription
- Monitor interactions for each patient
- Counsel patients on taking medication, potential side effects, and the importance of compliance
- Oversee the work of the pharmacy technician staff
- Work with other professionals and practitioners about medication therapies
- Administer specific vaccines as permitted by each State Board of Pharmacy

HISTORY OF PHARMACY LAWS

Just as there are considerable advances in drug therapy, drug delivery, and drug information, so too are there constant changes in the specificity and complexity of the laws and rules which govern the profession of pharmacy. It is the responsibility of the pharmacy technician to understand the legal boundaries of practice. It is important to remember that the following are federal laws, and these laws take precedence over state law, unless the state law is stricter. Pharmacy technicians must be aware of the laws of each individual state, as they vary in regards to certification, registration, and licensing. A summary of pharmacy laws is found in Table 2-1.

TABLE 2-1. Federal Laws and Regulations		
Year of Enactment	Name of Law/Regulation	Description
1906	The Pure Food and Drug Act	Prohibited foreign transport of misbranded or adulterated drugs
1938	The Food, Drug, and Cosmetic Act	Created the FDA and clearly defined adulterated and misbranding
1951	Durham-Humphrey Amendment	Defined legend drug Allowed verbal orders and refills
1962	Kefauver-Harris Amendment	Required medications to be both safe and effective
1970	Controlled Substances Act	Defined categories for controlled substances Established the DEA
1970	The Poison Prevention Packaging Act	Required child-resistant packaging to help prevent accidental poisoning
1970	Occupational Safety and Health Act	Established OSHA and helped protect employees from workplace injuries
1972	Drug Listing Act	Required each drug be assigned NDC number
1983	Orphan Drug Act	Provided tax incentives for manufacturers of orphan drugs
1987	Prescription Drug Marketing Act	Prohibited the sale and distribution of samples to anyone other than those licensed to prescribe them
1990	The Omnibus Budget Reconciliation Act (OBRA)	Established standards for records, DUR, and counseling
1994	Dietary Supplement Health and Education Act (DSHEA)	Dietary supplements were not required to prove safety or effectiveness, but must have proper labeling
1996	The Health Insurance Portability and Accountability Act (HIPAA)	Protected patient confidentiality by ensuring the safe collection, distribution, and usage of all protected health information (PHI)
2003	Medicare Prescription Drug Improvement and Modernization Act of 2003	Created Medicare Part D—a voluntary prescription drug program for Medicare patients
2004	Anabolic Steroid Control Act	Designated anabolic steroids as schedule-III narcotics
2005	Combat Methamphetamine Epidemic Act	Restricted quantity and frequency of ephedrine, pseudoephedrine, and phenylpropanolamine sales

PHARMACY LAWS

The **Pure Food and Drug Act of 1906** required that drugs not be mislabeled. Drugs were required to meet the standards set by the industry for purity and strength. Manufacturers could still make false claims regarding the therapeutic benefit of the medication, but the exact amount of active ingredient was required to be labeled. This act also prohibited the interstate transportation or sale of any adulterated or misbranded drug.

The **Food, Drug, and Cosmetic Act of 1938 (FDCA)** was passed to legally define a drug and establish policies to determine safety. Drugs are defined as the following:

- Items listed in the official United States Pharmacopoeia (USP), the National Formulary (NF), or the Homeopathic Pharmacopoeia of the United States
- Anything intended for use in the prevention, treatment, cure, diagnosis, or mitigation of disease
- Anything that is intended to affect the structure or function of the body of man or other animal

This act also created the FDA and required that any manufacturer producing a new drug must file a new drug application (NDA).

Finally, the FDCA clearly defined the difference between adulteration and misbranding. According to the FDA, adulteration and misbranding include drugs that contain the following features:

Adulteration
- Consists in whole or in part of any filthy, putrid, or decomposed substance.
- Have been prepared, packed, or held under insanitary conditions.
- Container is composed of any poisonous or deleterious substance which may render the contents injurious to health.
- Contains a color additive which is unsafe.

Misbranding
- Labeling is false or misleading in any particular way.
- Packaging that does not have a label containing (1) the name and place of business of the manufacturer, packer, or distributor; and (2) an accurate statement of the quantity of the contents in terms of weight, measure, or numerical count.
- If its container is so made, formed, or filled as to be misleading.
- Drugs are within a container that does not bear a label indicating "warning, may be habit forming" if the drug is habit forming.

Durham-Humphrey Amendment of 1951 was an amendment to the FDCA. This created 2 distinctly separate categories of medications. The 2 classes are OTC medicines and prescription (Rx) medications. Thus, the federal legend, "Caution: Federal Law prohibits dispensing without a prescription" was added to the labels of all prescription medications. This is how prescription drugs became known as "legend drugs."

In addition, the Durham-Humphrey Amendment required pharmacists to obtain authorization (verbal or written) to dispense a prescription drug.

Kefauver-Harris Amendment of 1962

The Kefauver-Harris Amendment of 1962, an addition to the FDCA, required all medications to be both safe and effective. This act was passed in response to the severe birth defects seen in children outside the United States after pregnant women took thalidomide for morning sickness.

TABLE 2-2. **DEA Drug Schedules**	
Schedule	*Definition*
I (C-I)	Have no currently accepted medical use in the United States, have a high potential for abuse, include crack cocaine, heroin, lysergic acid diethylamide (LSD), phencyclidine palmitate (PCP), and opium
II (C-II)	Have a high potential for abuse which may lead to severe psychological or physical dependence
III (C-III)	Have a potential for abuse less than substances in schedules I or II and abuse may lead to moderate or low physical dependence or high psychological dependence
IV (C-IV)	Have a lower potential for abuse relative to substances in schedule III
V (C-V)	Have a lower potential for abuse relative to substances in schedule IV and consist primarily of preparations containing limited quantities of certain narcotics

This amendment required drug manufacturers to prove that medications were both effective and safe prior to approval.

The **Comprehensive Drug Abuse Prevention and Control Act of 1970** was also known as the Controlled Substances Act (CSA). The CSA created the DEA, which is a division of the Department of Justice. The CSA also defined categories for certain medications due to addictive properties. There are 5 schedules of medications, each with its own definition of abuse potential and subsequent restrictions on prescribing (Table 2-2).Examples of schedules II to V medications are shown in the tables below (Tables 2-3 through 2-6).

Pharmacies that engage in the practice of dispensing controlled substances must register with the DEA. A pharmacy registers with the DEA by completing a DEA form 224. This registration must be renewed every 3 years.

Physicians and other practitioners who engage in the practice of writing prescriptions for controlled substances are also required to register with the DEA. The list of practitioners who are legally responsible for writing prescriptions is also growing. The following are permitted to prescribe medications, although this authority may be limited depending on the state:

* Medical doctor (MD)
* Osteopath (DO)

★ *TECH ALERT: The label of scheduled medications will be clearly marked with the designation of C-II, C-III, C-IV, or C-V.*

TABLE 2-3. **Examples of Schedule-II Drugs**	
Generic	*Brand*
Hydromorphone	Dilaudid
Methadone	Dolophine
Meperidine	Demerol
Oxycodone	Oxycontin, Percocet
Fentanyl	Duragesic
Morphine	MS Contin, MS IR, Roxanol
Cocaine	
Codeine	
Amphetamine	Adderall
Methylphenidate	Ritalin

TABLE 2-4. Examples of Schedule-III Drugs

Generic	Brand
Hydrocodone combinations (<15 mg/dose)	Norco, Vicodin
Codeine combinations (<90 mg/dose)	Tylenol with codeine
Buprenorphine	Suboxone
Ketamine	
Anabolic steroids	

- Physician assistant (PA)
- Certified nurse practitioner (CNP)
- Dentist (DDS)
- Optometrist (OD)
- Podiatrist (DPM)
- Veterinarian (DVM)—can only prescribe for animals

The DEA assigns a specific number to any pharmacy or practitioner. That number is formatted as 2 alpha characters followed by a series of 6 digits and 1 check digit, for example, AB1234563.

The first alpha character designates the type of practitioner. The letters A, B, or F are assigned to physicians, pharmacies, and hospitals. The letter M is assigned to midlevel practitioners such as nurse practitioners and physician assistants. The second alpha character matches the first letter on the licensee's application or the first letter of the last name of the individual. The series of numbers is also a very specific pattern. The first 6 numbers combine to give the last number which is a check digit. Let us review how to evaluate a DEA number.

AB 1 2 3 4 5 6 3

Add together the first, third, and fifth digit in the sequence.

1 + 3 + 5 = 9

TABLE 2-5. Examples of Schedule-IV Drugs

Generic	Brand
Alprazolam	Xanax
Carisoprodol	Soma
Clonazepam	Klonopin
Diazepam	Valium
Lorazepam	Ativan
Temazepam	Restoril
Tramadol	Ultram
Phentermine	Adipex
Zolpidem	Ambien

TABLE 2-6. Examples of Schedule-V Drugs

Generic	Brand
Codeine cough preparations <200 mg/100 mL	Robitussin AC, Phenergan with Codeine
Diphenoxylate with atropine	Lomotil
Pregabalin	Lyrica

Add together the second, fourth, and sixth digit in the sequence.

$$2 + 4 + 6 = 12$$

This total is doubled.

$$12 + 12 = 24$$

This sum is added to the sum of the first sequence.

$$24 + 9 = 33$$

The check digit in the ones place of the answer is the seventh digit in the DEA number sequence.

3**3**

QUICK QUIZ 2-1

Complete the blanks in the following questions:

1. BD328433_

2. AP062511_

3. MC034209_

4. Morphine is an example of a schedule _____ drug.

5. Ativan (lorazepam) is an example of a schedule _____ drug.

The DEA number of the prescriber is required to be on any prescription for a controlled substance. Many practitioners have preprinted prescription forms with their required information already contained on the prescription. This speeds up the prescribing process and ensures that the pharmacist has all information necessary to fill the prescription. Medical residents are also assigned a very specific DEA number. Any medical resident who is working within a hospital will be assigned a DEA number that includes the facility's DEA number and a suffix that is specific to that resident.

Ordering and Transferring Controlled Substances

The DEA number is used by the pharmacy to consistently track the purchasing, dispensing, and destruction (if necessary) of **controlled substances.** Every order form used to purchase a scheduled drug must contain the pharmacy DEA number. The DEA form 222 is used for purchasing schedule-II controlled substances. These forms are serially numbered and tracked by the DEA. Only a pharmacist is permitted to order schedule-II drugs through a form 222. If this form is marked incorrectly, it must be voided and returned to the DEA for proper documentation.

    The DEA form 222 has 3 separate, color-coded pages. The blue (back) page stays with the pharmacy. The 2 top copies are sent to the supplier, who fills in the correct information on the top copy and retains this for their records. The middle (green) copy is sent to the local DEA office. The sold product is then transported to the pharmacy. Upon receipt, a pharmacist must sign off on the form 222 by verifying each C-II was received which was ordered indicating a date of receipt on each line. This form 222 is kept as an official document for the pharmacy, and must be retained for a minimum of 2 years. Schedule-III and -IV medications can be ordered through any method, and a pharmacy technician is permitted to do so.

    Today many pharmacies are using the *Controlled Substances Ordering System* (CSOS) which is also enforced by the DEA. The CSOS allows for a secure transfer of schedule-II orders without all of the steps involved using the paper form 222. The CSOS system is fast, efficient, secure, and a true time-saver for pharmacies.

★ TECH ALERT: Authority to sign DEA form 222 and to use the CSOS system may be granted by assigning power of attorney.

Theft of Controlled Substances

DEA form 106 is used to report the loss of controlled substances. Whether by accident, theft, or other form of loss, a pharmacy is required to report to the DEA the following information:

1. Name and address of the pharmacy
2. DEA registration number
3. Date of theft
4. Local police department notified
5. Type of loss (theft, spill, etc)
6. A list of missing controlled substances
7. Cost information or specific markings on the bottles, if available

★ TECH ALERT: The DEA does not consider 1 or 2 missing or broken tablets to be a loss. However, these instances are worth documenting and should be clearly marked in the inventory of C-II substances.

Destruction of Controlled Substances

DEA form 41 is used to document destruction of schedule-II medications. Each tablet, milliliter of solution or transdermal patch is highly regulated. Therefore, if a dose is adulterated, broken, or unsuitable for patient consumption the DEA requires form 41 to be used to document the destruction of the schedule-II drug. This helps prevent diversion and holds the responsible pharmacist accountable for any medication that does not reach the patient.

Filling Controlled Substance Prescriptions

Table 2-7 summarizes the use of each form required by the DEA.

    A prescription written for a medication in schedule-II requires the full quantity of the prescription to be dispensed and must be written in numerical form (eg, 30)

TABLE 2-7. Summary of DEA Forms Filling Controlled Substance Prescriptions

DEA Form Number	Purpose
41	Destruction of outdated or damaged controlled substances
106	Theft of controlled substance
222	Ordering and transferring of schedule-II narcotics
224	Registering a pharmacy with the DEA

as well as in alpha form (eg, thirty). Schedule-II prescriptions are also not to have any refills and therefore the patient is required to present a new prescription for each dispensing. All prescriptions for schedule-II drugs must be handwritten or typed, have a legible signature.

Schedule-III, -IV, and -V prescriptions may be phoned in or faxed, depending on state laws. Schedule-III and -IV prescriptions are able to be refilled up to 5 times within 6 months and schedule-V prescriptions can be refilled as authorized by the prescriber (Table 2-8).

The Poison Prevention Act of 1970 required prescription medications, and most OTC medications should be packaged in child-resistant containers. It is important to note that there are some exceptions to this law. The following represent medications that do not require a child-resistant container:

- Aerosolized medications, such as inhalers
- Oral contraceptives
- Cholestyramine powder
- Sublingual nitroglycerin tablets
- Methylprednisolone tablets with no more than 85 mg per package

Patients may also request medications to be dispensed in a container that does not have child-resistant properties. This should be documented with a signed statement to be kept on file within the pharmacy.

The **Occupational Safety and Health Act of 1970** established the Occupational Safety and Health Administration (OSHA) who works to create a safe workplace for all employees. OSHA requires reporting of injuries sustained while on the job, as well as helping to set policies to minimize the risk of injuries. An example in the pharmacy is helping to prevent inadvertent needle sticks during sterile compounding. OSHA also addresses air contamination and protection from hazardous drug exposure, such as chemotherapy agents.

TABLE 2-8. Refills Permitted on Controlled Substance Schedules

Controlled Substance Schedule	Refills Permitted
I	Not able to be prescribed
II	None
III and IV	Up to 5 times within 6 months of date written
V	As authorized by prescriber

The **Drug Listing Act of 1972** required each drug be assigned a number known as the national drug code (NDC). This is an 11-digit number specific to each product. The first 5 numbers identify the manufacturer, the next 4 digits distinguish the drug product, and the last 2 numbers identify the package size for that particular product.

An orphan drug is a medication used to treat a disease which afflicts less than 200,000 people. Because incentive is not always there for drug manufacturers to invest in a therapy for a condition which does not affect a large part of the population, the **Orphan Drug Act of 1983** provided tax breaks and incentives for manufacturers to create orphan drugs.

The **Prescription Drug Marketing Act of 1987** prohibited the sale and distribution of samples to anyone other than a licensed practitioner. It also prohibited bringing drugs into the United States by anyone other than the manufacturer.

More recently, the federal law has focused more closely on the way business in the pharmacy is conducted in order to protect patients. The **Omnibus Budget Reconciliation Act of 1990 (OBRA '90)** requires pharmacies to establish standards regarding patient records, prospective drug utilization review (DUR), and patient counseling.

A pharmacy must make a reasonable effort to obtain and record information regarding the patient including the following:

- The patient's name
- Address
- Telephone number
- Age and gender
- History including disease states
- Allergy information and reactions
- An updated list of other medications including OTC medications

All of this information should be used during the dispensing of a prescription to detect any potential problems.

Upon dispensing the finished product to the patient, it is a requirement to make an offer to counsel the patient. A technician is permitted to ask the patient if they would like to speak to the pharmacist. The following are items a pharmacist must attempt to discuss with a patient:

- Name of drug and description of drug type
- Route of administration, dose, and dosage form of medication
- Storage information
- Potential side effects
- What to do in the event of a missed dose

★ TECH ALERT: Pharmacy technicians are not legally allowed to counsel a patient, but they are usually the one who will make the offer to counsel which is required by law. Any questions which require professional judgment should be directed to the pharmacist.

The **Dietary Supplement Health and Education Act of 1994 (DSHEA)** required all herbal products be labeled as a dietary supplement and identify all ingredients, including quantities of each. Dietary supplements are required to meet quality and purity specifications, but are not required to prove safety or effectiveness. The FDA does not have to approve a dietary supplement before it is produced. This is why the following message appears on packaging for herbal products and other dietary supplements:

> This statement has not been evaluated by the FDA.
> This product is not intended to diagnose, treat, cure,
> or prevent any disease.

The purpose of the **Health Insurance Portability and Accountability Act of 1996 (HIPAA)** was to set standards in the protection of privacy of a patient's **protected health information (PHI).** Specific regulations include how to store the information to how and when it is appropriate to access the information. As a pharmacy technician, it is necessary to understand that HIPAA standards create privacy protection for the patient.

Patients are given a "notice of privacy practices." Many patients are presented with this information upon picking up their prescription or entering a health care facility. An important component of HIPAA is understanding what information is needed to access in order to perform your job correctly. As a pharmacy technician you will have access to information beyond the scope of your professional practice, but only what is required to complete the task at hand should be viewed.

Beyond your access to information is the opportunity for others, generally the public, to obtain PHI. Follow several simple rules in order to protect the pharmacy from HIPAA violations:

1. Use a cover sheet when faxing information.
2. Ask other patrons to step back from the counter or counseling area when assisting in the dispensing process.
3. Move closer to the patient or a coworker when discussing sensitive information in order to protect privacy.
4. Access PHI only for a patient that has a valid prescription.
5. Keep up with your employee training as policies and procedures may change from year to year.

★ *TECH ALERT: HIPAA rules and regulations are designed to protect the public. Accessing a patient's profile should only occur if you need to do so to perform the usual functions of your job.*

The **Medicare Prescription Drug Improvement and Modernization Act of 2003 (MMA)** established prescription drug benefits for Medicare patients, known as Medicare Part D. These prescription benefits are voluntary, and patients must enroll in Medicare Part D during a designated period during each year.

Because of the continued abuse of anabolic steroids by athletes, the **Anabolic Steroid Control Act of 2004** classified anabolic steroids as schedule-III controlled substances.

The **Combat Methamphetamine Epidemic Act of 2005** was passed to restrict the sale of ephedrine, pseudoephedrine, and phenylpropanolamine, and placed these drugs and products that contain these drugs into the "scheduled listed chemical products" category. Any sales of these medications are subject to restrictions and record keeping requirements. Patients are limited to purchasing a maximum of 3.6 g per day and 9 g every 30 days. The pharmacy must keep written or electronic records of the sales including the product name, quantity sold, name and address of the purchaser, and date and time of sale.

Restricted Drug Programs

Some specific drug programs have been developed for particular drugs to help ensure safety of patients.

Clozapine is a drug approved for the treatment of schizophrenia and, although a useful treatment, has the potential to cause very serious side effects. Patients must be registered with a clozapine registry in order to fill a prescription for this medication. White blood cell counts (WBCs) and absolute neutrophil counts (ANCs) are required to stay within a designated limit to continue usage of clozapine. Patients must also start at a certain level before beginning this therapy.

Isotretinoin (Accutane) is used for the treatment and prevention of severe nodular acne. Due to the extremely high risk of birth defects, this drug cannot be taken in women who are or may become pregnant. The iPLEDGE program requires both prescribers and patients to be registered with the program, and the prescription can only be filled at a registered pharmacy. Female patients must take monthly pregnancy tests while on isotretinoin, and must also be utilizing 2 effective forms of birth control. Additionally, there is a 30-day waiting period before a female patient can begin therapy, and a negative pregnancy test is required before initiating treatment. Male patients and female patients who cannot get pregnant are also required to register with the program and see their doctor monthly for prescriptions.

Thalidomide, as discussed previously, causes severe birth defects in pregnant women. However, it is indicated for the treatment of multiple myeloma. Because of its continued use, a program known as System for Thalidomide Education and Prescribing Safety (STEPS) was developed and approved by the FDA as a means to prevent pregnant women from taking thalidomide.

QUICK QUIZ 2-2

1. How much pseudoephedrine may a patient purchase in 1 day?
   a. 3.6 g
   b. 6.3 g
   c. 9 g
   d. 100 mg

2. Which act created Medicare Part D?
   a. Medicare Prescription Drug Improvement and Modernization Act of 2003
   b. OBRA' 90
   c. HIPAA
   d. Prescription Drug Marketing Act

3. The CSA established how many schedules of controlled substances?
   a. 3
   b. 4
   c. 5
   d. 6

4. Which of the following forms is required to order C-II narcotics?
   a. DEA 224
   b. DEA 106
   c. DEA 41
   d. DEA 222

5. Which drug used to treat severe acne, requires the registration with the iPLEDGE program?

    a. Clozapine

    b. Thalidomide

    c. Isotretinoin

    d. Warfarin

~~~~~~

PHARMACY REGULATORY AGENCIES

Federal Agencies

The **Food and Drug Administration (FDA)** is part of the US Department of Health and Human Services. The FDA protects the public by assuring safety, effectiveness, and control of drugs, cosmetics, food, dietary supplements, and other medical products and devices. The FDA is even responsible for the advertising of drugs and medical devices.

    Today, the profession of pharmacy looks to the FDA for answers to very specific questions related to the approval and safety of new medications. Also, FDA policies address common issues such as personal importation of drugs from other countries as well as transparency for the public regarding the drug and food industry.

    The FDA collects and validates patient complaints, safety warnings and information provided by the general public in order to determine the need for further prescribing restrictions, recalls, market withdrawals, or modifying medication package inserts to include more warnings or cautions. The FDA works for the safety of the public.

    The Joint Commission (TJC) is an accrediting body for many hospitals, meaning it gives its "stamp of approval" on health care institutions after they have met specific requirements and standards. If a facility does not meet certain standards, it can be deemed ineligible to receive Medicare reimbursement and funding.

    The *Drug Enforcement Administration (DEA)* is responsible for enforcing the controlled substances laws of the United States. The DEA provides protection for the public by bringing to justice any person or organization responsible for illicit controlled substance drug trade and traffic in the United States.

    The *State Boards of Pharmacy (BOP)* have specific standards to follow in regards to pharmacy requirements. Each state BOP oversees pharmacy practice in that particular state and some things BOPs are responsible for include the following:

- Defining certification, registration, and licensing requirements for technicians
- Defining duties and expectations of the pharmacist—have authority to discipline for inappropriate behavior
- Setting standards for space, storage, and equipment requirements
- Establishing the criteria for continuing education for both pharmacists and technicians

All of the state BOPs together comprise the **National Association of the Boards of Pharmacy (NABP).** This organization has no regulatory authority over pharmacies, but helps identify trends in the field that may affect the practice of pharmacy.

    The *United States Pharmacopeia (USP)* is an organization which sets the standards for purity, quality, and strength of medications, including OTC drugs

★ *TECH ALERT: The FDA has oversight on all aspects of drug development including clinical trials, public complaints, safety reviews, and even television commercials for medications.*

and additional health care products. USP has 2 chapters which affect pharmacy practice extensively. USP <795> is the chapter which addresses nonsterile compounding, and USP <797> addresses sterile compounding guidelines. Both of these chapters help protect patients by providing pharmacies with guidance and standards for the safe practice of compounding. The pharmacy environment must be kept clean and organized in order to prevent contamination of medication and to keep patients safe.

Pharmacists and technicians should practice proper hand hygiene and garbing as defined by USP <795>, USP <797>, and per facility policy. Additionally, counting trays, spatulas, and the work area should be maintained and cleaned frequently in order to prevent **cross contamination** and facilitate accurate counting. Cross contamination is the unintentional transfer of one drug onto another through powder residue or insufficient cleaning practices. A visibly dirty counting tray could potentially transfer powder from one medication to another, which could potentially cause an allergic reaction in a patient sensitive to that drug and its residue. The workspace countertop should also be wiped down with appropriate cleaners as defined in the pharmacy policies.

Pharmacies with a sterile compounding area which includes a laminar or vertical flow hood or compounding device, must be familiar with USP <797> guidelines for cleaning, verification, and maintenance of all equipment used. There are additional requirements for personnel who use the equipment, including proper aseptic technique, which includes hand washing, garbing, and appropriate technique when compounding sterile products.

Additionally, personnel must undergo competencies designed to maintain compounding skills. Media fill transfer tests are designed to measure aseptic technique, and utilize the transfer of a medium broth from vial to additional vials or bags. These vials or bags are then incubated to see if bacteria growth occurs. Proper hood cleaning and personnel cleanliness should be obtained when compounding is assessed through the use of touch plates. These plates contain an agar, and when personnel complete a compounding activity, they touch the pads of the fingers in the plate. The agar plates are then incubated, and if growth of bacteria occurs, the employee must repeat the activity and be aware of improper or incomplete cleaning processes.

Sterile work environments must be kept clean from all particulates in order to maintain the quality of the final product. Introduction of any bacteria, fungi, or other particles from the air or contact with contaminated surfaces may lead to severe unintended infection for a patient.

Daily cleaning and equipment maintenance is the responsibility of everyone in the pharmacy. USP <797> provides specific recommendations for the type of cleaners, cleaning equipment, and maintenance of equipment and supplies for pharmacists and technicians to follow. This is an enforceable section of the USP and unless your workplace does not engage in any sterile compounding it is the responsibility of the pharmacy to follow these standards.

PHARMACY FACILITIES

In addition to adequate space for sterile compounding requirements, the pharmacy should have space dedicated for nonsterile compounding. This may vary depending on the amount of nonsterile compounding performed at a specific pharmacy. This space should be separated from the rest of the pharmacy, so calculations can be performed, and careful measuring and mixing can be completed.

Pharmacies must also have adequate space for pharmacists to perform professional clinical activities, such as counseling patients. For the sake of privacy and compliance with HIPAA, outpatient pharmacies need to create a private area for consultation and counseling. All of these areas are to be well lit, clean, and provide adequate security for personnel safety and medication storage. All work areas should be organized in order to promote efficiency as well as reduce the risk of contamination of products.

DRUG REFERENCES

Drug information resources must be up-to-date in order to promote the best patient care. Resources are found online in many pharmacies; however, there are several large texts and references that may be required by individual state boards.

EXAMPLES OF REFERENCE TEXTS	
Reference	*Description*
Drug Facts and Comparisons	Reference of drug information, both online and printed version, contains approximately 16,000 prescriptions and 6000 OTC **monographs** **(Note: A monograph lists information about a drug, eg, name of ingredient/s, package, label, and storage information)**
Physicians' Desk Reference (PDR)	Published twice a year, contains information from drug's package inserts
FDA Orange Book	An online reference for all therapeutically equivalent products
Trissel's Handbook on Injectable Drugs	Provides information on the stability and compatibility of injectable drugs

RECORD RETENTION

The pharmacy also needs space to store all of the required documents that must be readily retrievable upon the request of a governing body or during an inspection. A pharmacy must also have a place to file prescriptions, drug recall notices and resolutions, inventory counts and invoices, MSDS, and equipment maintenance logs. Controlled substance prescriptions must be filed separately from noncontrolled prescriptions. These must be readily retrievable (within 72 hours) when requested. Some examples of record retention requirements are as below:

- Documentation of a narcotic inventory count if pharmacist in charge changes.
- Form 222 and schedule-III and -IV order forms must be kept for at least 2 years.
- Documentation of complete narcotic inventory conducted every 2 years.
- Hard copies of prescriptions with a copy label on the back of the information regarding prescription filling must be kept for a minimum of 2 years.
- Log of repackaged medication must be maintained for a minimum of 2 years.
- Compounding records for nonsterile products must be maintained for a minimum of 2 years.

It is important to never throw away any documentation unless the 2-year minimum has been reached. Most facilities store documents off-site, and will retain records for 3 to 5 years to be safe. Also remember, documentation that contains any patient's PHI must be shredded, and not thrown in the trash.

HAZARDOUS SUBSTANCES

A hazardous substance is a drug or chemical stored or compounded in the pharmacy which has the ability to be the following:

- Carcinogenic (cancer causing)
- Teratogenic (producing birth defects)
- Cytotoxic (causes cell death)
- Genotoxic (manipulates or destroys DNA)

OSHA has set requirements to help minimize employee exposure to hazardous drugs, as well as instructions on how to handle spills, storage, and waste. Appropriate proper personal protective (PPE) must be worn when handling hazardous drugs. Additionally, disposing of hazardous drug waste is the responsibility of the pharmacy, and all local, state, and federal environmental regulations must be followed.

Certain hazardous drug products, such as chemotherapy, require specific procedures for disposal. It is not acceptable for a pharmacy to dispose of any hazardous medication (expired, wasted, or spilled) into any municipal solid waste. Instead, pharmacies are responsible for managing the disposal through proper sorting of waste into appropriate containers. Chemotherapy waste, needles and sharps, solid packaging waste/recycling, and chemical hazardous product waste along with others, all have their own waste receptacles. This helps keep the pharmacy in line with regulations and also prevents unwanted hazards from polluting the environment. Products such as nicotine patches, epinephrine, and warfarin are also listed as hazardous materials and health care organizations, including pharmacies, are responsible for determining the proper procedures to dispose of this waste.

Every pharmacy has access to the Material Safety Data Sheets (MSDS) for all chemicals used within the pharmacy. MSDS describes the chemical product and provides information such as toxicity, storage requirements, and procedures to follow in case of a spill or leak. MSDS references may be available in an online version or in many cases in printed form where it can be quickly accessed during an emergency.

New products or chemicals that are brought into the pharmacy should be reviewed for any potential hazardous issues such as skin irritation, eye irritation, flammability, etc. It is the responsibility of everyone in the pharmacy to understand how to use the emergency spill kit, the eyewash station, and how to contact the poison control center in case of accidental exposure to a chemical. The MSDS contains information on all risks and treatment procedures for the chemical product.

In the event that a pharmacy worker or other employee of the organization comes into contact with a hazardous substance, specific processes must be followed to prevent harm. Chemotherapy spill kits are available in the case of accidental spills of any antineoplastic agent. Additionally, if a hazardous substance comes into contact with the skin, it must be washed immediately, and for contact with the eyes, the emergency eyewash station should be utilized for immediate flushing.

QUICK QUIZ 2-3

1. Which of the following USP chapters outlines the requirements for sterile compounding?
   a. <795>
   b. <797>
   c. <61>
   d. <1056>

2. Which of the following USP chapters outlines the requirements for nonsterile compounding?
   a. <795>
   b. <797>
   c. <61>
   d. <1056>

3. Which reference can be used to check therapeutic equivalency?
   a. *PDR*
   b. *Drug Facts and Comparisons*
   c. *FDA Orange Book*
   d. *Trissel's Handbook on Injectable Drugs*

4. All the State Boards of Pharmacy together comprise which of the following?
   a. FDA
   b. DEA
   c. BOP
   d. NABP

5. Which organization can make decisions regarding licensure, certification, or continuing education requirements for each state?
   a. FDA
   b. BOP
   c. NABP
   d. DEA

PHARMACY MEDICATION RECALLS

Every pharmacy and patient is in some way affected by a medication recall. The product manufacturer will notify the public and pharmacy professionals when a medication is not to be dispensed but rather returned to a wholesaler, waste removal company, or manufacturer in order to prevent the product from reaching a patient and potentially causing harm. Everything from OTC pain relief medication to cancer chemotherapy agents has the potential to be recalled.

TABLE 2-9. Drug Recall Classifications	
Class 1 recall	Products those are dangerous or defective with a reasonable chance that usage will cause serious health problems or death. Example: an antibiotic that is found to be contaminated with a fungus resulting in increased harm to a patient
Class 2 recall	Products that may cause temporary or medically reversible consequences. Example: medication that is found to have less than the labeled amount of active ingredient
Class 3 recall	Products those are not likely to cause any health problems for the patient but still violate FDA regulations Example: a bottle of atorvastatin that only contains 80 tablets instead of the labeled 90 tablets

Recalls are classified based on the level of danger to the public. The recalls are categorized in Table 2-9.

The FDA expects all manufacturers of medications, food, and medical devices to take responsibility for their own recalls and to manage the notification, documentation, and resolution of the recall on their own. In all cases of recalls, the pharmacy should also maintain and keep all documentation of recalls received as well as the steps taken to comply with the recall and any follow-up action that was necessary.

CASE STUDY REVIEW

A customer, John Smith, enters your pharmacy and presents a prescription to you. You recognize the customer but the name on the prescription is for Ted Turner. He tells you that Ted is his neighbor. The prescription is written for alprazolam tablets to be used as needed for restlessness. The prescription is from Paige Turner, DDS. You see that the DEA number on the prescription is BT1578395. The prescription was written 3 weeks ago.

John really wants to get this script filled and give it back to his neighbor. You take the prescription back to the pharmacist for some clarification prior to entering the information into the computer. After reviewing the prescription, the pharmacist decides to ask Mr. Smith a few more questions and then makes a phone call to Dr. Paige Turner's office.

The pharmacist has decided not to fill the prescription and informs Mr. Smith that a full explanation of the reason for not filling the script will be reviewed with Mr. Turner over the phone.

The pharmacist makes a call to Mr. Turner. While there is nothing inherently wrong with Mr. Smith bringing Mr. Turner's prescription to the pharmacy to be filled, and for that matter, there is nothing wrong with Mr. Smith picking up Mr. Turner's prescription and returning it to him that is not why the script is rejected.

The reason for not filling the prescription is that Paige Turner, DDS, is Mr. Turner's daughter. Also, there is no reason for a dentist to prescribe for a family member. The medication which was prescribed is also outside of the scope of practice for a dentist and therefore the prescription is not going to be filled by the pharmacist.

```
Dr. Ina Rush          AR1234563        Date: 2/5/2013
123 Main St.
Anytown, ST 12345
555-123-4567

Patient: Helen Waite
         456 South St.
         Anytown, ST 12345


         Ciprofloxacin 500-mg Tablet
         Take 1 tablets bid x 10 days
         #20 tablets


0 refills                            Ina Rush M.D.
```

CHAPTER SUMMARY

- State and federal laws are enacted to protect the public.
- When faced with different state and federal laws, the stricter law is the right choice.
- Scheduled medications are categorized according to their addiction potential as well as their acceptable medical uses.
- Every patient has the right to speak with a pharmacist regarding their prescription on every occasion of dispensing.
- HIPAA rules and laws are in place to prevent the sharing of protected information without the patient's knowledge or permission.
- The FDA oversees medication approval, development, testing, and use.
- The DEA enforces controlled substance medication rules and laws.
- State agencies provide licensing requirements for pharmacy personnel as well as a set of rules and laws to govern the practice of each individual in the state. These agencies protect the general public.
- A valid prescription may be presented to you by the patient, faxed by the physician's office, e-prescribed, and phoned in to the pharmacy. In every case, the same basic requirements are necessary.

ANSWERS TO QUICK QUIZZES

Quick Quiz 2-1

1. 6   **2.** 7   **3.** 2   **4.** 2   **5.** 4

Quick Quiz 2-2

1. 3.6 g

2. Medicare Prescription Drug Improvement and Modernization Act of 2003

3. 5

4. DEA 222

5. Isotretinoin

Quick Quiz 2-3

1. <797> **2.** <795>   **3.** *Drug Facts and Comparisons*   **4.** NABP   **5.** BOP

CHAPTER QUESTIONS

1. USP refers to which of the following?
   a. United States Pharmacopeia
   b. United States Pharmacists
   c. Universal Sales Program
   d. United Service Plan

2. DEA form 106 is used to report which of the following?
   a. Order C-II medications
   b. Document destruction of C-II medications
   c. Document theft or loss of C-II medications
   d. None of the above

3. Which of the following medications is in schedule II?
   a. Diazepam
   b. Buprenorphine
   c. Midazolam
   d. Methadone
   e. Zolpidem

4. The Pure Food and Drug Act of 1906 required which of the following?
   a. That drugs not be mislabeled
   b. Industry purity and strength standards
   c. Therapeutic benefit documentation
   d. Both a and b

5. Drugs are intended for use in which of the following?
   a. Prevention of disease
   b. Treatment of disease
   c. Diagnosis of disease
   d. All of the above

6. Which of the following medications is with a low abuse potential and acceptable medical uses?
   a. Schedule II
   b. Schedule III
   c. Schedule IV
   d. OTC

7. The Durham-Humphrey Amendment created which of the following?
   a. Scheduled medications
   b. OTC medication class and Rx medication class
   c. Safety regulations
   d. Purity laws

8. The Drug Listing Act required which of the following?
   a. Tax incentives for orphan drugs
   b. Labeling of dietary supplements
   c. Is on all prescription medications
   d. All of the above

9. Pharmacies must make a reasonable effort to obtain which of the following?
   a. Patient's name
   b. Patient's physical address
   c. NDC numbers for medications
   d. Patient counseling

10. The Poison Prevention Act created which pharmacy dispensing standard?
    a. Patient counseling
    b. Child-resistant container use
    c. Counting tray use
    d. All of the above

11. Which of the following medications is in schedule III?
    a. Anabolic steroids
    b. Lorazepam
    c. Temazepam
    d. Morphine

12. Which of the following practices promotes protection of PHI?
    a. Faxing without a cover sheet
    b. Asking other patrons to step away from the counter during a counseling session

c. Looking up a neighbor's profile to "see what they are on"

d. Calling out a patient's name, drug that is ready, and reason for use

13. The "Combat Methamphetamine Epidemic Act" restricts the sale of which OTC medication?
    a. Acetaminophen
    b. Ibuprofen
    c. Guaifenesin
    d. Pseudoephedrine

14. The pharmacy must keep written or electronic records of ephedrine and pseudoephedrine including which of the following?
    a. Product name
    b. Date and time of sale
    c. Name and address of the purchaser
    d. All of the above

15. Which agency is responsible for enforcing the controlled substance laws of the United States?
    a. FDA
    b. DEA
    c. FBI
    d. OTC

16. USP refers to United States Pharmacopeia.
    a. True
    b. False

17. Which is a valid DEA number for Dr. John Smith?
    a. BS1234562
    b. MS1234564
    c. AS1234563
    d. All of the above

18. Which form is used to order C-II medication?
    a. DEA 41
    b. DEA 106
    c. DEA 222
    d. None of the above

19. Which of the following methods may be used to transmit a prescription to a pharmacy?
    a. Facsimile
    b. Telephone
    c. E-Script (electronic transfer)
    d. All of the above

20. Which of the following is not required on a valid prescription?
    a. Date of issue
    b. Name and address of the practitioner
    c. Name of the patient
    d. All of the above

21. A prescription for a C-II substance requires which of the following?
    a. Quantity in numerical form (30)
    b. Quantity in alpha form (thirty)
    c. Physician DEA number
    d. All of the above

22. HIPAA stands for Health Insurance Portability and Accountability Act.
    a. True
    b. False

23. FDA refers to which of the following?
    a. Federal Drug Administration
    b. Food and Drug Administration
    c. Food and Dental Agency
    d. Federal Drug Agency

24. Medication labels must contain at the very least which of the following?
    a. The name, address, and phone number of the pharmacy
    b. Name of the patient
    c. Date of next refill
    d. a and b only

25. When faced with different state and federal laws, which should be followed?
    a. The more strict law
    b. The state law
    c. It is the pharmacists discretion
    d. None of the above

26. OTC refers to over the counter.
    a. True
    b. False

27. The Pure Food and Drug Act of 1906 required which of the following?
    a. That drugs not be mislabeled
    b. Industry purity and strength standards
    c. The exact amount of active ingredient on the label
    d. All of the above

28. Which law was passed in 1938?
    a. Pure Food and Drug Act
    b. Health Insurance Portability and Account-ability Act
    c. Food, Drug, and Cosmetic Act
    d. OBRA '90

29. What did the Controlled Substances Act define?
    a. Labeling requirements
    b. Drug schedules
    c. Privacy laws
    d. Purity standards

30. Which of the following medications is in schedule IV?
    a. Morphine
    b. Anabolic steroids
    c. Clonazepam
    d. Heroin

31. Drugs are listed in which of the following?
    a. USP
    b. HIPAA
    c. DEA
    d. All of the above

32. Natural supplements are not drugs because they are not intended for use in which of the following?
    a. Prevention of disease
    b. Treatment of disease
    c. Diagnosis of disease
    d. All of the above

33. Which is the most restrictive class of medications defined by the Controlled Substances Act?
    a. C-V
    b. C-III
    c. C-II
    d. C-I

34. When referring to HIPAA, PHI stands for private hospital information.
    a. True
    b. False

35. Which of the following is *not* a factor when defining a medication schedule?
    a. Abuse potential
    b. Safety information
    c. Pharmacokinetics
    d. All of the above

36. Which law created the OTC class of medications?
    a. Durham-Humphrey Amendment
    b. Controlled Substances Act
    c. Poison Prevention Act
    d. OBRA '90

37. HIPAA refers to which of the following?
    a. Health Information Privacy Administration and Agency
    b. Hospital Infused Pure Antibiotic Adminis-tration
    c. Health Insurance Portability and Account-ability Act
    d. Health Insurance Privacy and Accountability Act

38. Which of the following is correct about "Caution: Federal law prohibits dispensing without a prescription"?
    a. Must never be shortened
    b. Is the federal legend
    c. Is on all OTC medications
    d. All of the above

39. Patient counseling became mandatory after which law was passed?
    a. 1970 Poison Prevention Act
    b. 1938 Food, Drug, and Cosmetic Act
    c. 1951 Durham-Humphrey Amendment
    d. 1990 Omnibus Budget Reconciliation Act

40. HIPAA sets standards to protect which of the following?
    a. USP
    b. PHI
    c. NF
    d. OTC

41. Which law sets standards for storing patient information?
    a. Poison Prevention Act
    b. Controlled Substances Act
    c. HIPAA
    d. All of the above

42. The "Combat Methamphetamine Epidemic Act" restricts the sale of which OTC medication?
    a. Acetaminophen
    b. Ibuprofen
    c. Guaifenesin
    d. None of the above

43. What does the DEA enforce?
    a. State-specific dispensing laws
    b. Pharmacist licensing
    c. Controlled substance laws of the United States
    d. OTC product labeling

44. Who licenses pharmacists?
    a. The DEA
    b. The State Board of Pharmacy
    c. The FDA
    d. All of the above

45. Which of the following medications is in schedule III?
    a. Zolpidem
    b. Lacosamide
    c. Hydromorphone
    d. Ketamine

46. NF refers to Natural Formulary.
    a. True
    b. False

47. DEA refers to which of the following?
    a. Drug Enforcement Administration
    b. Drug Enforcement Agency
    c. Drug Elimination Administration
    d. Drug Evaluation Agency

48. The Food, Drug, and Cosmetic Act of 1938 defined which of the following?
    a. Officially defined drugs
    b. Established policies to determine drug safety
    c. Created childproof cap laws
    d. Only a and b

49. Which of the following is an example of a medication that does *not* require child-resistant packaging?
    a. Birth control pills
    b. Lisinopril
    c. Hydrochlorothiazide
    d. Atorvastatin

50. Which of the following practices does *not* promote protection of PHI?
    a. Using a fax cover sheet
    b. Asking other patrons to step away from the counter during a counseling session
    c. Inviting more than one patient at a time into the counseling area
    d. Keeping up with training every year

Sterile and Nonsterile Compounding

CHAPTER
3

PTCB KNOWLEDGE AREAS

3.1 Infection control (eg, hand washing PPE)

3.2 Handling and disposal of hazardous waste (eg, receptacle, waste streams)

3.3 Documentation (eg, batch preparation, compounding record)

3.4 Selection and use of compounding equipment and supplies

3.5 Determination of compounded product stability (eg, beyond-use dating, signs of incompatibility)

3.6 Selection and use of equipment and supplies

3.7 Sterile compounding processes

3.8 Nonsterile compounding processes

KEY TERMS

Analytical balance: Uses electronic calibrations to determine the weight of a product

Aseptic technique: Technique necessary to minimize the risk of microbial contamination of a sterile product

Compounding: The act of reconstituting, mixing, or otherwise preparing a medication into a dosage form usable by the patient

Drip rate: The rate at which an intravenous (IV) medication is infused

Epidural: Injection of a medication directly into the epidural space, or the outermost part, of the spinal canal

Extemporaneous compounding: The preparation of pharmaceuticals in a nonsterile environment

Gauge (G): Thickness or diameter of a needle bore

Geometric dilution: A process in which ingredients are mixed together in equal proportions to ensure that the compounded substance results in an evenly mixed substance

Graduate: A cylindrical or conical-shaped container with clearly defined calibrations used for measuring liquids

Heterogeneous: A mixture that does not contain uniformly mixed ingredients

Homogeneous: A mixture of uniformly distributed ingredients. Homogeneous mixtures are the goal in pharmaceutical compounding

Intramuscular (IM): Medications administered into the muscle

Intravenous (IV): Medications administered into a vein

IV drip (also known as IV infusion): A medication administered slowly into a patient's vein

IV piggyback (IVPB): A small volume, generally less than 250 mL, of medication infused through the same IV line as a primary fluid

IV push (IVP): Rapid administration of a small volume of medication into the vein, usually over less than 5 minutes

Levigation: Reducing the particle size of a powder through the addition of a liquid in which the powder is not soluble

Meniscus: The curve in the surface of a liquid that occurs around the edge of the container due to surface tension

Parenteral: Medications administered which bypass the gastrointestinal tract

Patient-controlled analgesia (PCA): Allows a patient to bolus IV pain medication with the push of a button

Personal protective equipment (PPE): All items intended to reduce the risk of employee exposure to hazardous medication and possible contamination of a medication during the sterile compounding process. Examples of PPE include gloves, gowns, and hair covers

Precipitation: The process in which a solid forms from a chemical reaction in a solution, indicates incompatibility of 2 substances, and that a solution is not suitable for use

Reconstitution: Mixing a diluent into a preweighed powder to form a solution or suspension

Solubility: The ability of a substance to be dissolved

Solute: A solid ingredient dissolved in a solvent

Solution: A homogeneous mixture in which the active ingredient is completely dissolved within the liquid

Solvent: The liquid in which a solute is dissolved

Spatulation: The process of mixing 2 semisolid products, such as ointments or creams, together with a spatula to form a homogeneous mixture

Subcutaneous (sub-Q): Medications injected into the fatty layer below the skin

Suspension: A heterogeneous mixture in which the active ingredient is not completely dissolved, but rather suspended, in the liquid

Torsion balance: Uses weights on a counterbalance to determine the weight of a product

Total parenteral nutrition (TPN): Also known as hyperalimentation; IV administration of nutrition required to sustain life when a patient is unable to obtain nutrition orally

Trituration: The process of grinding particles into fine powders, usually using a mortar and pestle

Troche: A dosage form similar to a lozenge which is placed in the mouth and allowed to slowly dissolve, releasing the medication to absorb through the oral mucosa

Viscosity: Thickness of a substance

CASE STUDY

You are working as a pharmacy technician in an ambulatory care pharmacy. A pharmacist hands you the prescription (Figure 3-1) and asks you to compound the product based on the pharmacy's written protocol.

Patient: *Rebecca Watson*

Address: *1256 South Street Springfield, OH 43215 A*

DOB: *2/1/1955*

Lorazepam 1 mg / haloperidol 3 mg suppository

Sig i q6h PR PRN

Disp #120

Refills: 3

J Anderson, MD

Dr. John Anderson, MD

FIGURE 3-1 Sample prescription.

Self-Assessment Questions

- What equipment will you use in the extemporaneous compounding of this prescription?
- How many milligrams of lorazepam and haloperidol will you need?
- What type of suppository base should be used?
- What else do you need to consider during the compounding process?

INTRODUCTION

Not all prescriptions for patients are available in concentrations or doses prepared by pharmaceutical manufacturers. When a medication order is received that is not available commercially from the manufacturer, it will need to be compounded by the pharmacy staff. Compounded medications are prepared using either nonsterile (extemporaneous) or sterile (aseptic) techniques. Both nonsterile and sterile compounding are an important component to a pharmacy technician's duties. This chapter discusses compounding practices and procedures used to compound various medication orders and drug forms.

NONSTERILE COMPOUNDING PROCESSES

Nonsterile (extemporaneous) compounding includes all compounding of dosage forms not prepared in a sterile environment. Dosage forms compounded in a non-sterile environment often include topical, oral, rectal, vaginal and nasal products; whereas, products for intravenous or ophthalmic use are compounded in a sterile environment, such as a laminar flow hood or clean room.

Compounding is the act of reconstituting, mixing, or otherwise altering a commercially available product into a medication dosage form prescribed by a practitioner for a particular patient's specific medication needs. Medications such as oral powders for reconstitution, topical solutions, and gels are examples of common dosage forms compounded by a pharmacy. Recipes are created for each compounded drug order and are maintained on file in the pharmacy along with required compounding procedures. There are a number of reasons for a patient to require a compounded medication. The most common reasons are that the medication ordered is not commercially available in the required strength, route, or combination of ingredients. Additionally, there may be a situation when a patient cannot tolerate, or is allergic to, a component of the commercially available product, such as the dye or coloring used. Pharmacy technicians are permitted to compound medications under the supervision of a pharmacist. Ultimately, the pharmacist is responsible for the final product produced, and therefore, must verify all calculations are correct before the product is compounded.

Guidelines published by the United States Pharmacopeia (USP) for nonsterile compounding are defined in USP Chapter <795>. The Food and Drug Administration (FDA) declares that compounding is an integral part of pharmacy practice and essential to the provision of health care. Each State Board of Pharmacy (BOP) sets specific regulations for the compounding process, quality control, and required documentation. Additionally, each State BOP interprets and regulates compounding differently, and pharmacy technicians must be aware of each state's laws.

Selection and Use of Equipment and Supplies

Before beginning the compounding process, a pharmacy technician must prepare the compounding area. This includes clearing the area of all unnecessary clutter and wiping down the surface with an antimicrobial cleaning solution or 70% isopropyl alcohol.

The first step in the compounding process is gathering all required ingredients and equipment. The next section outlines the equipment used in various types of nonsterile compounding.

Equipment for Liquid Measurement

Liquid ingredients can be measured in a variety of ways. The best choice for measuring equipment largely depends on 2 factors: the volume being measured and the **viscosity** of the liquid. The volume being measured is the most important factor in determining the type and size of equipment should be used. For optimal accuracy in measuring liquids, the volume being measured should be no less than 20% of the total volume capacity of the selected equipment. That is, if 20 mL of a liquid needs to be measured, the largest equipment size that should be used is a 100-mL graduate (20% of 100 mL = 20 mL). It is best to use an even smaller graduate or a

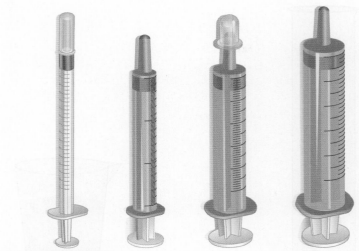

FIGURE 3-2 Oral syringes.

20-mL syringe as the smaller the capacity of a container, the more accurate is the measurement calibrations. In other words, choose the size of the equipment closest to the volume to be measured whenever possible.

Syringes are the ideal equipment for measuring small volumes of liquids. Syringes are available in a variety of sizes and types, and are used in both sterile and nonsterile compounding. Syringes offer exceptional accuracy, but can be difficult to use to withdraw a liquid from a container without a syringe adapter. For this reason, 10-mL graduates are often the equipment of choice for measuring volumes less than 10 mL.

Syringes are available in a number of sizes and varieties. Oral syringes (Figure 3-2) are used in nonsterile compounding.

A **graduate** is a container with clearly defined calibrations used for measuring liquids, and are available in cylindrical and conical shapes. Graduated cylinders (Figure 3-3) are the most common equipment used for measuring liquids. Conical graduates (Figure 3-4) are useful for measuring viscous liquids because the slope of the side of the container allows the liquid to be poured out more easily.

Beakers are cylindrical containers used to measure and mix liquid products. Beakers generally have less accurate calibrations than graduates and should only be used when precise measurements are not required, or in mixing liquids that have already been measured with more accurate equipment.

When using a graduate or a beaker, it is important to remember that the volume of the liquid must be read at the bottom of the curved liquid line, known as the meniscus (Figure 3-5). The **meniscus** is defined as the curve in the surface of a liquid that occurs around the edge of the container. This phenomenon occurs because of surface tension between the graduate or beaker and the liquid. To ensure accuracy, the container must be at eye level when determining the volume.

Characteristics of each specific liquid must also be taken into consideration when selecting the proper measuring equipment to use. For example, some liquids and pharmaceutical ingredients react with plastic. Hot liquids should be measured in glass to avoid warping and damaging equipment, whereas very cold liquids should be measured in plastic to avoid shattering glass equipment. These factors influencing product selection should be dictated in the pharmacy's compounding protocol written by a pharmacist.

★ *TECH ALERT: The meniscus is more pronounced in containers made of glass, as well as those in smaller diameters, because of greater surface tension.*

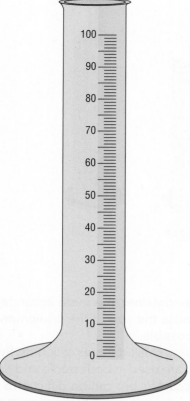

FIGURE 3-3 Graduated cylinder.

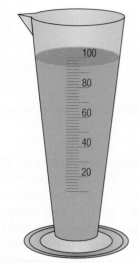

FIGURE 3-4 Conical graduate.

Equipment for Solid Measurement

Solid ingredients are measured by weight on a balance or scale. There are 2 types of balances typically used in pharmacies. A **torsion balance** (Figure 3-6a and b) uses weights on a counterbalance to determine the weight of a product. These are required in all pharmacies and known as class A balances because of the sensitivity

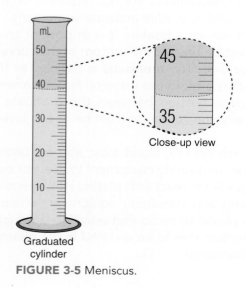

FIGURE 3-5 Meniscus.

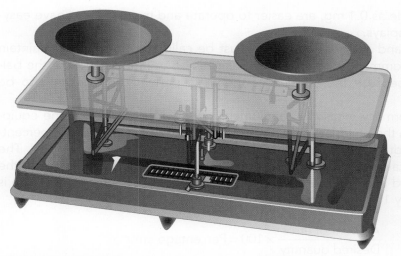
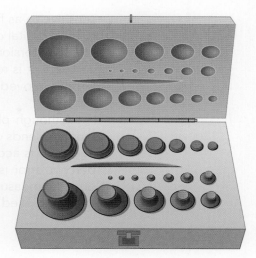

FIGURE 3-6a and b Torsion balance with counterweight set.

in measurement. Class A torsion balances are sensitive to as little as 6 mg and able to measure up to 120 mg. When using a torsion balance, it is essential that the counterweights and the product being weighed both be in the center of their respective weighing pans to achieve accurate measurement. Also, torsion balances are so sensitive that dust from the air and oils and dirt from fingers left on counterweights can affect the accuracy of the measurement. For this reason, the counterweights should be handled with forceps. The lid of a torsion balance should be closed at all times when the balance is not in use.

An **analytical balance** (Figure 3-7) uses electronic calibrations to determine the weight of a product. Analytical balances are also known as electronic balances and are generally preferred because they are able to measure heavier substances, are

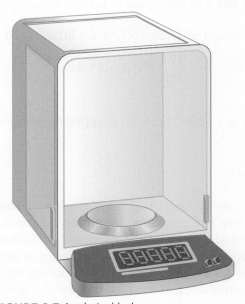

FIGURE 3-7 Analytical balance.

sensitive to as little as 0.1 mg, are easier to operate and maintain, and have easy-to-read digital displays.

Both torsion and analytical balances must be calibrated in order to maintain accuracy. It is recommended that torsion balances be calibrated anytime the balance is moved because these balances require a perfectly level setting to be accurate.

Although pharmacy measuring equipment is very accurate, use of the equipment depends on the pharmacy staff, thus is subject to human error. Some percentage error is acceptable in compound, up to 10% error is generally allowed. The percent error is calculated by dividing the amount of error (the difference in the quantity measured and the desired quantity) by the desired quantity. This value is then multiplied by 100 to obtain a percentage of error.

$$\frac{\text{Amount of error}}{\text{Desired quantity}} \times 100 = \text{Percentage error}$$

EXAMPLE

You are compounding an oral powder to fill capsules and the compounding recipe calls for 50 g of lactose powder. You are using an analytical balance to measure the quantity. Although you are trying to measure 50 g exactly, you are having difficulty getting perfect accuracy. The balance currently reads 50.74 g. What is the percentage error in your measurement?

SOLUTION

$$\frac{\text{Amount of error}}{\text{Desired quantity}} \times 100 = \text{Percentage error}$$

Amount of error equals the difference between what you were trying to measure and what you actually measured. Subtract the 2 values in a way that ensures a positive number results (ie, it does not matter which one is first in the equation, as long as you do not get a negative value for the amount of error).

$$\text{Amount of error} = 50.74 \text{ g} - 50 \text{ g} = 0.74 \text{ g}$$

$$\frac{0.74 \text{ g}}{50 \text{ g}} \times 100 = 1.48\%$$

The percentage error is 1.48%. This is an acceptable amount of error.

Mixing Techniques

A mortar and pestle can be used to triturate solids. **Trituration** is the process of grinding particles into fine powders. Mortar and pestles (Figure 3-8) made of ceramic and wedgewood are generally preferred for triturating solid products. Glass mortars and pestles are used for preparing liquid or semisolid products, such as ointments and creams. **Levigation,** or further reducing the particle size of a powder through the addition of a liquid in which the powder is not soluble, is generally performed in a glass mortar and pestle.

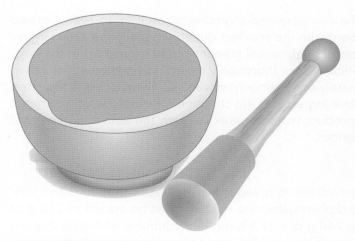

FIGURE 3-8a Wedgewood mortar and pestle.

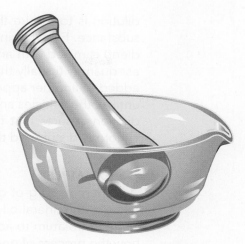

FIGURE 3-8b Glass mortar and pestle.

Mortars and pestles are available in a variety of different types. Typically, glass mortars and pestles are used for mixing wet ingredients and wedgewood or ceramic mortars and pestles are used for mixing dry ingredients.

Spatulation is the process of mixing 2 ingredients together with a spatula to form a **homogeneous,** or uniform, mixture. Generally, spatulation is used to fully incorporate 2 semisolid products, such as ointments or creams. Spatulation is typically performed on a large piece of smooth glass known as an ointment slab or pill tile.

NONSTERILE COMPOUNDING PROCEDURES

Once all the necessary ingredients and equipment are gathered in a clean, clutter-free environment, the compounding process may begin. The first step in every compounding process is to wash hands with antibacterial soap or clean with an alcohol-based hand sanitizer. Personal protective equipment (PPE), such as gloves or a gown, must then be donned. Gloves should always be worn when compounding. A gown may not be necessary in nonsterile compounding unless an ingredient or the final product is known to be corrosive, toxic, or otherwise hazardous.

Topical Preparations

Topical products can be prepared in a number of dosage forms. Ointments are defined as topical preparations containing 80% oil. Creams contain 50% oil, and lotions contain less than 50% oil. Most products can be compounded in any of these 3 topical dosage forms. Generally the properties of the active ingredient, the indication of the final product, and the body area being treated determine which topical preparation is preferred.

The key to preparing a homogeneous final product is the proper use of compounding equipment and techniques. Trituration and levigation must be completed as necessary until the desired particle size of the active ingredient(s) is reached. Then the ingredients are added to the designated ointment, cream, or lotion (also called the vehicle) by a process known as **geometric dilution.** The purpose of geometric

★ *TECH ALERT: Many topical products are referred to as semisolids. Semisolids include creams, gel preparations, and ointments. Because they are largely made of water, lotions are considered liquid products, not semisolids.*

dilution is to ensure that the compounded ingredients result in an evenly mixed substance. First, the ingredient with the smallest quantity (usually the active ingredient) is mixed with an approximately equal amount of the ingredient in the largest quantity (usually the vehicle). Once thoroughly mixed, this combination is then added to another approximately equal amount of vehicle. The process is repeated until all the vehicles and active ingredients are combined. Proper use of geometric dilution ensures that final product is homogeneous, with the active ingredient(s) uniformly distributed throughout.

EXAMPLE

There is 30 g of diphenhydramine powder that has been triturated and levigated with mineral oil. This diphenhydramine mixture must be added to 210 g of white petrolatum to achieve 240 g of a 12.5% diphenhydramine ointment. Explain how the process of geometric dilution will be used to incorporate the active ingredient into the ointment base.

Step 1: Add 30 g of active ingredient to an equal amount (30 g) of petrolatum and mix well. Result is 60 g of active ingredient or petrolatum mixture.

Step 2: Add the 60 g of active ingredient or ointment mixture obtained in step 1, to an equal amount of petrolatum (60 g) and mix well. Result is 120 g of active ingredient or petrolatum mixture. We have now used 90 g of the petrolatum base.

Step 3: Add 120 g of active ingredient or petrolatum mixture obtained in step 2 to the remaining 120 g of petrolatum base and mix well. Result is 240 g of final product.

Liquids

Liquid preparations are made up of 2 primary components: solutes and solvents. A **solute** is a solid ingredient dissolved in a liquid, and a **solvent** is the liquid in which the solute is dissolved. In pharmacy practice, the solute is generally the active ingredient and the solvent is the vehicle for the dosage form. Depending on the chemical properties of the active ingredient, a solute may or may not be completely soluble in the solvent. **Solubility** is the ability of a substance to dissolve in a particular solvent. For example, Kool-Aid powder is soluble (dissolves) in water, but oil is not (separates).

If an active ingredient is soluble in the given solvent, then the final dosage form is a **solution.** Solutions are homogeneous mixtures in which the active ingredient is completely dissolved in the liquid. Examples of solutions are shown in Table 3-1. If an active ingredient is not soluble in the given solvent, then the final dosage form is a **suspension.** Suspensions are **heterogeneous** mixtures in which the active ingredient is not completely dissolved, but rather suspended, in the liquid.

TABLE 3-1. **Examples of Solutions**	
Solution	Description
Elixir	Clear and sweet liquid, contains an alcoholic base
Enema	Solution administered rectally generally for cleansing of the bowel before a procedure
Syrup	Water-based solution containing sugar
Tincture	Solution of a pure chemical or extract with an alcoholic base

When compounding suspensions, it is important to remember that there will be visible particles in the final product. This is acceptable and should not be mistaken for a flaw in the product. However, if there are visible particles in a solution, it may indicate that the product has **precipitated** (a solid has formed from a chemical reaction in the solution) or is otherwise adulterated.

★ TECH ALERT: Suspensions must always be shaken well before use.

Oral Solutions From Powder for Reconstitution

Many medications are available in a dosage form known as powder for reconstitution. **Reconstitution** involves mixing a diluent into a preweighed powder to form a solution or suspension. Antibiotics for oral suspension are often manufactured as powders for reconstitution to preserve stability. These products are often only stable for days after reconstituted, but can be stored for years in their powder state.

★ TECH ALERT: Many oral solutions made from powder for reconstitution must be refrigerated after reconstituting.

The directions to prepare an oral liquid from a powder for reconstitution are clearly marked on the manufacturer's label. A specific amount of diluent is to be added to the powder in order to create a final product with the intended concentration. When adding the diluent to a powder for reconstitution, one should add half of the total amount, mix or shake, and then add the remainder of the diluent. This helps to ensure that the powder is evenly suspended in the liquid and does not overflow the bottle. Generally, distilled or sterile water should be used as the diluent for reconstituting because tap water may have impurities that can affect the stability of the product or the health of the patient.

Other Oral Dosage Forms

Sometimes patients are not able to tolerate a commercially available solid oral dosage form, such as a tablet or capsule, because of an allergy to an excipient, which are the inactive ingredients or fillers, used in medications, or to dyes in the product. In these cases, special capsules can be extemporaneously compounded. The required pharmaceutical ingredients are mixed together, added to a specified amount of filler powder such as lactose, and packed into empty capsules. The capsule consists of 2 pieces, the longer portion is the body, and the small portion is the cap. Capsules are available in varying sizes, ranging from 000 to 5. Size 000 capsules are the largest, measuring approximately 2.5 cm in length. Size 5 capsules are the smallest, measuring just over 1 cm. The most commonly used capsule sizes are 0, 00, and 4. Figure 3-9 depicts the various capsule sizes.

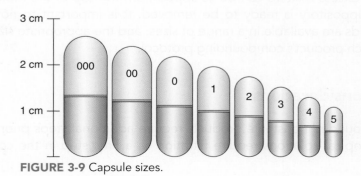

FIGURE 3-9 Capsule sizes.

Capsules can be produced through the punch method (smaller quantity) or through the use of a capsule filling machine (for a larger quantity). The punch method utilizes triturated powder placed on an ointment slab. The height of the powder should be about half the length of the capsule body. The empty capsule is then held vertically above the powder and the open end is "punched" into the powder, filling the capsule. The cap is placed on the capsule, and then each one must be weighed to add or remove powder as needed. This process can be time consuming and should only be used if a small number of capsules are needed.

An alternative method, when greater quantities are required, is through the use of a capsule filling machine. The designated amount of capsule bodies are placed in the machine and the triturated powder is spread over the top, filling the capsules evenly. Next, the caps are placed on the capsules, completing the filling process much more quickly and efficiently.

Tablets are prepared through compression, or molding of ingredients, and are the easiest dosage form to administer. Tablets are compounded in various shapes to help enable swallowing.

Troches are an additional oral dosage form which may be compounded. **Troches** contain the medication dispersed into a solid or wax-matrix, similar to a lozenge. Troches are placed in the mouth and allowed to slowly dissolve, releasing the medication to absorb through the oral mucosa. Since troches are absorbed directly through the mucosa and not swallowed, they bypass the digestive system and allow for rapid absorption of drug into the blood stream. Troches are commonly used for hormone replacement therapy, pain management, and to treat oral conditions such as oral yeast infections.

Suppositories

Suppositories are a dosage form used to administer medications through the rectum, vagina, or urethra. Suppositories are made of a base that is solid at room temperature or refrigerated, but are designed to melt at body temperature or in bodily fluids. The medication is through the mucosa of a particular body cavity when melted. Suppositories are mostly used for patients in whom oral administration of a medication is not possible, such as patients who are experiencing nausea or vomiting.

Suppositories can be prepared using either a fat- or water-soluble base. All suppositories are compounded in a similar manner regardless of the type of base used. First the active ingredients are triturated in a mortar and pestle. Then the mixture of active ingredients is added to the melted suppository base. Once fully dissolved or suspended, the mixture is poured into suppository molds (Figure 3-10). The molds should be slightly overfilled because the mixture will contract as it cools. Once fully cooled, any excess mixture can be scrapped from the top of the molds and each individual suppository is ready to be removed. It is important to note that suppository molds are available in a range of sizes, and the appropriate size should be noted on each product's compounding protocol.

Special Considerations

★ TECH ALERT:
Nonaqueous means a product does not contain water.

Some compounded nonsterile products require additional steps prior to dispensing. Some topical solutions require filtration as a final step in the compounding

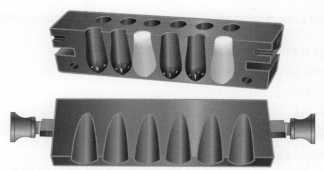

FIGURE 3-10 Suppository mold.

process. Filtering removes all particulate matter, including impurities and precipitants. Compounded preparations intended for nasal use generally require filtration.

Product Stability

The final step in **extemporaneous compounding** is to label the final product with an appropriate beyond-use date (BUD). BUDs differ from expiration dates in that BUDs relate specifically to the pharmacy-prepared final product, whereas expiration dates are assigned by manufacturers and relate to each individual ingredient used in the product. Still, the assigned BUD of a compounded product cannot be longer than the expiration date of any ingredient used in the preparation of that product. USP Chapter <795> guidelines for BUD of nonsterile compounded products are outlined in Table 3-2. Because mold, bacteria, and other microbes can grow easily in water, the beyond-use dating of a preparation depends on whether or not it contains water.

Compounding Documentation

USP Chapter <795> and State Boards of Pharmacy regulate the requirements for compounding documentation. All the necessary information must be included in a compounding log. The compounding log ensures that products can be traced in the event of a quality assurance issue, such as contamination, or FDA drug recall. Extemporaneously compounded medications must each be assigned a unique pharmacy lot number. The pharmacy lot number is the link between the dispensed product and the compounding log, which details all the included ingredients.

TABLE 3-2. USP Chapter <795> Guidelines for Beyond-Use Dating of Nonsterile Compounded Products	
Type of Product	*Beyond-Use Date Guidelines*
Topical nonaqueous liquid preparations	Not later than the earliest expiration date of any ingredient, or 6 months, whichever is earlier.
Topical liquid or semisolid preparations containing water	Not later than 30 days.
Oral preparations	Not later than 14 days. Must be refrigerated.

The following information should be included in a compounding log:

- Pharmacy lot number assigned
- Patient's name (and medical record number if applicable)
- Date compounded
- Date dispensed
- All ingredients used (including active and inactive ingredients)
- Manufacturer of each ingredient
- Lot number of each ingredient
- Expiration date of each ingredient
- Amount of each ingredient used
- Beyond-use date
- Technician and pharmacist initials

QUICK QUIZ 3-1

1. The major difference between trituration and levigation is that _____ uses the addition of a liquid to reduce particle size.
   a. Trituration
   b. Levigation
   c. Neither techniques involves the addition of a liquid
   d. Both techniques involve the addition of a liquid

2. A product has 50 g of dry ingredients to be added to 300 g of an ointment base. In the first phase of geometric dilution, how much ointment base should you add to the dry ingredients?
   a. 25 g
   b. 50 g
   c. 150 g
   d. 300 g

3. Amoxicillin 250 mg/5 mL liquid contains amoxicillin particles dispersed, but not dissolved, in the liquid. What type of liquid is this?
   a. Solution
   b. Solvent
   c. Suspension
   d. Solute

4. If white particles are found undissolved upon final inspection of a solution, it is likely that a _____ has formed.
   a. Complex
   b. Compound
   c. Suspension
   d. Precipitant

5. What is the beyond-use date of an extemporaneously compounded amiodarone 100 mg/10 mL oral solution?

   a. 7 days

   b. 14 days

   c. 30 days

   d. Equal to the expiration of the amiodarone powder

~~~~~~

Compounding Calculations

In the math review chapter, basic calculations required for dosage calculations were reviewed. These basic calculations related mostly to medications that are commercially available. That is, the desired concentration or strength of the medication is available from a manufacturer. There may be times when the desired concentration of a solution, lotion, ointment, or other liquid preparation ordered by a prescriber is not commercially available. The desired concentration may need to be compounded by mixing specific amounts of a higher concentration preparation and a lower concentrated preparation. The amounts of each concentration needed to compound the desired concentration can be calculated using the **alligation method.** When working with alligations the acronym **SAMD** can be used to recall the basic math operations used to perform the calculations.

★ TECH ALERT: *A memory by association tip can be used to remember SAMD when working with alligations; Sam is the lead pharmacist and he had a PharmD degree "Sam D."*

S—Subtraction: Subtract diagonally to determine the number of parts needed for each concentration.

A—Addition: Add the parts needed for each concentration to determine the total number of parts in the final solution or preparation.

M—Multiplication: Multiply the number of parts *per* concentration by the total volume ordered.

D—Division: Divide the answer from the multiplication equation by the total number of parts in the final solution.

The alligation method uses a grid, similar to that of a tic-tac-toe box, to set up and solve the calculations used to determine the amount of each concentration needed to compound the total volume of the desired concentration ordered.

🄴 EXAMPLE

A physician has ordered 60 mL of 3% lidocaine topical solution for a patient. The available concentrations on hand in the pharmacy are 2% lidocaine topical solution and 5% lidocaine topical solution. How much lidocaine 2% and lidocaine 5% must you mix together to make 60 mL of 3% lidocaine topical solution?

The first step in the alligation method is to set up the calculation grid in a specific format. Looking at the example, the desired concentration ordered is 3%.

	Desired concentration 3%	

Next, the concentrations on hand are inserted into the grid. The concentrations available are 2% and 5% lidocaine topical solution. The higher concentration of 5% is placed in the upper-left corner of the grid (Tip: higher box = higher concentration), and the lower concentration of 2% is placed in the lower-left corner of the grid (Tip: lower box = lower concentration).

Higher concentration 5%		
	Desired concentration 3%	
Lower concentration 2%		

Next, we set up the basic math skills needed to work the calculation using the acronym SAMD.

The first is subtraction **S**AMD.

Subtract diagonally, this will determine how many parts of each preparation are needed. Subtract the lower concentration from the desired concentration and record the answer in the upper-right corner.

Higher concentration 5%		3 – 2 = **1 part**
	Desired concentration 3%	
Lower concentration 2%		

Next, subtract the desired concentration from the higher concentration and record that answer in the lower right corner.

Higher concentration 5%		3 – 2 = **1 part**
	Desired concentration 3%	
Lower concentration 2%		5 – 3 = **2 parts**

The number of parts in the top right square correlates to the concentration in the top left square. In this case, the final product will contain **1 part** of **5% lidocaine solution.** The number of parts in the bottom right square correlates to the concentration in the bottom left square. The final product will contain **2 parts** of **2% lidocaine solution.**

Higher concentration 5%		3 – 2 = **1 part of 5% needed**
	Desired concentration 3%	
Lower concentration 2%		5 – 3 = **2 parts 2% needed**

Next, the basic math skill of addition is needed to work the calculation (S**A**MD).

Add vertically: Add the parts of each concentration to determine how many total parts are in your final product. In this example, 1 part + 2 parts = 3 parts.

Higher concentration 5%		3 – 2 = **1 part** of 5% needed
	Desired concentration 3%	+
Lower concentration 2%		5 – 3 = **2 parts** 2% needed
		1 part + 2 parts = 3 total parts

Next, multiply SA**M**D.
Multiply the number of parts needed per concentration by the total volume ordered.

Higher concentration 5%		3 – 2 = **1 part** of 5% needed Total volume ordered 60 mL 1 × 60 mL = 60 mL
	Desired concentration 3%	
Lower concentration 2%		5 – 3 = **2 parts** 2% needed Total volume ordered 60 mL 2 × 60 mL = 120 mL
		1 part + 2 parts = 3 total parts

The last SAM**D** math application is division.
Divide the answers from the multiplication equations by the total number of parts in the final solution or preparations.

Higher concentration 5%		3 – 2 = **1 part** of 5% needed Total volume ordered 60 mL 1 × 60 mL = 60 mL ÷ 3 total parts = 20 mL of 5% lidocaine topical solution is needed
	Desired concentration 3%	
Lower concentration 2%		5 – 3 = **2 parts** of 2% needed Total volume ordered 60 mL 2 × 60 mL = 120 mL ÷ 3 total parts = 40 mL of 2% lidocaine topical solution is needed
		1 part + 2 parts = 3 total parts

So, if you mix together 20 mL of 5% lidocaine topical solution and 40 mL of 2% lidocaine topical solution, you will make 60 mL of 3% lidocaine topical solution.

To check your work, simply add the 2 volumes needed to ensure that the 2 totals add up to the final volume ordered (20 mL + 40 mL = 60 mL).

The alligation method can also be used to determine how much water should be added to a concentrated product to make a certain volume of a less concentrated product. For any ingredient in the mixture which does not have strength, such as water, 0 is always used as the percent strength.

EXAMPLE
Isopropyl alcohol (IPA) is readily available as a 70% solution. What if you were cleaning a very sensitive pharmacy instrument that needed to be soaked in 50% IPA?

How much **water (0%)** and **70% IPA solution** would you mix together to make 100 mL of 50% IPA?

SOLUTION
First, set up the alligation grid.

Write the **desired concentration** (50% IPA) in the center square.

Write the **higher concentration** (70% IPA) available preparation in the upper left corner.

Write the **lower concentration** (water = 0%) available preparation in the lower left square.

Higher concentration 70%		
	Desired concentration 50%	
Lower concentration 0%		

Subtract diagonally and write the difference of the numbers in the appropriate square. This will determine how many parts of each preparation are needed.

Higher concentration 70%		50 – 0 = **50 parts**
	Desired concentration 50%	
Lower concentration 0%		

And

Higher concentration 70%		50 – 0 = **50 parts**
	Desired concentration 50%	
Lower concentration 0%		70 – 50 = **20 parts**

The number of parts in the top right square correlates to the concentration in the top left square. In this case, the final product will contain **50 parts** of **70% IPA.** The number of parts in the bottom right square correlates to the concentration in the bottom left square. The final product will contain **20 parts** of **water (0%).**

Then, add the parts of each concentration to determine how many total parts are in your final product. In this case, 50 parts + 20 parts = 70 parts.

Higher concentration **70%**		50 – 0 = **50 parts of 70% IPA**
	Desired concentration **50%**	+
Lower concentration **0%**		70 – 50 = 20 parts **of** **0% (water)**
		50 parts + 20 parts = 70 total parts

Next, multiply the number of parts needed per concentration by the total volume ordered.

Higher concentration **70%**		50 – 0 = **50 parts** of 70% IPA Total volume ordered **100 mL** **50 × 100 mL = 5000 mL**
	Desired concentration **50%**	
Lower concentration **0%**		70 – 50 = **20 parts** of 0% (water) Total volume ordered **100 mL** **20 × 100 mL = 2000 mL**
		50 parts + 20 parts = 70 total parts

Last, divide the answers from the multiplication equations by the total number of parts in the final solution or preparations.

Higher concentration **70%**		50 – 0 = **50 parts** of 70% IPA Total volume ordered **100 mL** **50 × 100 mL = 5000 mL ÷** **70 total parts = 71.42, which** **rounds to 71.4 mL of 70% IPA**
	Desired concentration **50%**	
Lower concentration **0%**		70 – 50 = **20 parts** of 0% (water) Total volume ordered **100 mL** **20 × 100 mL = 2000 mL ÷** **70 total parts = 28.57, which** **rounds to 28.6 mL**
		50 parts + 20 parts = 70 total parts

If you mix together 71.4 mL of 70% IPA and 28.6 mL of water, you will make 100 mL of 50% IPA. If you add these 2 volumes together, you will get 100 mL, an easy check to see if we calculated correctly (71.4 + 28.6 = 100).

QUICK QUIZ 3-2

1. How much of a 5% solution and a 12% solution do you need to mix together to get 30 mL of a 8% solution?

2. How much of a 20% solution and a 70% solution do you need to mix together to get 500 mL of a 40% solution?

3. How many grams of a 10% w/w powder and a 30% w/w powder do you need to mix together to get 50 g of a 25% w/w powder?

4. How many grams of a 15% ointment and a 30% ointment do you need to mix together to get 480 g of a 25% ointment?

5. How many milliliters of a 1:100 solution and a 5:100 solution do you need to mix together to get 60 mL of a 4:100 solution? (Hint: Remember that a percentage means amount per 100).

★ TECH ALERT: Since the eyes are also vulnerable to contaminants, ophthalmic preparations are compounded in a sterile environment.

STERILE COMPOUNDING

★ TECH ALERT: The abbreviations SQ and SC for subcutaneous are part of The Joint Commission's forbidden abbreviation list. Only sub-Q is an acceptable abbreviation.

Sterile compounding encompasses all preparation of dosage forms in a sterile environment, such as a laminar flow hood or clean room. Most **parenteral** medications, or medications administered by any means other than orally, must be sterile. Parenteral medications are most often administered by injection. The 3 most common administration routes for injection are intravenous, intramuscular, and subcutaneous. **Intravenous (IV)** medications are administered directly into a vein, **intramuscular (IM)** medications are injected into the muscle, and **subcutaneous (sub-Q)** medications are injected directly into the fatty layer below the skin. Sterility is important for these medications because parenteral administration bypasses the body's natural defenses of the gastrointestinal system.

Intravenous medications can be administered in a number of different methods. An **IV push** is the rapid administration of a small volume of medication into the vein. An **IV piggyback,** or intermittent IV, is a small volume (generally <250 mL) of medication that is infused through the same IV line as a primary IV fluid. An **IV drip,** or IV infusion, contains a medication that is administered slowly into a patient's vein.

Guidelines for sterile compounding are defined in the USP Chapter <797>. Before USP <797> standards, there were no guidelines for compounding sterile products. Although this chapter of USP is not regulated or enforced by the government, State Boards of Pharmacy examine the overall compounding processes at each facility and enforce the requirements of USP <797> specific to each state. As with nonsterile compounding, each State Board of Pharmacy sets specific requirements for the sterile compounding process, quality control, and documentation. Each state interprets and regulates compounding differently, and pharmacy technicians must be aware of the laws for state in which they are working.

Sterile Compounding Calculations

The final calculations involved in IV infusions are related to drip rates. The **drip rate** of an IV is the rate at which the medication is infused. Drip rates can be defined as the amount (mg, mcg, units, etc.) of drug infused over a period of time or as the volume of solution infused over a period of time. Also, physicians and nurses may refer to the drip rate in drops per minute. This is determined by the drop factor (DF) of the IV tubing used and is generally dictated by the physician's order or by nursing protocol.

Drip rate calculations are useful in determining the amount of medication given over a period of time, how much solution is needed to last a defined period of time, or how much time remains until an IV bag is empty.

IV Flow Rates

To determine a flow rate, the volume to be infused and amount of time of infusion must be known. The infusion rate can then be found using the following formula:

$$\frac{\text{Volume of infusion}}{\text{Time}} = \text{Infusion rate}$$

Infusion rates can be used to determine how many bags of IV solution a patient will need or how long each bag will last.

EXAMPLE

What is the infusion rate in mL/h of a 1000-mL IV being infused over 6 hours?

$$\frac{1000 \text{ mL}}{6 \text{ h}} = 166.67 = \text{round to } 167 \text{ mL/h}$$

EXAMPLE

If a patient is receiving a 1000-mL infusion at 125 mL/h and the infusion started at 0700 hours, at what time would the patient need another bag of IV solution?

First determine how many hours one bag will last.

Set up using ratio-proportion method.

$$\frac{X \text{ h}}{1000 \text{ mL}} = \frac{1 \text{ h}}{125 \text{ mL}}$$

Cross multiply and divide.

$$1 \times 1000 = X \text{ h} \times 125$$

$1000 = 125X$

Solve for X.

$1000 \div 125 = 8 \text{ h}$

$$X = 8 \text{ h}$$

Solve using dimensional analysis.

$$\frac{1000 \text{ mL}}{1} \times \frac{1 \text{ h}}{125 \text{ mL}}$$

Cancel the like units to leave hours remaining. Multiply the fractions, then divide the numerator by the denominator.

$1000 \times 1 = 1000$, *and* $1 \times 125 = 125$

$1000 = 125$

$1000 \div 125 = 8\ h$

The bag will last the patient 8 hours.
Now add 8 hours to the time when this infusion started = 0700 hours.
The patient will need a new bag at 1500 hours or 3 PM.

EXAMPLE

If a patient is receiving an infusion at a rate of 250 mL/h, and the IV is made in a 1000-mL bag, how many bags will be needed to last this patient 24 hours?
First determine how many hours one bag will last.

$$\frac{X\ h}{1000\ mL} = \frac{1\ h}{250\ mL}$$

Cross multiply and solve for X.

$1 \times 1000 = X \times 250$

$1000 = 250\,X$

$1000 \div 250 = 4\ h$

Solve using dimensional analysis.

$$\frac{1000\ mL}{1} \times \frac{1\ h}{250\ mL}$$

Cancel the like units to leave hours remaining. Multiply the fractions, then divide the numerator by the denominator.

$1000 \times 1 = 1000$, and $1 \times 250 = 250$

$1000 \div 250 = 4\ h$

One bag will last 4 hours.
To determine how many bags the patient will need for 24 hours, divide 24 hours by 4.

$$\frac{24\ h}{4} = \textbf{6 total bags.}$$

So, 6 bags will be neded to last the patient 24 hours.

IV Drip Rates

Drip rates are measured in drops/min and calculations should be rounded to the nearest whole drop. The following formula will allow you to calculate a drip rate easily.

$$\frac{total\ volume \times drop\ factor}{total\ minutes}$$

EXAMPLE

An order for a patient is 250 mL of a drug over a 3-hour period at a drip factor of 15 gtt/mL. What is the drip rate in drops/min?

First convert hours to minutes.

$3\ h \times 60\ min = 180\ min$

Then multiply your total volume by the drip factor.

$250\ mL \times 15 = 3750$

Divide by the total minutes.

$3750 \div 180 = 20.83$ (round to 21)

The rate is 21 drops/min.

QUICK QUIZ 3-3

1. A patient is to be given 800 mL of a drug over 5 hours at 20 gtt/mL. What will be the drip rate?

2. 700 mL is ordered using a 10-gtt/mL set running over 6 hours. What is the rate in drops/min?

3. If a patient receives a 500-mL infusion at 50 mL/h at 0900 hours, at what time will a new bag be needed?

4. If a patient is receiving a 1500-mL infusion at 500 mL/h, how many bags will be needed for a 24-hour supply?

5. If a patient receives a 1250-mL infusion at a rate of 250 mL/h, when will a new bag be needed if the patient started the infusion at 0700 hours?

Alternative Units of Measurement (mEq and Units)

Calculating doses using milliequivalent is done the same way as if a medication was measured in milligrams.

EXAMPLE

A patient has an order for 20 mEq of potassium chloride (KCl) and the pharmacy has a vial in stock of 2 mEq/mL. How much volume is needed to fill this order?

$$\frac{X\ mL}{20\ mEq} = \frac{1\ mL}{2\ mEq}$$

Cross multiply and then divide: $2 \times X = 2X$, and $20 \times 1 = 20$
$2X \div 2 = X$, and $20 \div 2 = 10$

$X = 10\ mL$

TABLE 3-3. Common IV Electrolytes	
Sodium chloride	mEq
Calcium chloride	mg
Potassium chloride	mEq
Magnesium sulfate	mg
Sodium acetate	mEq
Potassium acetate	mEq
Sodium bicarbonate	mEq

Cancel same units.

$$\frac{20\ mEq}{1} \times \frac{1\ mL}{2\ mEq}$$

Multiply the fractions and then divide the numerator by the denominator.

$$1 \times 20 = 20,\ and\ 1 \times 2 = 2,\ then\ 20 \div 2 = 10$$

$$X = 10\ mL$$

In addition to potassium chloride, there are other IV electrolytes measured in milliequivalent used for TPN dosing. Some common IV electrolytes are listed in Table 3-3.

For each electrolyte added into a TPN, the calculation is completed in the same way as the previous example with KCl.

Practice Problems

A patient is to have a TPN compounded with the following additives. Complete the chart with the quantity required for each additive, based on the dose prescribed.

Each of the following medications is available in a **20-mEq/mL vial.**

Additive	Dose	What is the volume dispensed?
Sodium chloride	35 mEq	1.
Potassium chloride	20 mEq	2.
Potassium acetate	30 mEq	3.

An additional measurement system used in dispensing insulin and heparin is **units.**

For most insulin dosages, a conversion that is important to remember is that there are **100 units of insulin in every 1 mL of solution,** although the vial size may vary. This value is important for ensuring the patient will have a sufficient quantity for therapy.

EXAMPLE
A patient is prescribed 36 units of insulin before breakfast. How many milliliters will be injected into the patient?

Remember insulin is available as 100 units/1 mL.

$$\frac{X \text{ mL}}{36 \text{ units}} = \frac{1 \text{ mL}}{100 \text{ units}}$$

Cross multiply and then divide.

X × 100 = 100X, and 1 × 36 = 36

100X ÷ 100 = X, and 36 ÷ 100 = 0.36

X = 0.36

Cancel same units.

$$\frac{36 \text{ units}}{1} \times \frac{1 \text{ mL}}{100 \text{ units}}$$

Multiply the numerators, then divide the answer by the product of the denominator.

1 × 36 = 36, and 1 × 100 = 100, then 36 ÷ 100 = 0.36

X = 0.36 mL

Answer = 0.36 mL

EXAMPLE
This patient has 1 vial of insulin (10 mL). What is the estimated days' supply? The patient is taking 36 units of insulin (0.36 mL) each morning and the vial contains 10 mL.

Remember there are 100 units of insulin in every 1 mL of solution.

$$\frac{X \text{ days}}{10 \text{ mL}} = \frac{1 \text{ day}}{0.36 \text{ mL}}$$

Cross multiply and then divide.

1 × 10 = 10, and X × 0.36 = 0.36 X

10 ÷ 0.36 = 27.777, and 0.36 X ÷ 0.36 = X

X = 27.7777 days

Note: Round down to 27 days because the patient does not have enough insulin to last a full 28 days.

X = 27 days

Cancel same units.

$$\frac{10 \text{ mL}}{1} \times \frac{1 \text{ day}}{0.36 \text{ mL}}$$

Multiply the fractions, then divide the numerator by the denominator.

Answer = 27 days

Note: Round down because the patient does not have enough insulin to last a full 28 days.

QUICK QUIZ 3-4

1. Heparin is available in a 10-mL vial with 5000 units/mL. A patient has an order for 25,000 units of heparin, how much volume is needed?

2. A patient needs 26 units of insulin in the morning and 35 units in the evening. How many milliliters will the patient inject total daily?

3. Using the answer from question 2, how long will a 10 mL vial last this patient?

4. If a patient is to receive 15,000 units of heparin and the pharmacy stocks 5000 units/mL, how many milliliters are needed for the dose?

5. A patient requires a medication for irrigation at a dose of 50,000 units in 0.9% normal saline (NS) 1000 mL. This is available after reconstitution as a 5000 units/mL vial. How much must be drawn up to prepare this solution?

IV push, IM, and Subcutaneous Dose Calculations

Some parenteral medications intended for IV push, IM, or subcutaneous administration are supplied from the manufacturer as injectable solutions. Generally these solutions do not require further dilution and are available in unit dose vials. However, many medications have short stability once diluted, and thus are supplied as a sterile powder for reconstitution. The manufacturer's label or package insert most often contains instructions for dilution of the product, including the amount and type of diluent needed.

EXAMPLE
Vancomycin is supplied as a sterile powder for reconstitution. The vial of vancomycin 1 g reads "add 20 mL sterile water for injection."
What is the resulting concentration of the dilution?

1 g vancomycin/20 mL final volume = 50 mg/mL

Some powders for reconstitution expand to occupy a certain volume in the final product. The manufacturer label or package insert will define how much volume the powder adds, and the resulting final volume and concentration when diluted as directed.

ⓔ EXAMPLE

Cefazolin is supplied as a sterile powder for reconstitution. The vial of cefazolin 500 mg reads "add 2 mL sterile water for injection or 0.9% sodium chloride for injection. Provides an approximate volume of 2.2 mL."

What is the resulting concentration of the dilution?

ⓢ SOLUTION

500 mg cefazolin / 2.2 mL final volume = approximately 225 mg/mL

ⓔ EXAMPLE

There is a patient in the Emergency Department without IV access. A physician orders cefazolin 150 mg IM q6h. How many mL would need to be drawn up to dispense the appropriate dose?

ⓢ SOLUTION USING CROSS-MULTIPLICATION

Set up the ratios.

$$\frac{225 \text{ mg}}{1 \text{ mL}} = \frac{150 \text{ mg}}{X \text{ mL}}$$

Cross-multiply.

$$225 \times X = 1 \times 150$$

Solve.

$$225 \times X = 150$$

$$X = \frac{150}{225}$$

$$X = 0.67 \text{ mL}$$

0.67 mL of the cefazolin injectable solution contains a 150 mg dose.

ⓢ SOLUTION USING THE CANCEL OUT METHOD

Set up the equation so that like units cancel out.

$$150 \; \cancel{mg} \times \frac{1 \text{ mL}}{225 \; \cancel{mg}} = 0.67 \text{ mL}$$

The units mg cancel out and the desired unit of measure, mL, is left.
0.67 mL of the cefazolin injectable solution contains a 150 mg dose.

QUICK QUIZ 3-5

1. A physician writes "phenobarbital gr ii IM STAT." Phenobarbital is supplied from the manufacturer in a 200 mg/mL injectable solution. How much phenobarbital should be dispensed?

2. Famotidine is available in 200 mg/20 mL injectable solution. How many 40-mg doses are contained in one 20-mL vial?

> ★ *TECH ALERT: In adults, IM injection volume should be no more than 2 mL in the deltoid or thigh muscles, and no more than 5 mL in the gluteus maximus. If more volume is necessary, multiple injections must be dispensed.*

3. Caffeine citrate injectable solution is supplied in a 60 mg/3 mL concentration. The infant dose of caffeine citrate is 5 mg/kg. How many milliliters should be dispensed for an 11-lb infant?

4. If a patient requires a 30-mg dose of morphine, and it is available as a 15-mg/mL injection, how many milliliters will be drawn up into the syringe?

5. If a patient receives a 3.5-mL dose of gentamicin 40 mg/mL, how many milligrams were in the dose?

IV Piggyback and IV Drip Calculations

An IV piggyback is an injectable medication diluted in a small amount, generally less than 250 mL, of intravenous solution. It is also known as small-volume parenteral, or SVP. An IV drip or IV infusion is an injectable medication diluted in a large amount, generally more than 250 mL, of intravenous solution. It is also known as large-volume parenteral, or LVP.

The most common intravenous base solutions are shown in Table 3-4. These base solutions are prepackaged in IV bags or vials of various sizes.

If a medication is supplied as a sterile powder for injection, the first step in compounding an IV piggyback or IV drip is to dilute the medication as described in the package insert or on the manufacturer's label, as outlined in the previous section. This step is not necessary if the medication is already supplied as a solution. The second step in compounding an IV piggyback or IV drip is to ensure the medication is added to the appropriate amount of solution needed to equal the desired (ordered) concentration. Each medication has specific concentration or range of concentrations that are acceptable for IV administration. These concentrations may be defined in the medication package insert. Many hospitals also set standardized concentrations per their Pharmacy and Therapeutics Committees. Standardized concentrations allow a hospital to standardize drip rates, program IV pumps, and limit the amount of errors associated with IV infusions.

Infection Control in Sterile Compounding

★ TECH ALERT: Artificial nails are not allowed in sterile compounding environments as they can harbor bacteria and lead to contamination.

Guidelines for sterile compounding are defined in the United States Pharmacopeia (USP) Chapter 797. USP <797> outlines specific regulations for PPE, hand washing, cleaning requirements, and sterility standards.

TABLE 3-4. Common Base Solutions for IV Medications	
Base Solution	*Abbreviation*
0.9% sodium chloride (normal saline)	NS
0.45% sodium chloride (half normal saline)	1/2 NS
0.225% sodium chloride (quarter normal saline)	1/4 NS
Dextrose 5% in water	D5W or D_5W
Dextrose 10% in water	D10W or $D_{10}W$
Lactated Ringer	LR
Sterile water	SWFI

TABLE 3-5. Infection Control in Sterile Compounding

Location	Infection Control Step
Prior to entering the sterile compounding area	Remove all personal outer garments Remove all cosmetics and jewelry and tie back long hair
Anteroom or designated gowning area	1. Put on shoe covers 2. Put on hair/head covers 3. Put on face mask/eye shield 4. Aseptically wash hands for at least 30 seconds with antimicrobial soap and water 5. Put on nonshedding gown (at least knee-length) 6. Put on sterile gloves 7. Cleanse gloves with antimicrobial hand sanitizer or sterile isopropyl alcohol

Hand washing prior to sterile compounding is extremely important. Hands must be washed for at least 30 seconds with antimicrobial soap and water. **Personal protective equipment (PPE)** includes all items intended to reduce the risk of employee exposure to hazardous medication and to reduce the risk of contamination from employee to medication during the sterile compounding process. PPE in sterile compounding environment includes shoe covers, hair covers, face masks/eye shields, full gowns, and gloves. Table 3-5 outlines the order in which PPE should be donned prior to sterile compounding.

PPE should be donned in the ante area, which is the location prior to the clean room where supplies are gathered and gowning occurs.

The actual process of sterile compounding may occur in different locations based on the facility type. Many hospitals have an entire room designated as the clean room designed for sterile product compounding. Clean rooms utilize special filters to produce very clean air with extremely low levels of particulate matter. An additional option is having an area where microbial counts are kept to a minimum, designated as a clean space. The first space would be an ante area which is where garbing and hand washing occur. This is the least clean space (in terms of air particles). The next space is known as the **buffer** or **clean room.** This space is where supplies used in the compounding process are stored, as well as the laminar flow hood and/or glove box isolators. Each compounding device uses a high-efficiency particulate air (HEPA) filter to remove 99.97% of all air particles.

The area where sterile compounding is performed must meet specific criteria regarding air quality. The International Organization for Standardization (ISO) has created standards for maintaining a clean and safe environment. The lower the ISO class, the cleaner the air. Below are the standards for ISO class as it applies to sterile compounding (Table 3-6).

TABLE 3-6. ISO Standards in Sterile Compounding

ISO Class	Required in
5	Air within the hood or glove box
7	Clean room and buffer area
8	Ante area

Laminar flow hoods constantly draw air through a HEPA filter to be blown into the work area creating a sterile environment for compounding. Horizontal laminar flow hoods draw air first into a prefilter, which helps filter large particles from the outside air. This air is then filtered again through the HEPA filter from the back of the hood and blown out horizontally toward the user. Because of this airflow direction, objects must not be placed in front of each other, to ensure they receive proper HEPA-filtered air. They should be placed horizontally or side by side, instead of lining up supplies vertically toward the compounding technician. Horizontal airflow hoods are the most common type of laminar flow hoods and are used in sterile compounding of nonhazardous medications.

Vertical airflow hoods follow the same mechanism with the prefilter as do horizontal airflow hoods. The difference in this type is that air is pulled from the top of the hood vertically down to the compounding surface and into a vent at the front of the hood. Vertical flow hoods usually have shields to provide additional protection for the user against exposure. Since vertical flow hoods minimize exposure to the user, they are used for the sterile compounding of hazardous medications, such as chemotherapy. A biological safety cabinet (BSC) is an example of a vertical flow hood. There are several different types of BSCs used in different facilities depending on the type of compounding being completed.

Horizontal and vertical laminar flow hoods are illustrated in Figures 3-11 and 3-12.

An additional compounding device is known as a glove box isolator, or aseptic isolator. There are 2 different types of glove boxes. A compounding aseptic isolator (CAI) utilizes positive pressure to keep out all unclean air particles and ensures a sterile environment for compounding. Like horizontal laminar flow hoods, positive-pressure glove boxes can be used for compounding with nonhazardous medications. A compounding aseptic containment isolator (CACI) utilizes negative pressure to ensure a sterile compounding environment while protecting the user from exposure. Like vertical laminar flow hoods, negative-pressure glove boxes are used for compounding of hazardous medications. Figure 3-13 depicts an aseptic glove box isolator.

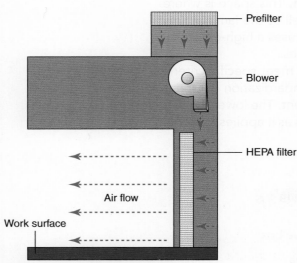

FIGURE 3-11 Horizontal laminar flow hood.

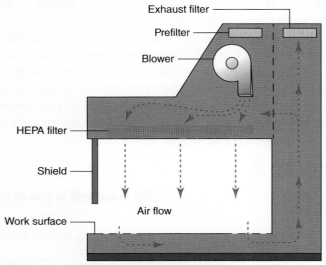

FIGURE 3-12 Vertical laminar flow hood.

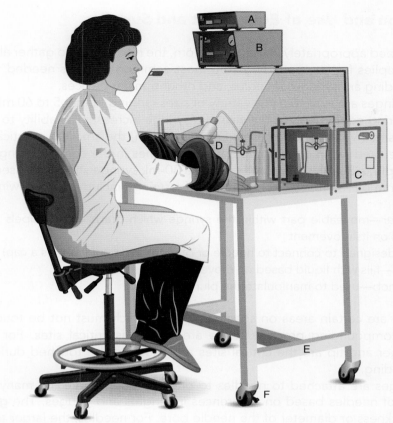

FIGURE 3-13 Glove box isolator.

Laminar flow hoods and glove box isolators must be cleaned frequently with antimicrobial cleaning solution or isopropyl alcohol. USP <797> requires the cleaning of a compounding device to occur in the following:

- At the beginning of every shift
- Before the start of any batch compounding
- No longer than 30 minutes following the previous cleaning when ongoing compounding is occurring
- When a spill has occurred

When cleaning the sterile compounding environment, it is important to clean from the cleanest to the dirtiest part of the area. This includes both the sterile compounding device, as well as the clean room and ante area. This ensures that contamination is not pulled into a clean area during the cleaning process.

For laminar flow hoods, this means that cleaning should take place in the direction in which the clean HEPA-filtered air flows. A horizontal flow hood should be cleaned from back to front, and a vertical flow hood should be cleaned from top to bottom.

Each cleaning is to be documented on a Hood Cleaning Log, as well as monthly decontaminations required for any device used for compounding chemotherapy or other hazardous drugs.

Selection and Use of Equipment and Supplies

Once garbed appropriately in the clean room, the next step is to gather all the necessary supplies for compounding. The most common supplies needed for sterile compounding are syringes, needles, and other transfer devices.

IV syringes are available in a variety of sizes ranging from 0.5 to 60 mL. As with all measuring equipment, as the size of a syringe increases, its ability to precisely measure small volumes decreases. For this reason, the smallest practical syringe should be used when drawing up specific volumes in the compounding process. For example, a 20-mL syringe rather than a 30-mL syringe should be used to draw up a volume of 15 mL. The components of a syringe include the following:

- Plunger—moveable part within the syringe which draws in or propels liquid out based on its movement
- Tip—designed to connect to needle or other attachment (such as a cap)
- Barrel—fills with liquid based on movement of the plunger
- Flat knob—used to manipulate the plunger

There are certain areas on specific supplies which must not be touched during the compounding process. These are known as critical sites. For syringes, the plunger and tip are the critical sites and must not be touched during sterile compounding.

Syringes are attached to needles to draw up fluid. There are many different varieties of needles based on differences in lengths and gauges. The **gauge (G)** is the thickness or diameter of the needle bore. For needles, the larger the gauge number, the smaller the needle. Large-bore needles of 16 and 18 gauges are typically used for IV compounding. Figure 3-14 illustrates the components of a syringe and needle. The entire needle is a critical site and must not be touched during the compounding process. The parts of the needle include the following:

- Bevel—slanted, opening of the needle
- Lumen—hollow part of the needle
- Hub—end of needle which attaches to a syringe
- Tip—end and sharpest point of needle

Each needle comes supplied with an individual cap. This cap should be left on when attaching to syringe and until ready to begin compounding.

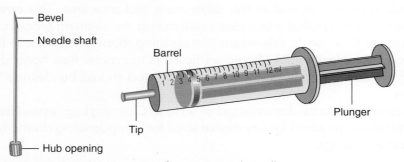

FIGURE 3-14 Components of a syringe and needle.

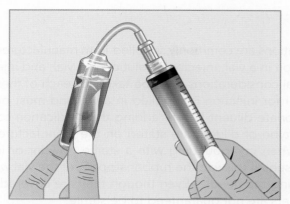

FIGURE 3-15 Use of a filter straw with ampule.

Although most medications are drawn from vials, occasionally medications are packaged in an ampule. An ampule is a glass container which must be broken to withdraw the medication. Because of the potential for glass shards to fall into the liquid, filter needles and straws are used to withdraw medication from an ampule. This ensures that any glass shards produced when the ampule was cracked will not be transferred into the final product. A filter needle should be used only once. It should be used to either withdraw the fluid from the vial, or if a regular need is used to withdraw the fluid, a filter needle should replace the regular needle prior to injection into the IV bag. If you draw up a solution with a filter needle and use the same needle to inject the solution, any particles captured in the filter may be injected out with the solution. The product label and protocol at the hospital should dictate if a filter is required. Figure 3-15 illustrates the use of an ampule and filter straw.

Vented needles are also used for reconstituting powder medications. These needles have openings on the sides which help in air pressure to prevent spraying or foaming when reconstituting medications.

STERILE COMPOUNDING PROCEDURES

Aseptic Technique

Aseptic technique encompasses all precautions and procedures undertaken to minimize the risk of microbial contamination of a sterile product. Contamination of sterile products can be extremely dangerous, even fatal, since most sterile medications are given directly into a patient's circulatory system. In pharmacy practice, aseptic technique begins with proper hand washing and PPE as described earlier in this chapter.

Several practices must be considered to maintain sterility during compounding in a laminar flow hood. First, no extraneous materials should be stored in a laminar flow hood. Any unnecessary materials increase the risk of disturbing the flow of clean, filtered air and jeopardize sterility. Second, nothing should pass between the sterile product and the source of clean air. In a horizontal flow hood, this means nothing should pass behind the sterile product. In a vertical flow hood, nothing should pass above the product. Third, all manipulations of sterile products should occur at least 6 inches from the sides and front of the laminar flow hood to ensure proper air flow and maintain sterility.

IV Admixtures

IV additive medications are commonly supplied from manufacturers in 3 ways: sterile powder for injection in a vial, injectable solution in a vial, and injectable solution in an ampule. Special considerations must be taken for each of these products.

Sterile powder for injection is supplied in a vial and must be diluted with the amount of appropriate diluent before adding the medication to an IV admixture. The amount and type of diluent are stated on the manufacturer's label or in the package insert. When compounding with a sterile powder or injectable solution from a vial, it is essential to swab the rubber stopper of the vial with isopropyl alcohol prior to inserting the needle. Even though they are covered with a plastic flip top, rubber stoppers are not guaranteed to be sterile.

Injectable solutions are supplied in either multidose or single-dose vials (SDVs). Multidose vials (MDVs) contain preservative to inhibit microbial growth. For this reason, MDVs are considered sterile for 28 days after the initial entry with a needle. A beyond-use date should be clearly marked on the vial after first use. SDVs do not contain preservatives and should be discarded immediately after use.

Since large-bore needles are typically used in compounding, there is a risk that the needle could dislodge a piece of the rubber stopper upon insertion; this is called coring. To prevent coring, the needle should always be inserted into the rubber stopper with bevel up as shown in Figure 3-16. Also, when drawing up solution from a vial, an equal amount of air must be first injected into the vial. This prevents the formation of a vacuum, which makes the solution very difficult to withdraw from the vial. Caution must be used not to inject too much air into the vial such that a positive-pressure system is created. Positive pressure can cause the rubber stopper to dislodge from the vial or the contents to spray out of the area where the needle is inserted.

Ampules are composed entirely of glass and must be broken prior to use. Before an ampule is opened, tap the ampule gently to dislodge any injectable solution in the top part of the ampule to the bottom. Although there are several types of tools available for snapping ampules, they are generally broken easily and

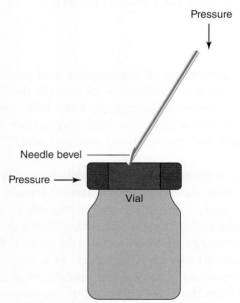

FIGURE 3-16 Aseptic technique.

can be done without the use of any aids. The neck of the ampule is a critical site and must be swabbed with isopropyl alcohol prior to snapping. As described earlier in this section, a filter needle or filter straw must be used to withdraw medication from an ampule. This ensures that any glass shards produced when the ampule was broken will not be transferred into the final product.

Most sterile products intended for use in adults are dispensed in a bag of IV fluid. Since children generally receive a smaller dose of medications, some hospitals prefer to dispense pediatric IV piggybacks and infusions in syringes. These syringes are hung on syringe pumps and are infused exactly as an IV bag would be. Prior to injecting medication into an IV fluid bag, the rubber port of the IV bag (injection port) must be swabbed with sterile isopropyl alcohol. Just as the plastic flip top cover does not guarantee sterility for a vial, the plastic overwrap does not guarantee sterility for an IV fluid bag.

Chemotherapy

Aseptic technique for chemotherapy (or biohazardous) products is more detailed than standard requirements. Chemotherapy PPE gowns are denser to reduce the risk of exposure in the case of a spill. Also, specific gloves designed to reduce exposure must be worn. Gloves must extend over the arm cuff of the gown to ensure that no skin is exposed.

Because chemotherapy agents are hazardous chemicals, special precautions must be taken during sterile preparation. First, chemotherapy should always be prepared in a vertical flow (BSC), or CACI to protect the compounder from exposure. Second, special care must be taken to avoid spills. Since inserting air into a vial can produce a positive-pressure system and lead to sprays or leaks, the volume of air injected into a chemotherapy vial should be no more than 75% of the amount of medication being withdrawn. This will prevent positive pressure from building up and decrease the risk of spill and exposure.

An additional method of protection is through the use of closed system transfer devices (CSTDs). These devices produce a complete chain—no environmental contaminants can get into the system and hazardous drug or air exposure can be released. These are very useful in the compounding of chemotherapy to protect compounding personnel from accidental exposure.

Special Preparations

Total parenteral nutrition (TPN), also known as hyperalimentation, is the IV administration of nutrition required to sustain life. The base components to a TPN include the following:

- Amino acids—for protein
- Lipids—for fat
- Dextrose—for carbohydrates
- Sterile water—for hydration

There are other additives that may be added depending on the patient and individual needs. These include the following:

- Electrolytes
- Trace elements and minerals
- Certain drugs—insulin, heparin, H_2 antagonist (e.g, famotidine, ranitidine)

TPN is generally used for patients who are not able to eat to maintain their nutritional status for extended periods of time. TPNs must be compounded in a specific order to prevent **precipitation** from occurring. First the base fluids are added, except the lipids. Lipids will turn a TPN white and will make it difficult to observe any incompatibilities. Some facilities administer lipids separate from the TPN altogether.

After the base fluids are added, phosphate must be added first and calcium last, to prevent precipitation from occurring. After the phosphate is added, the rest of the additives can be mixed as long as calcium is always the last to be added. Any colored additives (e.g., multivitamin) should be added at the end to prevent difficulty in observing precipitation.

It is not uncommon for TPNs to contain more than 20 ingredients in order to provide specialized nutrition to a patient. For this reason, many hospitals contract the preparation of TPNs to specialty pharmacies. Technicians in these specialty pharmacies will become uniquely familiar with the equipment, process, and quality measures used in TPN compounding.

Patient controlled analgesia (PCA) is a method of medication administration that allows a patient to bolus IV pain medication with the push of a button. PCAs may also provide a basal rate of the pain medication. **Epidural** administration is the injection of medication directly into the epidural space, or the outermost part of the spine. It is generally used for analgesia, anesthesia, or steroid injections. Special care must be taken with PCA and epidural preparation. Some methods require that all excess air be removed from the IV bag to reduce the risk of an air embolism. The hospital and pharmacy's protocols will dictate if measures must be taken to remove excess air prior to dispensing.

Sterile compounding may be necessary for some noninjectable products also. For example, ophthalmic preparations are compounded in a sterile environment because microbial contamination can be dangerous if instilled into the eye. Sterility may also be required for topical preparations intended for use on lacerated or burned skin because compromised skin provides little defense against microbial contaminants.

Product Stability

Before compounding, all products must be inspected for signs of precipitates, discoloration, or other incompatibilities. Also, be sure that no product has passed its assigned expiration date. The pharmacy technician must also inspect the final sterile product after compounding for precipitates, discoloration, container integrity, and other signs of contamination.

Beyond-use dating for sterile products is outlined in USP Chapter <797>. Sterility depends on the environment in which a product was compounded and the risk of contamination. Contamination risk is increased with each manipulation of the sterile product (Table 3-7).

Low-risk products involve minimal manipulations, generally limited to the addition of not more than 2 medications to an IV bag. Medium-risk products include multiple manipulations (ie, the addition of many medications into a TPN). High risk applies to any sterile products that are prepared with a nonsterile ingredient. High-risk products must be sterilized prior to use. Table 3-8 describes the guidelines for beyond-use dating of sterile products.

It is important to note that the beyond-use date guidelines outlined in Table 3-8 are based on *sterility* of a final product. The *stability* of the final product must

TABLE 3-7. Risk Levels of Sterile Products

Sterile Product Contamination Risk Level

Low risk	• Compounded within an ISO 5 environment • Transfer and mixing of no more than 3 packaged sterile drugs • Example: drawing an antibiotic from a sterile vial and injecting into a sterile IV bag
Medium risk	• Multiple doses combined to prepare a sterile product, or it will be administered to multiple patients • Example: addition of medications into a TPN
High risk	• Uses nonsterile ingredients that are not intended for sterile routes of administration • Compounding personnel not properly garbed • Example: compounding a drug outside of an ISO 5 environment must be filtered and sterilized before use
Immediate use	• Used only for emergency and administered immediately • Example: IV drip made during a code blue

also be considered. Stability is specific to the medication or combination of medications used in the product. Stability for medications can be found in the manufacturer's package insert or in a drug reference such as *Trissel's Handbook on Injectable Drugs* or the *King Guide to Parenteral Admixtures*.

Additional Considerations

When the compounding process is complete, all materials and wasted medication must be disposed of properly. Paper products, plastic syringe caps, and vial flip tops can be disposed of in a regular waste receptacle. Needles, empty glass ampules, and vials must be disposed of in a sharps container. In the United States, sharps containers are made of heavy-duty red plastic. The red color and appropriate labeling designate that the containers may contain biohazardous waste. Sharps containers must be handled by a licensed biohazardous waste removal company. This waste is autoclaved (sanitized), ground into fine particles, and disposed of in a landfill.

TABLE 3-8. Beyond-Use Dating of Sterile Products

Compounding Location	Beyond-Use Date Guidelines	
Nonsterile environment (emergency preparations only)	Product is intended for immediate use only. No extended beyond-use date is applied.	
Sterile environment (clean room or laminar flow hood)	Low risk	Beyond-use date: Room temp = 48 hours Refrigerated = 14 days
	Medium risk	Beyond-use date: Room temp = 30 hours Refrigerated = 7 days
	High risk	Beyond-use date: Room temp = 24 hours Refrigerated = 3 days

All pharmaceutical waste should be disposed of per the hospital or pharmacy's protocols. The Environmental Protection Agency (EPA) has developed guidelines related to the proper disposal of pharmaceutical waste. Also, many states enforce more stringent pharmaceutical waste regulations. These guidelines aim to protect human health and the environment from potential hazards of waste disposal. Specific efforts are directed toward limiting the amount of pharmaceutical waste disposed of through the sewer system. Intact pharmaceuticals have the ability to leach into drinking water in potentially hazardous concentrations. EPA and state regulations dictate that pharmaceutical waste be disposed of in special waste receptacles and removed by a licensed pharmaceutical waste removal company. Pharmaceutical waste is incinerated and the ashes are disposed of in a landfill. Incineration destroys all pharmaceutical activity and limits the potential hazard of the components leach into drinking water.

Pharmaceutical waste removal programs can be costly and many hospitals struggle to designate the resources required for proper waste removal. One way to minimize pharmaceutical waste, and therefore decrease the expense of waste removal, is by using reverse distribution. Reverse distribution is a process in which unused or expired medications are returned to the manufacturer. Proper documentation is required to transfer ownership of these medications back to the manufacturer. Many manufacturers will not accept controlled medications through reverse distribution because additional Drug Enforcement Administration (DEA) documentation and licensure is required.

QUICK QUIZ 3-6

1. Which of the following should not be prepared in a horizontal laminar flow hood?
    a. Vancomycin 1-g IV piggyback
    b. Bupivacaine 0.2% epidural
    c. Docetaxel chemotherapy 80-mg IV piggyback
    d. Morphine 100-mg/mL PCA

2. Which of the following represents the smallest-diameter needle?
    a. 16 gauge
    b. 18 gauge
    c. 19 gauge
    d. 22 gauge

3. A filter must be used in which scenario?
    a. Using a 1% lidocaine ampule to prepare an injection
    b. Using a morphine 10-mg/mL multidose vial to prepare an IV push
    c. Using a potassium chloride 40-mEq/mL single-dose vial
    d. Using a morphine 10-mg/mL multidose vial to prepare an epidural

4. Which of the following is part of aseptic technique?

    a. Proper hand washing

    b. Wearing appropriate PPE

    c. Not letting anything pass between clean, filtered air and the sterile product in a laminar flow hood

    d. All of the above

5. If you are drawing 10 mL of methotrexate (a chemotherapeutic agent) out of a vial, you should first inject 10 mL of air into the vial to equalize the pressure.

    a. True

    b. False

CASE STUDY REVIEWED

You are working as a pharmacy technician in an ambulatory care pharmacy. A pharmacist hands you the prescription (see Figure 3-1) and asks you to compound the product based on the pharmacy's written protocol.

Patient: *Rebecca Watson*

Address: *1256 South Street Springfield, OH 43215* A

                DOB: *2/1/1955*

Lorazepam 1 mg / haloperidol 3 mg suppository

Sig i q6h PR PRN

Disp #120

Refills: 3　　　　　　　　　　　*J. Anderson, MD*

                      Dr. John Anderson, MD

Self-Assessment Questions
- What equipment will you use in the extemporaneous compounding of this prescription?
    - A torsion or analytical balance for weighing lorazepam, haloperidol, any inactive ingredients, and suppository base
    - A wedgewood or ceramic mortar and pestle for trituration of lorazepam and haloperidol powders
    - Suppository molds
- How many milligrams of lorazepam and haloperidol will you need?
    - This will depend on the pharmacy's compounding protocol. It is customary to prepare 10% extrasuppository mixture because some mixture can be lost in the pouring, cooling, and final handling process. If you prepare 10% extra, you are preparing 12 extrasuppositories, for a total of 132 suppositories. You will need 132 mg of lorazepam and 396 mg of haloperidol.
- What type of suppository base should be used?
- Since these suppositories are intended for rectal administration, a fatty base such as cocoa butter would be ideal. The compounding protocol should indicate this.
- What else do you need to consider during the compounding process?
    - Storage conditions (refrigerate if cocoa butter base is used), beyond-use dating (not later than the earliest expiration date of any ingredient, or 6 months, whichever is earlier), and any other patient-specific factors such as allergies, knowledge of suppository use, etc.

CHAPTER SUMMARY

- Compounding equipment should be selected based on the characteristics of the ingredients used. The smallest practical liquid measuring equipment should be used to ensure accuracy.
- Nonsterile compounding may be performed by a pharmacy technician pursuant to a standard compounding protocol written by a pharmacist.
- Nonsterile compounded product stability depends on the expiration dates of the ingredients used, the intended route of administration, and whether or not the product contains water. Sterile compounded product beyond-use dating largely depends on the number of manipulations of the product, and indication of the risk of contamination.
- Compounded product must always be labeled with an appropriate beyond-use date and documented according to pharmacy protocol.
- Allegations are a means of computing the amount of 2 specific concentrations of a product that must be mixed together to create the desired concentration of the product. Allegations can also be used to determine how much water should be added to a product to create a desired dilution.
- Aseptic technique begins with proper hand hygiene. Aseptic technique is essential in sterile compounding.
- Sterile products must be prepared in a clean room or laminar flow hood to promote sterility and limit the risk of contamination. Contaminated sterile products can be fatal to patients.
- Hazardous waste must be disposed of pursuant to EPA regulations and hospital protocols. A licensed waste removal company must dispose of hazardous waste.

ANSWERS TO QUICK QUIZZES

Quick Quiz 3-1

1. Levigation   **2.** 50 g   **3.** Suspension   **4.** Precipitant   **5.** 14 days

Quick Quiz 3-2

1. 17.1 mL of 5% solution and 12.9 mL of 12% solution

2. 300 mL of 20% solution and 200 mL of 70% solution

3. 12.5 g of 10% powder and 37.5 g of 30% powder

4. 160 g of 15% ointment and 320 g of 30% ointment

5. 15 mL of 1:100 (1%) solution and 45 mL of 4:100 (4%) solution

Quick Quiz 3-3

1. 53 drops/min

2. 19 drops/min

3. 1900

4. 8 bags

5. 1200

Quick Quiz 3-4

1. 5 mL   **2.** 0.61 mL   **3.** 16 days   **4.** 3 mL   **5.** 10 mL

Quick Quiz 3-5

1. 10 mL   **2.** 490 mL   **3.** 60 mg   **4.** 2 mL   **5.** 140 mg

Quick Quiz 3-6

1. Docetaxel chemotherapy 80-mg IV piggyback

2. 22 gauge

3. Using a 1% lidocaine ampule to prepare an injection

4. All of the above

5. False. Since methotrexate is chemotherapy, not more than 7.5 mL of air should be injected to avoid spraying or spilling.

CHAPTER QUESTIONS

1. _____ is the act of grinding particles into fine powders with the use of a mortar and pestle.
   a. Geometric dilution
   b. Trituration
   c. Solubility
   d. Spatulation

2. Levigation is the process of reducing the particle size of a powder through the addition of a (n) _____.
   a. Excipient
   b. Liquid
   c. Precipitant
   d. Solid

3. A _____ is a homogeneous mixture in which the active ingredient is not completely dissolved, but rather suspended, in liquid.
   a. Solution
   b. Solvent
   c. Solute
   d. Suspension

4. _____ medications are injected directly into the fatty layer below the skin's surface.
   a. Intramuscular
   b. Subcutaneous
   c. Intravenous
   d. Epidural

5. IV piggybacks are a small volume of medication, typically less than _____, which is infused through the same lines as a primary IV fluid.
   a. 50 mL
   b. 250 mL
   c. 500 mL
   d. 1000 mL

6. The _____ _____ is the rate at which an IV medication is infused.
   a. IV push
   b. Solubility rate
   c. Drop factor
   d. Drip rate

7. _____ graduates are best suited for viscous liquids.
   a. Conical
   b. Cylindrical
   c. Small
   d. Large

8. The volume of a liquid in a graduate should be read at the _____ of the meniscus.
   a. Top
   b. Middle
   c. Bottom
   d. Any of the above, the meniscus does not really affect the volume level

9. Which of the following preparations does not require extemporaneous compounding?
   a. Amoxicillin (400 mg/5 mL) powder for reconstitution
   b. Lorazepam 1 mg and haloperidol 3-mg suppositories
   c. Morphine 100 mg/100 mL PCA
   d. Bupivacaine 0.2% epidural

10. What is the proper procedure for cleaning a horizontal laminar flow hood?
    a. Wipe with isopropyl alcohol from back to front
    b. Wipe with isopropyl alcohol from top to bottom
    c. Wipe with soap and water from back to front
    d. Wipe with soap and water from top to bottom

11. Compounding should always take place _____ in from the front and sides of a laminar flow hood?
    a. 3
    b. 6
    c. 9
    d. 12

12. If there is 5 mg of epinephrine to be combined into 240 mg of lidocaine topical jelly, how much lidocaine topical jelly should be initially mixed with the 5 mg of epinephrine using the principle of geometric dilution?
    a. 2.5 mg
    b. 5 mg
    c. 120 mg
    d. 240 mg

Use the following information for questions 13 to 16:

You receive a prescription for losartan 12.5 mg/5 mL oral suspension, 20 mL bid, dispense a 30-day supply. Losartan oral suspension is not available commercially and must be extemporaneously compounded.

13. Where should the product be compounded?
    a. At patient's bedside
    b. Anywhere in the pharmacy
    c. In a nonsterile compounding area
    d. In a sterile compounding area

14. What is the dose of the prescription as written?
    a. 12.5 mg bid
    b. 25 mg bid
    c. 50 mg bid
    d. 250 mg bid

15. Assuming all ingredients have expiration dates beyond 1 year, what is the beyond-use date of the compounded suspension?
    a. 14 days
    b. 30 days
    c. 6 months
    d. 1 year

16. Can a 30-day supply be dispensed to the patient?
    a. Yes
    b. No
    c. Yes, only if stored in the refrigerator
    d. Yes, only if stored in the freezer

17. _____ is the process in which unused or expired medications are returned to the manufacturer.
    a. Geometric dilution
    b. Hazardous waste
    c. Reverse distribution
    d. DEA form 222

18. What is the beyond-use date of product prepared at a patient's bedside in an emergent situation?
    a. Immediate use only
    b. 48 hours
    c. 30 hours
    d. 24 hours

19. What is the room temperature of beyond-use date of a TPN prepared in a horizontal laminar flow hood?
    a. 24 hours
    b. 30 hours
    c. 36 hours
    d. 48 hours

20. You finish compounding a TPN and notice that there are white, solid formations floating in the solution. What does this mean?
    a. A precipitant has formed in the solution, and the bag should not be dispensed.
    b. A precipitant has formed in the solution, but it will dissolve over time and the bag is okay to dispense.
    c. The TPN is actually a suspension, so it is okay to dispense.
    d. A nonsterile ingredient was used in the TPN and it is okay to dispense.

21. Ophthalmic preparations should be compounded in a _____ environment.
    a. Nonsterile
    b. Nontoxic
    c. Sterile
    d. Quiet

22. In which of the follow scenarios should a filter be used?
    a. Preparation of an IV push with a lidocaine ampule
    b. Preparation of an IV push with a lidocaine vial
    c. Preparation of an epidural with a lidocaine vial
    d. Preparation of an epidural with a morphine vial

23. Special PPE must be worn while compounding chemotherapy due to the potential hazards of the medications.
    a. True
    b. False

24. Which of the following is not a typical component in a TPN?
    a. Amino acids
    b. Dextrose
    c. Lipids
    d. Acetic acid

25. Which of the following products should not be prepared using a multidose vial of morphine?
    a. IV push
    b. IV piggyback
    c. PCA
    d. Epidural

26. Which of the following steps is not part of infection control in sterile compounding?
    a. Remove all personal outer garments
    b. Take off shoes
    c. Remove all cosmetics
    d. Put on hair cover

27. What is the purpose of aseptic technique?
    a. To limit dosing errors
    b. To limit the amount of rework necessary
    c. To limit the risk of microbial contamination
    d. To limit the risk of precipitation

28. Why are vertical flow hoods used to compound chemotherapy medications?
    a. Because the downward flow of air protects the user from exposure to the potentially hazardous medication
    b. Because chemotherapy medications are more expensive and need to be better contained
    c. Because the outward flow of air protects the user from exposure to the potentially hazardous medication
    d. Because chemotherapy medications are at risk for drug shortages and need to be better contained

29. Appropriate hand washing means washing for at least _____ seconds with antimicrobial soap and water.
    a. 15
    b. 30
    c. 60
    d. 120

30. USP Chapter _____ defines guidelines for nonsterile compounding.
    a. <795>
    b. <797>
    c. <979>
    d. <959>

31. _____ is the rapid administration of a small volume of medication into the vein.
    a. IV piggyback
    b. IV push
    c. Epidural
    d. Subcutaneous injection

Use the following information to answer questions 32 to 36:

Doxycycline is available as a powder for reconstitution. After reconstitution, the concentration is 25 mg/5 mL and the total volume is 60 mL. The volume of the powder occupies 12.4 mL. The pediatric dose of doxycycline is 2.2 mg/kg.

32. What volume of water should be added to achieve the appropriate final concentration?
    a. 12.4 mL
    b. 37.6 mL
    c. 47.6 mL
    d. 60 mL

33. A physician orders 100 mg bid × 7 days for an adult. How many teaspoons will be given for each dose?
    a. 2
    b. 3
    c. 4
    d. 5

34. Will the 60-mL bottle last the entire treatment course?
    a. Yes
    b. No

35. What is the dose of doxycycline for a 15-lb patient?
    a. 5 mg
    b. 15 mg
    c. 31.3 mg
    d. 72.6 mg

36. What is the volume of the dose of doxycycline for a 15-lb patient?
    a. 3 mL
    b. 5 mL
    c. 12 mL
    d. 15 mL

37. What is the abbreviation for dextrose 10% in water?
    a. 10DW
    b. D10W
    c. DW10
    d. Dex10

38. The drip rate of Vaprisol infusion is 4.2 mL/h. If the concentration of the infusion is 20 mg/100 mL, how much Vaprisol will be infused in a 12-hour infusion?
    a. 10 mg
    b. 12 mg
    c. 14 mg
    d. 16 mg

39. The drip rate of diltiazem is 0.25 mL/min. The standard diltiazem concentration is 1 mg/mL. How many milligrams of diltiazem will be infused in a 6-hour period?
    a. 15 mg
    b. 60 mg
    c. 90 mg
    d. 120 mg

40. What is the term for the process in which ingredients are mixed together in equal proportions to ensure a homogeneous final product?
    a. Spatulation
    b. Levigation
    c. Sterile compounding
    d. Geometric dilution

41. What is another term for TPN?
    a. Hypercalcemia
    b. Hypomagnesemia
    c. Hyperalimentation
    d. Sustaination

42. Which of the following products can be compounded in a nonsterile environment?
    a. Rectal suppository
    b. TPN
    c. Epidural
    d. Ophthalmic solution

43. Beakers are _____ accurate in measuring volume than graduated cylinders.
    a. More
    b. Less
    c. Equally as
    d. None of the above

44. Which of the following must be shaken well before use?
    a. Solution
    b. Solvent
    c. IV piggyback
    d. Suspension

45. Assuming all ingredients have a 6-month or longer expiration dates, what is the beyond-use date of an extemporaneously compounded topical ointment?
    a. 14 days
    b. 30 days
    c. 60 days
    d. 6 months

46. What is the primary benefit of a vertical laminar flow hood versus a horizontal laminar flow hood?
    a. The air is more sterile
    b. They are easier to use
    c. They are larger
    d. The vertical flow of air protects the user from exposure to hazardous chemicals
    e. Never inject any air into the vial first

47. Which of the following should not be used in compounding a neonatal product?
    a. Morphine multidose vial
    b. Morphine single-dose vial
    c. Fentanyl ampule
    d. Fentanyl single-dose vial

48. Which of the following items must be disposed of in a sharps container?
    a. Needles
    b. Ampules
    c. Broken glass vials
    d. All of the above

49. Why is pharmaceutical waste regulated by the EPA?
    a. Because intact pharmaceuticals can leach into drinking water and cause toxicity
    b. To control for diversion
    c. Because landfills are too full
    d. Pharmaceutical waste is not regulated

50. In which location should you put on PPE?
    a. Anteroom or designated gowning area
    b. Clean room
    c. Outside the pharmacy
    d. Anywhere, as long as it's prior to compounding

Medication Safety

CHAPTER
4

PTCB KNOWLEDGE AREAS

4.1 Error prevention strategies for data entry (eg, prescription or medication order to correct patient)

4.2 Patient package insert (PPI) and medication guide requirements (eg, special directions and precautions)

4.3 Identification of issues that require pharmacist's intervention (eg, drug utilization review [DUR], adverse effect [ADE], over-the-counter [OTC] recommendation, therapeutic substitution, misuse, missed dose)

4.4 Look-alike-sound-alike medications

4.5 High-alert or risk medications

4.6 Common safety strategies (eg, tall-man lettering, separating inventory, leading and trailing zeros, limit use of error-prone abbreviations)

KEY TERMS

Apothecary: Historical system of measurement

Competency: The quality of being able to perform

Computerized physician order entry (CPOE): Electronic entry of physician orders

Illegible: Unreadable

Interdisciplinary: Involves 2 or more disciplines (ie, physicians, nurses, and pharmacists)

Narrow therapeutic range: Small difference between therapeutic and toxic effects

Near miss: Unplanned event that did not result in injury, illness, or death, but had the potential to do so

Nomenclature: List of names or terms

Nonpunitive: Not involving the infliction of punishment

Order sets: Predefined groupings of standard orders for a condition, disease, or procedure

Patient identifiers: A unique characteristic of the patient that allows a health care provider to identify them (ie, name, birthday, social security number, etc)

Protocol: Plan for the course of treatment

CASE STUDY

You are working in a retail pharmacy store that you have never worked at before, covering a shift as requested by your district manager. The pharmacy phone is ringing as a new patient, Kim Thomas, brings in 3 new prescriptions. She is talking on her cell phone and appears to be rushed. The patient does not have her prescription insurance card with her and would like you to call the local competitor to obtain the information. She also informs you that she takes 2 other medications, "one blue pill, and one little white pill." When you ask her if she knows what the prescriptions are for, she shakes her head, no (Figure 4-1).

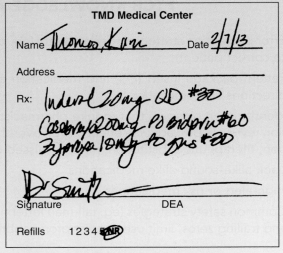

FIGURE 4-1 Patient's prescription.

As you work through this chapter, keep the above case study in mind. After completing this chapter you should be able to answer the following self-assessment questions.

Self-Assessment Questions
- What are the distractions occurring in the pharmacy?
- What elements of the prescriptions could potentially lead to an error?
- Are there any safety strategies that the pharmacy can utilize to help prevent errors with these prescriptions?

INTRODUCTION

In 2006, Emily Jerry began her last chemotherapy treatment. She had just turned 2 years old. Unfortunately, her chemotherapy had been prepared with 23.4% concentrated sodium chloride instead of 0.9% sodium chloride, a concentration error which would be fatal for an adult or a child. This chemotherapy was prepared by a pharmacy technician and double checked by a pharmacist. Emily Jerry died as a result of an avoidable medication error. As a result of this and other serious and fatal errors, laws, regulations, and safety efforts have been put in place to help identify and prevent system or process breakdowns which can lead to medication errors and negative patient outcomes. This chapter discusses the critical responsibility of medication safety required of all personnel working in the practice of pharmacy.

Ohio Case Spurs Legislation

Prior to the Emily Jerry case, Ohio had no laws regulating the testing or training of pharmacy technicians. After Emily's death in 2006, Senate Bill 203 was introduced in Ohio's General Assembly in July 2007. It was signed into law in 2009 by Ohio Governor Ted Strickland, known as "Emily's Law." The law establishes standards for qualified pharmacy technicians and requires them to undergo criminal background checks, pass a competency test, and it establishes penalties for activities (i.e. compounding, packaging, and preparing a drug) performed by an individual who is not a pharmacist, pharmacy intern, or qualified pharmacy technician. Emily's Law sets a standard for national pharmacy technician legislation.

MEDICATION ERRORS

What is the definition of a medication error? According to the National Coordinating Council for Medication Error Reporting and Prevention, a medication error is defined as below:

> "Any preventable event that may cause or lead to inappropriate medication use or patient harm while the medication is in the control of the health care professional, patient, or consumer. Such events may be related to professional practice, health care products, procedures, and systems, including prescribing; order communication; product labeling, packaging, **nomenclature;** compounding; dispensing; distribution; administration; education; monitoring; and use."

Medication errors result in significant patient harm and economic cost to both the health care system and the nation. In 1999, the Institute of Medicine (IOM) published the "To Err Is Human" report, which brought national attention to the problem of adverse events in health care. The report estimated that adverse events were causing up to 98,000 patient deaths per year. Medication errors are the cause of 1 out of every 131 outpatient deaths and 1 out of every 854 inpatients deaths. This number is probably underestimated due to the lack of poor documentation and reporting systems currently in place. The total costs of adverse events in the United States are estimated to be between $37.6 and $50 billion, when accounting for lost income, lost household production, disability, and health care costs.

There are many points at which a medication error can occur. Inattention to detail, staffing shortages, similar patient names, and similar medication names all contribute to medication errors. Even though pharmacists are ultimately responsible for all dispensed prescriptions, pharmacy technicians are an essential member of the patient safety team.

* TECH ALERT: Using the IOM estimate, a retail pharmacy that fills about 2,000 prescriptions per week may generate up to 2 clinically significant prescription errors per week.

MEDICATION USE PROCESS

Medication use is a complex, multistep process that involves multiple individuals at various locations. Every step in the medication use process has the potential for error and the risk for patient harm. Pharmacy technicians need to understand the medication use process and error prevention strategies.

* TECH ALERT: When taking a prescription for a child, obtain the patient's weight. The need for calculation of doses based on age and weight is especially important in pediatric patients.

MEDICATION USE PROCESS AND ERROR PREVENTION STRATEGIES

Patient Information

In order to choose the appropriate medication for a patient, health care professionals must know specific information about the patient. It is important for members of the pharmacy team to know basic demographic and clinical information (ie, age, weight, height, allergies, diagnoses, pregnancy status).

The patient's identity should be confirmed by checking 2 **patient identifiers** such as name, date of birth, phone number, or other patient identifiers. Stay alert for situations prone to patient mix-ups, such as between patients with the same name (ie, Tom Smith), family members with similar names (ie, John and Jack Black), or in patients whose last and first names can be easily inverted (ie, Carol Thomas and Thomas Carol).

In the inpatient setting, many health systems utilize bar coding technology on patient's wristbands and medications to ensure the appropriate medication is matched to the correct patient. A barcode scan helps provide the final check prior to medication administration. In the outpatient setting, standardized procedures help prevent errors at drop off and pick up, such as verifying a patient's first and last names and date of birth.

* TECH ALERT: When asking for patient identifiers, avoid asking questions that can be answered with a yes or no (ie, "Is your date of birth January 25th, 1976?"). Instead, ask the patient "What is your date of birth?"

PREVENTION STRATEGIES

- Verify height, weight, age, and pregnancy status of the patient.
- Obtain complete medication and allergy history from patient, including prescription and nonprescription medications prior to dispensing medications.
- If possible, acquire medication indication from patient.

Drug Information

To minimize the risk of error, accurate drug information (ie, drug references, protocols, and computer drug information systems) should be readily available to pharmacy personnel.

PREVENTION STRATEGIES

- Maintain up-to-date drug information resources.

Communication of Drug Information

Miscommunication between physician, nurses, pharmacists, and pharmacy technicians is a common cause of medication errors. Communication errors can occur in many different ways. It is always important to standardize methods of communication (ie, avoid handwriting errors, improper placement of decimal points or zeroes, improper use of abbreviations) in which drug information can be misinterpreted.

Handwriting

Unfortunately, illegible handwriting is commonplace in the health care field. With many medications being look-alike drugs, it is easy to understand how errors can occur. Preprinted orders, **order sets** and CPOE help minimize the errors from illegible handwriting.

PREVENTION STRATEGIES

- Evaluate entire order. The dose and route may help clarify the ordered medication.
- Clarify questionable orders with prescriber.
- Utilize order sets and CPOE.

Decimal Points and Zeros
Misplacing a decimal point by one point can result in errors of 10- to 100-fold greater or less than the intended dose. For drugs with **narrow therapeutic ranges,** which have a small range between therapeutic and toxic effects, (ie, warfarin, insulin) the results can be fatal. Failure to write a leading zero in front of a number less than 1 (ie, .1 mg instead of 0.1 mg) might be read as a whole number (1 mg). Writing trailing zeros can also be confusing and lead to an overdose (ie, 10.0 mg instead of 10 mg may be interpreted as 100 mg). Pharmacy technicians should be aware of the potential for decimal point errors and alert the pharmacist of questionable orders.

PREVENTION STRATEGIES

- Always use leading zeros when writing numbers less than one.
- Do not use trailing zeros.

Abbreviations
Drug names and medical terminology are frequently abbreviated which can lead to medication errors. There are many accepted abbreviations in health care. The Joint Commission (TJC) requires that institutions maintain an approved list of acceptable abbreviations and terms (Table 4-1). Creating new abbreviations or using "text" formatting is inappropriate.

TABLE 4-1. The Joint Commission's "Do Not Use" Abbreviation List

Do Not Use	Potential Problem	Use Instead
U, u (unit)	Mistaken for "0" (zero), the number "4" (four), or "cc"	Write "unit"
IU (international unit)	Mistaken for IV (intravenous) or the number "10" (ten)	Write "international unit"
Q.D., QD, q.d., qd (daily)	Mistaken for each other	Write "daily"
Q.O.D., QOD, q.o.d., qod (every other day)	Period after the Q mistaken for "I" and the "O" mistaken for "I"	Write "every other day"
Trailing zero (X.0 mg)	Decimal point is missed	Write "X mg"
Lack of leading zero (.X mg)		Write "0.X mg"
MS	Can mean morphine sulfate or magnesium sulfate	Write "morphine sulfate"
MSO_4 and $MgSO_4$	Confused for one another	Write "magnesium sulfate"

ISMP's complete list of error-prone abbreviations is available at http://www.ismp.org/tools/errorproneabbreviations.pdf.

PREVENTION STRATEGIES

- Avoid abbreviations on TJC's "Do Not Use" and the ISMP's "Error-Prone" lists.
- Do not use nonstandard abbreviations.
- Write out ambiguous abbreviations.
- The complete drug name, preferably the generic should be utilized.

TECH ALERT: The Joint Commission (TJC) is the organization that accredits health care organizations (i.e hospitals, nursing homes, etc).

Metric and Apothecary Systems

The metric system is the standard system of measurement used for prescriptions and orders. The apothecary system was used in the early practice of pharmacy and is now considered archaic. When a prescriber utilizes the apothecary system (ie, 1/200 grain = 0.3 mg), errors are common; therefore, the use of the apothecary system should be avoided.

PREVENTION STRATEGIES

- Double check calculations to confirm accuracy.
- Remind prescribers of the potential errors caused by utilizing the apothecary system.

Verbal Orders

Verbal orders can be a source of medications errors. Poor telephone connection, similar-sounding medications, language barriers, and unknown terminology can lead to medication errors from verbal orders. Verbal orders should be reserved for circumstances that make it impossible to write the order or submit it electronically. Most states limit the ability to accept a verbal order to pharmacists or pharmacy interns. The role of the pharmacy technician in transcribing verbal orders varies by state.

TECH ALERT: When documenting "read back telephone order," the abbreviation RBTO may be utilized.

PREVENTION STRATEGIES

- Read back order to prescriber to ensure clarity of order.
- Request prescriber to spell medication when there is difficulty understanding.
- Avoid the use of verbal orders for high risk medications (i.e. Chemotherapy agents).

Calculation Errors

There are many reports of medication errors, some fatal, that were caused by mathematical miscalculations. Calculation errors are made by prescribers, pharmacists, pharmacy technicians, nurses, and other allied health professionals. Calculation errors made by health care professionals occur frequently even with the use of calculators. Pediatric patients are at a higher risk since many medications are not available in a pediatric formulation, so an adult formulation must be diluted to obtain the appropriate dose. Health care professionals with many years of experience are just as likely to make these errors as inexperienced professionals. Calculation errors are often made by using the wrong concentration of stock solutions, misplacing a decimal point, or using a wrong conversion factor.

PREVENTION STRATEGIES

- Double check own work.
- Do not rely on memory for conversions.
- Ask "Does the answer seem reasonable?"
- Utilize a 2-person independent check of calculation prior to product preparation.

Drug Labeling, Packaging, and Nomenclature

Drug names that look alike or sound alike and products that visually look alike contribute to medication errors. When filling a prescription, it is important that a technician selects the correct medication prescribed.

Look-Alike-Sound-Alike Drugs
According to the ISMP, name mix-ups are the cause of more than one-third of medication errors (Table 4-2). Medications with similar names can also have similar indications and strengths. It is easy to understand how mix-up errors can occur, but these must be avoided to prevent medication errors.

* TECH ALERT: The ISMP is the nation's only nonprofit organization devoted entirely to medication error prevention and safe medication use.

TABLE 4-2. List of Commonly Used Confused Drug Names	
Drug Name	Confused Drug Name
Actonel	Actos
Adderall	Inderal
Avandia	Prandin, Coumadin
Bupropion	Buspirone
Celebrex	Celexa, Cerebyx
Celexa	Zyprexa, Celebrex, Cerebyx
Clonidine	Clozapine, Klonopin
Depo-Medrol	Solu-Medrol
Ephedrine	Epinephrine
Fentanyl	Sufentanil
Glipizide	Glyburide
Humulin	Humalog, Novolin
Hydromorphone	Morphine
Kapidex	Casodex, Kadian
Lamictal	Lamisil
Lasix	Luvox
Methadone	Metadate CD, Metadate ER
Metformin	Metronidazole
Nifedipine	Nicardipine, nimodipine
Prednisolone	Prednisone
Seroquel	Seroquel XR, Sinequan, Serzone
Tegretol	Tegretol XR, Trental
Topamax	Toprol XL, Topiramate, Tobradex
Zyprexa	Zestril, Zyrtec, Zelapar

ISMP's complete list of confused drug names is available at http://www.ismp.org/tools/confuseddrugnames.pdf.

TABLE 4-3. Suggested Tall-Man Letter Examples	
Drug Name With Tall-Man Letters	*Confused With*
bu**PROP**ion	bus**PIR**one
DAUNOrubicin	**DOXO**rubicin
DOBUTamine	**DOP**amine
Glipi**ZIDE**	gly**BURIDE**
hydr**ALAZINE**	hydroxyzine
ni**CAR**dipine	**NIFE**dipine
predniso**LONE**	predni**SONE**
ISMP's complete list of drugs with tall-man letters is available at http://www.ismp.org/tools/tallmanletters.pdf.	

Tall-man letters (mixed upper and lower case) can help distinguish look-alike drug names, potentially decreasing errors (Table 4-3). Many organizations dedicated to medication safety support the use of tall-man letters to reduce the confusion between similar drug names.

Look-Alike Packaging

Look-alike packaging also presents the possibility of potential medication errors. Many medications are packaged in bottles with similar size, colors, and labeling leading to confusion. Often pharmacy staff chooses a product based on memory of what a product looked like instead of what a product actually said. Physically separating inventory that has look-alike packaging can decrease medication errors.

High-Alert Medications

High-alert medications have an increased risk of causing significant patient harm when they are used in error (Table 4-4). Although mistakes may or may not be more common with these drugs, the consequences of an error are more devastating to patients.

PREVENTION STRATEGIES

- Review ISMP look-alike-sound-alike drug list to keep alert of potential errors.
- Alert Food and Drug Administration (FDA) of potentially dangerous mix-ups.
- Highlight medications that have similar names by using "tall-man" lettering.

TABLE 4-4. High-Alert Medication Examples	
Antiretroviral agents	Chemotherapeutic agents
Hypoglycemic agents	Immunosuppressant agents
Insulin	Opioids
Pediatric liquid agents	Pregnancy category X drugs
Anticoagulants	Concentrated electrolytes
ISMP's complete list of drugs with high-alert medications is available at http://www.ismp.org/Tools/highAlertMedicationLists.asp.	

- Use shelf dividers or separate inventory that with look-alike names or packaging in all storage areas, refrigerators, and narcotic shelves.
- Utilize ISMP tall-man lettering where recommended.
- Report hazardous labels to ISMP.

Drug Storage, Stock, Standardization, and Distribution

Medications prescribed to patients should be stored in a safe and secure manner. Medications and other supplies should be stored, dispensed, and returned to stock in a manner that decreases the incidence of a medication error.

Drug storage areas should be clean, organized, and of adequate size to avoid clutter. Refrigerators should only be used to store medications, and not for employee's personal use. There have been reported errors of accidental ingestion of medications when food and medications were stored together.

A standardized system for organization of medications is recommended, including a simple A to Z by brand or generic name without regard to dosage form. Shelf dividers should be utilized for medications that could lead to mix-up errors and reminder cards can be used for medication that must be refrigerated, mixed before dispensing, or have other special dispensing instructions.

Prevention Strategies

- Utilize a standardized practice to store medications.
- Utilize a form of notification which reminds staff of any special instructions upon dispensing.

Drug Device Acquisition, Use, and Monitoring

The potential for human error can be decreased through careful maintenance, use, and standardization of devices used to prepare and deliver medications. Patients often have to use a device (ie, oral or insulin syringe, inhaler) to administer a medication, and many times, require education on the use of the device prior to leaving the pharmacy.

Prevention Strategies

- Offer counseling from a pharmacist to a patient who utilizes a special device for medication use.

Environmental Factors, Workflow, and Staffing Patterns

Environmental factors such as poor lighting, cluttered work space, noise, interruptions, and nonstop pharmacy activity all contribute to pharmacy errors. Inefficiencies in workflow can also increase medication errors, including reduced staffing levels leading to increased workload.

Prevention Strategies

- Provide adequate lighting and space for work area.
- Arrange for work areas that are free from distractions when processing medications.

* TECH ALERT: Liquid prescriptions should be dispensed with a syringe or dosing spoon that closely matches the dose. A household teaspoon can hold anywhere from 3 to 7 mL.

- Allow for adequate staffing to cover meals and breaks.
- Evaluate workflow to ensure efficient and safe plan.

Staff Competency and Education

Staff education is an important error prevention strategy. Pharmacy staff education topics should include the following:

- New medications
- High-alert medications
- Protocols, policies, procedures
- Recent medication errors and the prevention strategies
- Competencies in specific skill sets

PREVENTION STRATEGIES

- Establish a quality assurance program which evaluates staff competencies for designated skills at least once a year.
- Take advantage of all educational opportunities to learn more about pharmacy and medication safety trends.

Patient Education

Patients can play a vital role in the prevention of medication errors. They should be offered counseling by a pharmacist when prescriptions are picked up and encouraged to ask questions about these prescriptions. Patients should be active members of their care, but it is an essential task of the pharmacist to educate on the importance of compliance and proper medication use.

PREVENTION STRATEGIES

- Technicians should encourage all patients to talk to the pharmacist about medication.
- Patients should be encouraged to read the PPI (discussed in the Drug Information for Patients section later in this chapter).
- Encourage patients to keep an active, written record of each prescription and nonprescription medications.

Quality Processes and Risk Management

In order to prevent errors, it is best to analyze the systems, processes, and behaviors that lead to the error, rather than focus on blame or punitive action after an error has occurred. A **nonpunitive** approach should be used and supported by management for medication error reduction. Pharmacy staff should be encouraged to report errors and "**near misses.**" A near miss is an unplanned event that did not result in injury, illness, or death, but had the potential to do so.

Interdisciplinary teams should conduct investigations after errors have been reported, to avoid the potential for the same error occurring again. Teams can utilize multiple medication safety resources (Table 4-5).

TABLE 4-5. **Medication Safety Resources**	
US Food and Drug Administration	www.fda.gov
Agency for Healthcare Research and Quality	www.ahrq.gov
Centers for Disease Control and Prevention	www.cdc.gov
Department of Veterans Affairs National Center for Patient Safety	www.patientsafety.gov
Institute for Safe Medication Practices	www.ismp.org
National Patient Safety Foundation	www.npsf.org
National Coordinating Council for Medication Error Reporting and Prevention	www.nccpmerp.org

PREVENTION STRATEGIES

- Information should be distributed throughout the organization to help prevent errors and investigate patterns.
- Encourage staff to report errors and "near misses."

Pharmacist Intervention

When processing prescriptions, pharmacist intervention will often be necessary. A pharmacy technician cannot make a clinical decision regarding drug therapy, but should alert a pharmacist regarding therapeutic interchange, drug utilization review, medication misuse, missed doses, or OTC recommendations.

Therapeutic Interchange

Therapeutic interchange (substitutions) between AB-rated medications (brand-generic) is common in order to contain drug costs. This activity can be performed in a pharmacy without a physician's approval. However, if a physician states that generic substitution is not permitted by writing "Brand Necessary," "Dispense as Written," "Medically Necessary," or other state-approved wording on the prescription a generic substitution may not be dispensed.

Additionally, therapeutic substitution between products from the same class of drug, even though they are not therapeutically equivalent (ie, Protonix for Prevacid), may be permitted in some states. States that allow therapeutic interchange do so only based on an approved **protocol**. Many hospital formularies allow for automatic therapeutic substitution without physician's authorization based on approval from the **Pharmacy and Therapeutics (P&T) Committee.** Additionally, in the retail setting prescription, insurance companies may require a therapeutic substitution. In this situation the pharmacist must be alerted to contact the prescriber and discuss a change in therapy covered by the patient's insurance provider.

Drug Utilization Review

The Omnibus Budget Reconciliation Act of 1990 (OBRA' 90) required pharmacies to perform a prospective drug utilization review on all prescriptions.

Computer programs are also used to assist the pharmacist in identifying potential drug utilization problems. However, it is up to the pharmacist's professional

* TECH ALERT: The P&T Committee actively manages the formulary system for the hospital, institution, or insurance company.

* TECH ALERT: OBRA '90 also mandates the offer to have a pharmacist counsel patients about their prescriptions and the documentation of all interventions. The technician should ask the patient "What questions do you have for the pharmacist?" This encourages the patient to think about their medication concerns.

judgment to decide the course of action to resolve the problem. A pharmacy technician should **always** notify a pharmacist to an alert during prospective drug utilization. The following are areas for drug therapy problems that the pharmacist must screen:

- Therapeutic duplication
- Drug-disease contraindications
- Drug-drug interactions
- Incorrect drug dosage
- Incorrect duration of treatment
- Drug-allergy interactions
- Clinical abuse or misuse of medication

Misuse

During prospective drug utilization review, sometimes an alert may be seen for medication misuse. The patient could be filling the medication too early, at multiple pharmacies, or from multiple prescribers. The pharmacist should be notified if there is a concern for medication misuse.

Missed Refill

The pharmacist should also be notified when patients are late for refilling maintenance medications that should be taken everyday (ie, hypertension, diabetes, etc). Pharmacists can then counsel patients about the importance of compliance and help identify any barriers that may be preventing the patient from taking the medication as prescribed.

OTC Recommendation

Patients will commonly ask questions regarding OTC medications. Pharmacy technicians cannot answer these questions within the scope of their practice. For example, a pharmacy technician may think that it is okay to recommend to Mrs. Smith to take ibuprofen for her arthritis but does not know that she has a gastric ulcer. Taking ibuprofen with a gastric ulcer could predispose the patient to excessive bleeding. Participation in drug selection and counseling of patients are 2 activities that **must** be performed by pharmacists, or pharmacy interns under the supervision of a pharmacist. Remember that a pharmacist is legally responsible for the pharmacy technician's actions. Alert the pharmacist if a patient is requesting advice regarding an OTC product.

Drug Information for Patients

When providing drug information to patients, it should contain information that is useful and written in a way that is easy to understand. The criteria for useful information have been determined by the FDA (Table 4-6).

Patient Package Inserts

Patient package inserts (PPIs) must be provided for oral contraceptives containing estrogen or progesterone. Required PPIs must be provided for each new prescription and all refill prescriptions. Manufacturers must provide the pharmacy with PPIs

* TECH ALERT: Patient information should be written at a sixth-grade reading level. Always assume that a patient knows nothing about their medication or how to take it.

TABLE 4-6. **Criteria for Useful Patient Oriented Drug Information**
1. Drug names, indications for use, and how to monitor for improvement
2. Contraindications
3. Specific directions about how to use and store the medicine, and overdose information
4. Specific precautions and warnings about the medicine
5. Symptoms of serious or frequent possible adverse reactions and what to do
6. Certain general information, including encouraging patients to communicate with health professionals, and disclaimer statements
7. Information that is scientifically accurate, unbiased in tone and content, and up to date
8. Information in an understandable and legible format that is readily comprehensible to consumers

to give the patient. As a technician, if you are unsure if a PPI should be given to a patient, consult with your pharmacist.

Medication Guide

There are over 240 medications that require guides to be distributed to patients (Table 4-7). Medication guides are paper handouts that are required to be issued with certain prescribed drugs. The FDA determines a medication guide to be distributed when the following is true:

* Certain drug information is necessary for the patient to know to prevent serious adverse effects.
* A patient should be informed about a known serious side effect.
* Patient adherence to directions for the use of a product is essential to its effectiveness.

* TECH ALERT: If a pharmacy does not provide a PPI with an oral contraceptive, the product is considered misbranded and the pharmacy in violation of a federal law.

TABLE 4-7. **Examples of Prescriptions That Require Medication Guides**		
Abilify	Klonopin	Seroquel
Adderall XR	Morphine	Strattera
Ambien	Opana ER	Suboxone
Celexa	Oxycontin	Tegretol
Coumadin	Paxil	Testosterone Gel
Effexor	Plavix	Thalomid
Fosamax	Pradaxa	Topamax
Janumet	Ritalin	Zyprexa
For a complete list visit http://www.fda.gov/Drugs/DrugSafety/ucm085729.htm		

QUICK QUIZ 4-1

1.

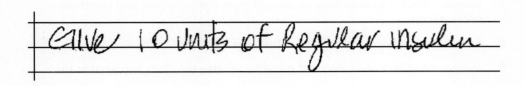

Give 10 units of Regular insulin

Interpret this order. _____

What is the appropriate way to write the order? _____

2.

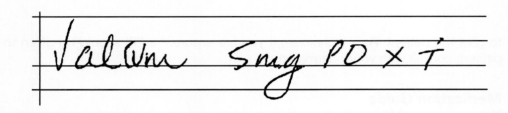

Valium 5mg PO × ī

Interpret this order. _____

What is the appropriate way to write the order? _____

3.

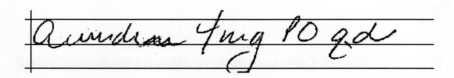

Quinidine 4mg PO qd

What 2 drugs could this order potentially be written for? _____

4. List 2 abbreviations that should be avoided and the suggested term/s to use instead.

_____

_____

5. List 3 examples of commonly confused drug names.

_____

_____

_____

~~~~~~

CASE STUDY REVIEWED

You are working in a store that you have never worked at before, covering a shift as requested by your district manager. The phone is ringing as a new customer Kim Thomas brings in 3 new prescriptions. She is talking on her cell phone and appears to be rushed. She does not have her prescription card and would like you to call the local competitor to obtain the information. She knows she takes some medications, "one blue pill, and one little white pill." When you ask her if she knows what the prescriptions are for, she shakes her head, no (see Figure 4-1).

Self-Assessment Questions
- What are the distractions occurring in the pharmacy for the technician?
  - New work environment
  - Ringing of phone
  - Patient on cell phone, rushed
  - Patient unsure of information
- What elements of the prescriptions could potentially lead to an error?
  - First and last names interchangeable
  - Illegible handwriting
  - Look-alike-sound-alike medications
  - Banned abbreviations
- Are there any safety strategies that the pharmacy can utilize to help prevent errors with these prescriptions?
  - Tall-man lettering
  - Shelf dividers
  - Staff education

CHAPTER SUMMARY

- Medication errors are a leading cause of preventable death in the United States.
- Errors can occur in any step of a complex medication use process.
- Pharmacy technicians can help prevent medication errors by following a systematic approach to practice, staying focused, double checking their work, and seeking help if needed.
- Alerting pharmacists to concerns that need potential intervention is an important part of a pharmacy technician's duty.
- There are a multitude of safety strategies that can be utilized by all pharmacy personnel to decrease medication errors.

ANSWERS TO QUICK QUIZ

Quick Quiz 4-1

1. Give 1 unit of regular insulin
2. Valium 0.5 mg PO × 1 dose
3. Avandia, Coumadin
4. Answers will vary (see Table 4-1)
5. Answers will vary (see Table 4-2)

CHAPTER QUESTIONS

1. Which of the following numbers could lead to a medication error due to a decimal point error?
   a. 1.5
   b. 0.5
   c. 3.4
   d. 6.0

2. Which of the following strategies can help decrease handwriting errors?
   a. Verbal orders
   b. CPOE
   c. Tall-man letters
   d. Bar code

3. Which of the following abbreviations is on The Joint Commission's (TJC's) "Do Not Use" list?
   a. IU
   b. IV
   c. IM
   d. IO

4. Which of the following abbreviations is on The Joint Commission's "Do Not Use" list?
   a. qid
   b. bid
   c. qod
   d. tid

5. What health care professional is ultimately responsible for all dispensed prescriptions?
   a. Physician
   b. Pharmacy technician
   c. Dispensing pharmacist
   d. Pharmacist manager

6. What clinical information should be obtained on a pediatric patient to help prevent medication errors?
   a. Date of birth
   b. Weight
   c. Height
   d. All of the above

15/50   35/50 = 70

7. A pregnant patient presents a prescription for Accutane to the pharmacy technician. What should the technician do?
   a. Alert the pharmacist that the patient is pregnant and filling a category X medication
   b. Contact the physician to discuss the patient's pregnancy status
   c. Return the patient's prescription without filling
   d. Fill the prescription without notifying the pharmacist

8. Which of the following are high-alert medications?
   a. Insulin, heparin
   b. Insulin, citalopram
   c. Heparin, citalopram
   d. Morphine, pantoprazole

9. Which of the following should not be used during prescribing in order to minimize errors?
   a. mg
   b. grain
   c. mL
   d. gm

10. What can contribute to a medication error during a verbal order?
    a. Poor cell phone connection
    b. Accent
    c. Similar-sounding medications
    d. All of the above

11. Which of the following strategies can be utilized during verbal orders to help minimize medication errors?
    a. Read back the order to the prescriber
    b. Guess at the prescriber's order
    c. Multitask during verbal orders
    d. All of the above

12. Which of the following patients are at the highest risk of a calculation error?
    a. A 7 week old
    b. A 14 year old
    c. A 28 year old
    d. A 56 year old

13. Which of the following prevention strategies can be used to help prevent look-alike-sound-alike errors?
    a. Computerized physician order entry
    b. Tall-man lettering
    c. Shelf dividers
    d. Adequate lighting

14. Which of the following organizations is devoted entirely to medication error prevention?
    a. Institute for Safe Medication Practices
    b. National Patient Safety Foundation
    c. The Joint Commission
    d. The American Heart Association

15. The use of shelf dividers can help prevent which of the following type of error?
    a. Calculation error
    b. Decimal point error
    c. Look-alike packaging error
    d. High-alert medication error

16. Which of the following is a high-alert medication?
    a. Insulin
    b. Heparin
    c. Morphine
    d. All of the above

17. Why are high-alert medications more dangerous than other medication categories?
    a. Commonly prescribed
    b. Uncommonly prescribed
    c. High cost
    d. Devastating adverse effects

18. Which of the following systems helps decrease medication errors when stocking medications?
    a. Sorting medications by brand name A to Z
    b. Sorting medications by generic name A to Z
    c. Sorting medications by dosage form A to Z
    d. Sorting medications by fast movers

19. Which of the following should be dispensed with a prescription for amoxicillin of 250 mg/5 mL—give 500 mg PO bid × 10 days?
    a. 2.5 mL syringe
    b. 5 mL dosing spoon
    c. 5 mL syringe
    d. 10 mL dosing spoon

20. Which of the following pharmacy personnel can counsel a patient on how to use a medication device?
    a. Cashier
    b. Pharmacy technician
    c. Certified pharmacy technician
    d. Pharmacist

21. Which of the following contributes to medication errors?
    a. Poor lighting
    b. Cluttered work space
    c. Loud noise
    d. All of the above

22. Which of the following prevention strategies can be implemented to decrease medication errors?
    a. Adequate lighting
    b. Dim lighting to save on electricity
    c. Spotlight each work area
    d. None of the above

23. Which committee develops a formulary for an institution?
    a. BOP
    b. FDA
    c. P&T
    d. TJC

24. Which of the following is the best method to reduce medication errors?
    a. Education of pharmacy staff
    b. Redesign systems and processes that lead to errors
    c. Correct individuals who make errors
    d. Overlook errors

25. When should a pharmacy technician alert a pharmacist to make a clinical decision?
    a. Therapeutic interchange
    b. Drug utilization review
    c. Medication misuse
    d. All of the above

26. The OBRA '90 required pharmacies to do which of the following?
    a. Perform a prospective drug utilization review on all prescriptions
    b. Provide drive-through service
    c. Therapeutically substitute brand to generic drugs
    d. Protect private information

27. Which of the following numbers could lead to a medication error due to a decimal point error?
    a. 1.00
    b. 1.01
    c. 0.11
    d. 0.01

28. Which of the following is required during a prospective drug utilization review?
    a. Therapeutic duplication
    b. Drug-disease contraindications
    c. Incorrect drug dosage
    d. All of the above

29. Which of the following committees manages the formulary system?
    a. Medical Executive Committee
    b. Nursing Council
    c. Pharmacy and Therapeutics Committee
    d. Pharmacy Administration Board

30. Which of the following is an example of a generic substitution?
    a. Norvasc-Amlodipine
    b. Lopressor-Toprol XL
    c. Protonix-Prevacid
    d. Prozac-Zoloft

31. Which of the following is an example of the therapeutic substitution?
    a. Protonix-Prevacid
    b. Norvasc-Amlodipine
    c. Prozac-Fluoxetine
    d. Ventolin-Albuterol

32. If a medication guide is required to be dispensed with a medication, when should it be given to the patient?
    a. First time only
    b. Refills only
    c. Every time dispensed
    d. Only if the patient is younger than 18 years

33. Mr. Smith is asking for an OTC recommendation. Who may answer his question?
    a. Pharmacy technician
    b. Certified pharmacy technician
    c. Pharmacist
    d. All of the above

34. Which of the following activities may be performed by a certified pharmacy technician?
    a. Patient counseling
    b. Generic substitution
    c. Prospective drug utilization review
    d. OTC medication recommendation

35. Which of the following abbreviations is on TJC's "Do Not Use" list?
    a. qd
    b. Daily
    c. bid
    d. Twice daily

36. Which law requires pharmacies to perform a prospective drug utilization review on all prescriptions?
    a. Food, Drug, and Cosmetic Act of 1936
    b. Durham-Humphrey Act of 1950
    c. Occupational Safety and Health Act of 1970
    d. Omnibus Budget Reconciliation Act of 1990

37. What does the FDA refer to?
    a. Free Drug Assistance
    b. Food and Drug Association
    c. Food and Drug Abuse
    d. Food and Drug Administration

38. Which of the following is not a task completed by pharmacy technicians?
    a. Refilling prescriptions
    b. Performing inventory
    c. Counseling patients
    d. Ordering medications

39. Pharmacy technicians may perform all of the tasks except which of the following?
    a. Drug utilization review
    b. Inventory review
    c. Laminar flow hood cleaning
    d. Repackaging medications

40. What should a certified pharmacy technician do when encountering an incorrect drug dosage during a prospective drug utilization review?
    a. Evaluate drug dose
    b. Contact the physician to change the dose
    c. Alert the pharmacist
    d. Return the prescription to the patient

41. Who may recommend an OTC medication to a patient?
    a. Pharmacy technician
    b. Certified pharmacy technician
    c. Certified pharmacy technician with OTC training
    d. None of the above

42. For which of the following reasons tall-man lettering is being used on medications?
    a. Easier to read for patients
    b. Reduces errors from look-alike drugs
    c. Enlarged to fit the size of the prescription bottle
    d. None of the above

43. Which of the following best defines a formulary?
    a. A set of rules for nurses on how to administer medications
    b. A list of medications that are approved by the medical council
    c. A list of medications that are approved by the P&T Committee
    d. A set of rules for the department of pharmacy

44. The requirement for pharmacists to counsel patients on a medication they have not taken before is listed under which law?
    a. Prescription Drug Marketing Act
    b. Kefauver-Harris Amendment
    c. OBRA '90
    d. Durham-Humphrey Amendment

45. Which of the following prevention strategies should be utilized to decrease medication errors?
    a. Two-person independent check of medication calculation
    b. Tall-man lettering
    c. Shelf separators
    d. All of the above

46. Which of the following strategies have been shown to decrease medication errors?
    a. Punitive strategies
    b. Staff education
    c. Redesign process
    d. All of the above

47. Which of the following strategies can help prevent illegible handwriting errors?
    a. Verbal orders
    b. Telephone orders
    c. Computerized physician order entry
    d. Handwriting Classes

48. Which of the following medications is a high-alert medication and can cause significant patient harm?
    a. Acetaminophen
    b. Citalopram
    c. Warfarin
    d. Fluticasone

49. Which of the following medications has a narrow therapeutic range?
    a. Fluticasone
    b. Acetaminophen
    c. Phenytoin
    d. Metoprolol

50. Tall-man lettering can help prevent which of the following type of error?
    a. Calculation error
    b. Decimal point error
    c. Look-alike-sound-alike drug error
    d. High-alert medication error

Pharmacy Quality Assurance

PTCB KNOWLEDGE AREAS

5.1 Quality assurance practices for medication and inventory control systems (eg, matching National Drug Code [NDC] number, bar code, data entry)

5.2 Infection control procedures and documentation (eg, personal protective equipment [PPE], needle recapping)

5.3 Risk management guidelines and regulations (eg, error prevention strategies)

5.4 Communication channels necessary to ensure appropriate follow-up and problem resolution (eg, product recalls, shortages)

5.5 Productivity, efficiency, and customer satisfaction measures

KEY TERMS

Bar code: An optical machine-readable representation of information related to the object to which it is attached

Continuous quality improvement (CQI): A process to ensure programs are systematically and intentionally improving services and increasing positive outcomes

Failure mode and effects analysis (FMEA): Proactive evaluation of a system or process that allows one to determine a mechanism of potential failures in advance

Medication error: Any variation from a prescription order not corrected prior to dispensing the medication to the patient

National Drug Code (NDC): Unique, 3-segment number that identifies drug products

Patient safety organizations (PSOs): A group of associations that share the goal of improving the quality and safety of health care delivery

that was created by the Department of Health and Human Services

Productivity: The quality of being productive or being able to produce. Typically measured as the amount of work, or number of tasks accomplished during a set period of time

Quality assurance (QA): The process used to ensure that a product or service meets appropriate or predetermined standards

Root cause analysis (RCA): Retrospective method for identifying the underlying factors that caused an error

Risk management: The identification, analysis, assessment, control, and avoidance, minimization, or elimination of risks

Sentinel event: An unexpected occurrence involving death or serious injury or psychological injury. Serious injury specifically includes loss of limb or function

CASE STUDY

Mr. Smith calls your pharmacy and has a question about the tablets in his prescription bottle. He tells you that there are 2 tablets, one is orange and the other is white. He is concerned that these are not the same medication and that an error has occurred which may be harmful to him.

You gather all the information from Mr. Smith. You ask him to describe the tablets and from his profile you verify the dispensing dates from his previous fills. All this information is given to the pharmacist to review.

Self-Assessment Questions
- What has occurred?
- What are the facts?
- What are the steps necessary for resolution?
- How can an error like this be prevented from happening again?

INTRODUCTION

Improving and sustaining the workflow process in order to provide the safest possible service to the patient is a challenge faced by every pharmacy technician and pharmacist. There are a variety of methods that when used correctly assist the technician and the pharmacist to avoid the most common pitfalls of dispensing medication. This chapter examines methods and procedures used to help protect the patient through pharmacy quality assurance.

QUALITY ASSURANCE PRACTICES

Quality assurance (QA) is a system created within an organization, that when used correctly, helps ensure the quality of the product produced. QA is process driven, meaning the focus is on preventing any defects in the product. This means having effective policies and procedures in place is imperative for a proper QA system. The goal of a successful QA system is to constantly testing and monitoring systems so that deficiencies do not arise, or are addressed immediately when discovered. An example of QA in the pharmacy is requiring competencies for all sterile compounding personnel, to confirm proper technique and cleaning methods are being utilized.

Quality control (QC) examines the product after it is completed. This is a system based more on identification of defects, rather than prevention methods used in QA systems. QC is a more reactive process by identifying problems when they arise. While QA is a more preventative process that discovers problems within the process itself possibly leading to a defective product.

There are many processes that pharmacies must examine for an effective QA program. Infection control procedures, medication safety practices, and effective communication are examples of processes monitored through audits and QA programs.

Infection Control

As discussed in Chapter 3, infection control is vital for the compounding of sterile products. Proper hand washing is important for this process, but for many other pharmacy practices to help prevent the spread of microorganisms to patients and pharmacy staff. In addition to sterile compounding garbing practices, hands should be washed after using the restroom, before and after interaction with a patient, before and after eating, or if they become visibly soiled. An alcohol-based sanitizer gel or foam may also be used, if hands are not visibly dirty.

Proper garbing is also essential for sterile compounding and other areas of pharmacy practice. The following is the order of donning PPE for sterile compounding (assuming the employee is already wearing scrubs):

1. Shoe covers
2. Hair covers
3. Beard covers (if needed)
4. Face mask
5. Wash hands
6. Gown
7. Eye shield (if needed)
8. Sterile gloves

Additionally, when compounding sterile products, it may be necessary for the compounding technician to recap a needle. Although it should be avoided, if a needle must be recapped, use the scooping method to avoid needle sticks and potential infection control issues. The scooping method is shown below in Figure 5-1. The cap of the needle should be on the surface of the hood or isolator glove box, and one hand is used to scoop the needle into the cap. This should avoid potential sticks.

★ **TECH ALERT:** *Stay alert while at work. Keep the computer screen 20-26 inches away from your eyes, regularly clean your areas, keep your area well lit, and focus on areas close to you and far away from you at frequent intervals. This will help decrease eye fatigue and keep you sharp!*

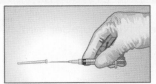
Step 1
Place the cap on a flat surface, then remove your hand from the cap.

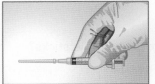
Step 2
With one hand, hold the syringe and use the needle to "scoop up" the cap.

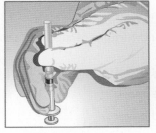
Step 3
When the cap covers the needle completely, use the other hand to secure the cap on the needle hub. Be careful to handle the cap at the bottom only.

FIGURE 5-1 Scooping method for recapping needles.

★ *TECH ALERT: The NDC consists of the labeler code (4 or 5 digits), the product code (3 or 4 digits), and the package code (1 or 2 digits). The labeler code is assigned by the FDA and the product and package code are assigned by the labeler.*

Correct Medication Selection

Choosing the correct product for a patient's prescription, although seemingly a simple task, is not void of the possibility for errors. Confirmation bias occurs when a pharmacy staff member chooses the wrong medication based on what he or she expected to see, rather than what was actually there. An example of this would be if a new medication was received and all the drugs were moved to create space for this new drug. Then, when the pharmacy staff member goes to retrieve a medication that was normally in the space where the new drug has been placed, an incorrect drug could possibly be retrieved if the pharmacy staff member failed to check if it is the correct product. The challenge for all pharmacies is providing tools and training to help each team member pick the correct product from the shelf.

A very simple solution to this problem is found printed on the manufacturer's bottle. The **National Drug Code (NDC)** is a unique identifier for each individual product, manufacturer, and strength, as well as size of the stock bottle.

The NDC number is matched with a reference number found on the prescription label or in many cases a **bar code** printed on the prescription label. A simple match procedure involves the technician visually verifying the NDC on the label matches the NDC on the manufacturer's bottle.

Using a barcode scanner with audible cues for the technician and pharmacist is a much more reliable way to determine the correct product has been chosen from the shelf of the pharmacy. Typically, these scanners are handheld and portable. This allows the technician to move freely through the pharmacy to the shelves. Usually the patient's prescription label is scanned first and then the stock bottle is scanned second. The user is notified if a selection is incorrect and does not scan. In many cases, the handheld scanner is tracking statistics for each unique user and pharmacies can measure workload, accuracy, and speed, and this information can be used to determine the individual needs for a technician's further training or coaching.

QUICK QUIZ 5-1

1. Which of the following is in the correct NDC number format?
   a. 12345-1234-12
   b. 1234-12-12345
   c. 12-1234-12345
   d. 2345-12-1234

2. Which of the following is used to prevent needle sticks?
   a. Scooping method of recapping needles
   b. Taking your gloves off before putting needle caps on
   c. Using both hands to recap the needle
   d. There are no situations that would require recapping a needle

3. Which of the following is the correct order of garbing PPE?
   a. Gown, gloves, shoe covers, face mask
   b. Face mask, gown, gloves, beard cover
   c. Wash hands, gown, gloves, face mask
   d. Shoe covers, face mask, wash hands, gown, and gloves

4. What can occur when a pharmacy worker selects a medication based on what they expect to see, but not what they actually see?

   a. Quality assurance

   b. Confirmation bias

   c. Quality control

   d. Bar coding

5. Which system focuses on the process and prevents defects in the product?

   a. Quality assurance

   b. Confirmation bias

   c. Quality control

   d. Risk mitigation strategy

Correct Medication Quantity

Pharmacies have adopted strategies utilizing technology to assist with accurate counting. The use of countertop counting machines in some retail or outpatient pharmacies, as well as automated dispensing cabinets in hospitals are all useful means to help dispense accurate counts of medication to patients.

Medication counting is a common task for pharmacy technicians, so the importance in accuracy and efficiency is apparent. Many pharmacies use a "double-count" process for counting narcotics, especially C-II medications. This process usually involves a double count by the technician, as well as an additional count by the pharmacist verifying the final product. In many states, the pharmacist must also count the quantity of the contents remaining in the bottle, to confirm it matches the inventory of the narcotic drug.

QUALITY IMPROVEMENT STANDARDS AND GUIDELINES

A commitment to continually improving the quality of your work will benefit each patient. Today, there are many organizations which have created guidelines to help pharmacies make informed choices on the creation and implementation of a quality improvement program that will meet or exceed the patient's expectation.

These organizations exist in large part due to the federal and state regulations regarding quality improvement. Payment for services, accreditation, and licensing of a pharmacy may all depend on the creation, implementation, and documentation of a quality improvement program. Not every state requires specific quality assurance standards in each pharmacy. It is therefore up to the pharmacy director or pharmacist in charge to be familiar with the particular standards for their state.

In 2008, the Federal Register published the rules associated with the 2005 Patient Safety and Quality Improvement Act. This regulation establishes a way for health care providers to voluntarily report information to Patient Safety Organization (PSO) in order to evaluate safety events. As a result of this Act, several patient medication safety organizations were created as official PSOs. These organizations help pharmacies and their teams understand the **best practices** and how workflow processes or design can lead to unintended patient errors. Best practices are accepted as the correct or most effective for a specific task.

★ *TECH ALERT: PSO information may be found on the Agency for Healthcare Research and Quality (AHRQ) website at www. pso.ahrq.gov.*

Medicare and other private insurance companies are asking pharmacies to provide documentation of their quality assurance and improvement program as a requirement for payment. The Medicare Modernization Act of 2003 specifically states that "Quality assurance measures and systems reduce **medication errors** and adverse drug interactions and improve medication use" will be in place.

PHARMACY QUALITY ASSURANCE ORGANIZATIONS

There are numerous pharmacy quality assurance organizations to help improve patient safety. These organizations all have slightly different goals, but all have a focus on improving patient safety.

Agency for Healthcare Research and Quality (AHRQ)

The AHRQ is in charge of developing research, reports, practical tools, and other resources to improve the quality, safety, effectiveness, and efficiency of health care. This agency is located within the Department of Health and Human Services. The information provided by the AHRQ is expansive. It includes data for patients, consumers, health care professionals, and policy makers.

Food and Drug Administration (FDA)

⋆ *TECH ALERT: Tall man letters used mixed case letter to help draw attention to the differences in their name. Example: glyBURIDE vs. glipZIDE.*

The FDA is responsible for protecting the public health by assuring that foods are safe, wholesome, sanitary, and properly labeled. They are also responsible for human and veterinary drugs, vaccines, biological products, and medical devices. The FDA ensures that those products are safe and effective for human use. The FDA is also responsible for monitoring the labeling of cosmetics and dietary supplements to ensure no misbranding. In addition, they regulate tobacco products.

Institute of Safe Medicine Practices (ISMP)

The ISMP is the only nonprofit organization dedicated solely to medication error prevention and safe medication use. It has a voluntary medication error reporting system that allows practitioners across the nation to report errors in hopes of preventing further errors or to examine trends in processes or workflows.

The ISMP also has the following multiple safety tools:

- "Do not crush list"—oral dosage forms that should not be crushed
- Abbreviations toolkit—resources to eliminate the use of error-prone abbreviations
- Black box warnings—listing and summary of products with black box warnings
- Error-prone abbreviations list—listing of abbreviations that are involved in harmful medication errors
- FMEA process—overview of the failure mode and effects analysis is a proactive risk assessment of a high-risk process that occurs before an event occurs
- ISMP confused drug name list—listing of all drugs that have been mistaken for one another
- ISMP high-alert medications—drugs that have a heightened risk of causing significant harm when used in error
- Tall-man letters—sets of look-alike drugs that have been modified using "tall-man" letters

ISMP operates 2 programs for error reporting: the National Medication Errors Reporting Program (MERP) and the National Vaccine Errors Reporting

TABLE 5-1. Medication Error Reporting Programs	
FDA Medwatch www.fda.gov	Voluntary reporting of serious adverse events, potential or actual product errors, and product quality issues
MedMaRx www.medmarx.com	Voluntary reporting system of adverse drug events
ISMP www.ismp.org	Voluntary reporting system of medication errors
TJC www.jointcommission.org	Organizational (hospital, nursing home, etc) reporting of sentinel events

Program (VERP). Both reporting programs are confidential so that errors can be examined from a process viewpoint and not a punitive approach. Additional medication error reporting programs are shown in Table 5-1.

Occupational Safety and Health Administration

OSHA is an agency of the US Department of Labor. The goal of OSHA is to assure safe and healthful working conditions. OSHA requires that material safety data sheet (MSDS) be available in the pharmacy for hazardous compounds.

State Boards of Pharmacy

The Board of Pharmacy (BOP) is responsible for administering and enforcing laws governing the legal distribution of drugs. It is also in charge of licensing pharmacists and pharmacy technicians. Each State BOP has different rules and laws regarding pharmacy quality assurance.

The Joint Commission

As discussed in Chapter 2, the goal of The Joint Commission (TJC) is to improve health care for the public by evaluating health care organizations. TJC has specific standards that an organization must meet to become certified. There are different levels of certification and disease-specific standards that an organization may obtain. They also encourage hospitals to report **sentinel events** and the root cause analysis performed to identify the lesson learned.

United States Pharmacopeia (USP)

The USP contains drug information on over 11,000 generic and brand name medications. Medications, biologics, medical devices, and compounded products must abide by the standards set forth by the USP. The USP established reference standards for nonsterile compounding (USP <795>) and sterile compounding (USP<797>).

VA National Center for Patient Safety (NCPS)

The NCPS was developed to create a culture of safety throughout the Veterans Health Administration. Their goal is to reduce and prevent hard to patients as a result of their healthcare. They provide support for healthcare professionals and patients on various safety topics.

★ *TECH ALERT: MSDS provides procedures for handling or working with substances in a safe manner including toxicity, disposal, protective equipment, and spill-handling procedures. Many workplaces keep MSDS information online for frequent updating and easy access.*

RISK MANAGEMENT GUIDELINES AND REGULATIONS

Although there are many measures to help prevent error, human error is inevitable in pharmacy practice. However, an organization with a commitment to quality will make every effort to prevent errors from occurring. A committed organization will also have policies and procedures in place and will be able to act quickly and effectively when faced with a potential problem that might include an error. This is the process of managing risk and if everyone on the team is involved, there is a greater likelihood that the workflow will be safe and effective for the patients being served.

Risk management programs in the pharmacy are generally multifaceted and are a great way to involve the technicians in the prevention and identification of potential errors. The program may be designed to reach an error level of zero, but actually the benefit of a risk management program extends beyond this goal. Many accrediting bodies and even insurance companies are requesting risk management programs and effective program development. The development of a risk management program requires input from everyone on the pharmacy team and typically follows a rigorous evaluation of every step of the medication workflow. This will require a detailed understanding of the entire process and the steps involved with each individual task along the way.

A risk management program allows the team to look very objectively at each step of the workflow and make a judgment on how likely it is to fail, how detrimental the impact will be, and how the probability of failure can be reduced.

Spending time with the pharmacy team brainstorming, assigning risk levels to workflow tasks, evaluating the probability of a problem surfacing, and evaluating methods to reduce the risk will keep your team engaged in a culture of quality (Table 5-2).

Analyzing Errors

When an error occurs, a health care organization should examine the error to investigate where the system failed, or if it was a product of human error. Two common methods to examine errors are RCA and FMEA.

A **root cause analysis (RCA)** is a retrospective approach after an event occurs. It helps identify a system or process a problem after an event occurs. A **failure mode and effects analysis (FMEA)** is a proactive risk assessment of a high-risk process that occurs before an event occurs.

Communication Channels

The purpose of effective communication is to disseminate information about a subject to an audience. Communication is crucial in pharmacy practice. It is used to ensure ongoing quality improvement through education about issues (ie, recalls, drug shortages, etc) and also problem resolution (ie, change in process due to an error, editing a policy to be in compliance, etc).

For example, wholesalers, professional pharmacy networks, national organizations, and word of mouth are some of the communication channels used to identify upcoming, current, and continuous medication shortages. These shortages must be communicated to specific patients and prescribers in order to set the expectation that a necessary medication may not be available for use for a period of time. Viable alternatives may or may not be available for a patient and in some cases the medication may not ever be available again.

TABLE 5-2. **Risk Management Recommendations for Retail Pharmacy**	
Generation of prescription	• Use computerized generated transmission of prescriptions and e-prescribing
Interpretation of prescriptions	• Obtain clarification with ambiguous orders • Be mindful of look-alike and sound-alike medications
Obtain patient data	• Obtain allergies and disease states • Ask for height and weight
Prescription data entry	• Use the NDC from the medication stock bottle during data entry
Medication storage	• Store all medications in alphabetical order A to Z • Indicate high-alert, look-alike, and sound-alike medications
Prescription filling	• Fill one prescription at a time • Verify the written prescription with the computer-generated label • Do not leave a medication container unlabeled • Place multiple prescriptions for a patient together to ensure the appropriate patient gets the correct medication • Utilize automation to decrease error potential
Medication delivery	• Ask the patient for 2 identifiers prior to dispensing (ie, name, birthday, address, etc) • Show the medication vials to the patient to verify the name and medication • Use the barcode scanner to verify the right patient is receiving the right medication

Regardless of the medication, every member of the pharmacy team should be apprised of the current shortages. Again, communication is a key component of the pharmacy's quality improvement process. Table 5-3 lists common communication methods.

For more information about pharmacy recall, please refer to Chapter 2: Pharmacy Law and Regulations for the Pharmacy Technician.

PRODUCTIVITY, EFFICIENCY, AND CUSTOMER SATISFACTION MEASURES

Every team needs to know how well it is performing and whether or not changes are necessary in order to perform at a higher level and to meet the expectations

★ *TECH ALERT: "Key performance indicators" as well as "dashboards" are ways to understand how much work is being done, by whom, and how efficiently. These tools can be very valuable when evaluating performance.*

TABLE 5-3. **Communication Methods**	
Face-to-face	Most effective method; allows for interactive discussion; best for complex messages
Broadcast media (TV, radio, loud speaker)	Used to address mass audience; may use visual aids to assist
Telephone	Mobile method; between 2 persons or small group
E-mail/social media/Internet	One-on-one, small group, or mass media; use caution with wording
Written memos/letters	No interpersonal interaction needed; policies, notices, announcements

of the business. Pharmacies are held to specific budgets and are required to meet expectations related to filling prescriptions as well as maintaining a level of quality and patient satisfaction in order to continue business.

Productivity

Productivity is a measure of the activities being performed during a period of time. In pharmacy, there are many common productivity measures. Pharmacies may measure prescriptions checked per hour worked, phone orders completed per hour worked, and prescriptions filled per hour worked. These numbers should be reviewed frequently with a pharmacy manager or team leader. Understanding individual goals and whether more training, coaching, or support is needed to reach a goal is a great way to get involved with improving your performance.

Productivity improvements may occur when new technology is introduced or when a process is modified in order to speed up a transaction or reduce a "bottleneck" in the workflow. Technology helps technicians choose the right medication the first time and therefore reduces the number of return trips to the shelves in order to find the correct bottle. A pharmacist using barcode readers with updated software will easily identify the tablet or capsule in the bottle instead of relying on opening a stock bottle or thumbing through catalogs of pictures to verify correct medications.

In the end, if productivity can be increased, there will be more time available to provide assistance to customers: answering questions, maintaining documentation requirements, and enhancing the overall experience.

Efficiency

Efficiency is the time, effort, or cost of producing an outcome. Pharmacies may measure efficiency by average wait time per patient, prescription turnaround time, number of prescription errors per month, or inventory turnover rates.

Similar to productivity, efficiency goals should be reviewed with each staff member. Efficiency can also be improved with technology and constant discussion with staff to improve goals.

Customer Satisfaction

The key piece of any business is maintaining a customer base that will recommend your service, store, people, and product and will keep coming back. The philosophy of high-quality customer satisfaction is simple, but the execution of this is a continuous challenge. Most pharmacies use a survey technique after a patient has visited that location. Hospital pharmacy services are typically reviewed by nursing staff and physicians through annual nursing or medical staff surveys. Inpatients are mailed a survey after a hospital stay, and although the questions are based on the whole experience of the hospital, some questions are directed at pharmacy services and the ability to provide drug information or counseling to a patient. It is important to examine the feedback received regardless.

Customer service is important for all pharmacy technicians, regardless of the practice setting. Keep in mind that the customer does not always need to be right, but the customer is your only source of information related to the perceived quality of your product and therefore deserves attention. Table 5-4 describes useful customer service skills.

TABLE 5-4. Customer Service Skills

1. **Patience:** Remember, many of your patients may be ill and may not feel well. Take the time to help them understand their medication, by offering counseling by a pharmacist.

2. **Pay attention:** Listen to your patient. Do not interrupt them and ask open-ended questions to get the most information.

3. **Clearly communicate:** Speak clearly so that your patients can understand what you are saying.

4. **Pleasant attitude:** Smile; use kind words; speak nicely about others.

5. **Handle surprises:** Be prepared for all situations; be adaptable to changes.

6. **Work under pressure:** The pharmacy is often busy and fast paced, be prepared.

7. **Know your product:** Be knowledgeable of medications, your job responsibilities, and your workplace procedures.

8. **Take the extra step:** Going one extra step to help your patient will help increase customer satisfaction.

9. **Caring:** Be compassionate and kind to your patients; treat them how you would like to be treated.

10. **Learn from mistakes:** Remember your own mistakes and use that information to improve on your skills.

CASE STUDY REVIEWED

Mr. Smith calls your pharmacy and has a question about the tablets in his prescription bottle. He tells you that there are 2 tablets, one is orange and the other is white. He is concerned that these are not the same medication and that an error has occurred which may be harmful to him.

You gather all the information from Mr. Smith. You ask him to describe the tablets and from his profile you verify the dispensing dates from his previous fills. All this information is given to the pharmacist to review.

Self-Assessment Questions

- What has occurred?
  - Mr. Smith does have 2 different tablets in his prescription bottle. Somewhere along the way there was a mix-up of tablets.
- What are the facts?
  - At this point, facts need to be gathered.
  - Mr. Smith should be asked if he had poured tablets from one bottle to another.
  - Stock bottles on the shelves should be checked for any tablets that are mixed in (which is why you should not return medication to stock bottles).
- What are the steps necessary for resolution?
  - In many cases it is not possible to determine the exact origin of the error, but through careful documentation of processes and positive identification of personnel responsible for each step along the way, it is possible to get further input directly from those who took care of Mr. Smith's prescriptions.
- How can an error like this be prevented from happening again?
  - Identifying potential problems in the workflow.
  - Evaluating processes not being followed according to policy.

CHAPTER SUMMARY

- Quality assurance and quality control help ensure appropriate standards are met and helps improve the safety of the patient.
- Basic pharmacy dispensing requires the correct patient to get the correct medication with the correct instructions in a timely manner. Efficient, accurate, and safe medication dispensing is aided by the use of product double check including the use of technology to guide and assist the technicians and pharmacists.
- **Patient safety organizations** help health care facilities and pharmacies perform their best by collecting, analyzing, and reporting data submitted by pharmacists and technicians and other health care professionals. Learning from the experiences of other organizations can prevent future errors and lead to efficient and productive workflow systems.
- Medication recalls and drug shortages are certainly botherations to the pharmacy enterprise. But, these annoyances, if properly planned for and communicated to patients and prescribers do not have to interrupt proper care of the patient. A well-written medication recall and drug shortage policy and procedure provide peace of mind that quality patient care will continue despite the challenges of recalls and shortages.
- Customer satisfaction is generally accomplished by maintaining integrity, responding to patient requests, and treating others with respect. Every patient has the right to get your best professional effort with every prescription filled. Errors will happen in the workplace. Pharmacy errors have the potential to be very dangerous and could result in serious harm for a patient. Minimize the risk of a serious error occurring by participating in risk management strategies with your pharmacy team. Evaluate your performance and hold everyone to the same high standards.

ANSWERS TO QUICK QUIZ

Quick Quiz 5-1

1. 12345-1234-12

2. Scooping method of recapping needles

3. Shoe covers, face mask, wash hands, gown, and gloves

4. Confirmation bias

5. Quality assurance

CHAPTER QUESTIONS

1. What is an NDC?
   a. An optical machine-readable representation of information related to the object to which it is attached
   b. A unique, 3-segment number that identifies drug products
   c. Issued by the DEA
   d. Issued by the State Board of Pharmacy

2. Which of the following organizations oversees MERP?
   a. ISMP
   b. FDA
   c. DEA
   d. TJC

3. What is the quality of being productive or being able to produce?
   a. Risk management
   b. Productivity
   c. CQI
   d. PSO

4. Which method of communication is most efficient for a policy announcement?
   a. Face-to-face
   b. Telephone
   c. Loud speaker
   d. Written memo

5. What does the acronym DEA stand for?
   a. Drug Enforcement Area
   b. Disease Enforcing Agency
   c. Department of Enforcement Agency
   d. Drug Enforcement Agency

6. Before a high-risk process is implemented, what type of risk analysis may be performed?
   a. Root cause analysis
   b. Productivity analysis
   c. Failure mode and effects analysis
   d. Efficiency analysis

7. What is the time, effort, or cost of producing an outcome?
   a. Efficiency
   b. Productivity
   c. Customer satisfaction
   d. Analysis

8. Which line of communication is a formal line of communication?
   a. Pharmacy technician to pharmacist
   b. Pharmacy technician to pharmacy technician
   c. Pharmacy technician to patient
   d. Pharmacy technician to hospital chief executive officer

9. Who sets standards for medications, biologics, medical devices, and compounded products?
   a. OSHA
   b. TJC
   c. USP
   d. P&T

10. Who issues a medication recall?
    a. TJC
    b. FDA
    c. DEA
    d. P&T

11. A drug company is required to remove its medication from market due to the risk of death. What type of recall is this?
    a. Class I
    b. Class II
    c. Class III
    d. Market withdrawal

12. Who created patient safety organizations?
    a. The FDA
    b. The Department of Health and Human Services
    c. The DEA
    d. The State Board of Pharmacy

13. What is the Agency for Healthcare Research and Quality (AHRQ)?
    a. An agency in the Department of Health and Human services
    b. An agency dedicated to improve quality, safety, and efficiency of health care
    c. Both a and b
    d. a only

14. Which segment of the NDC code represents the labeler code?
    a. The first 4 or 5 digits
    b. The second 3 or 4 digits
    c. The third 1 or 2 digits
    d. a and c

15. Which organization oversees Medwatch?
    a. FDA
    b. DEA
    c. USP
    d. TJC

16. When does quality control investigate a product?
    a. Before completion
    b. During manufacturing
    c. After completion
    d. None of the above

17. What is continuous quality improvement?
    a. The quality of being productive or able to produce
    b. The identification of risk and the avoidance or minimization of risk
    c. A process to ensure programs are intentionally improving services
    d. Only for large corporate businesses

18. How are evaluations of productivity usually measured?
    a. Amount of work accomplished during a set time period
    b. Organizations to determine efficiency
    c. Supervisors in order to thoroughly evaluate an employee
    d. All of the above

19. The Patient Safety and Quality Improvement Act established the PSO. What does the acronym stand for?
    a. Patient safety organization
    b. Patient satisfaction organization
    c. Pharmacist safety organization
    d. Pharmacist satisfaction organization

20. What is the unique, 3-segment number that identifies drug products?
    a. The bar code
    b. The NDC
    c. The federal legend
    d. The schedule

21. Which organization is solely dedicated to medication error prevention?
    a. OSHA
    b. FDA
    c. TJC
    d. ISMP

22. Name the process to ensure programs are intentionally improving service and increasing positive outcomes.
    a. Risk management
    b. Productivity
    c. Entrepreneurship
    d. Continuous quality improvement

23. Which of the following organizations is classified by the Department of Health and Human Services to improve quality and safety of health care services?
    a. PSO
    b. CQI
    c. HIPAA
    d. DEA

24. Risk management involves which of the following in order to eliminate or minimize risk?
    a. Analysis of workflow
    b. Identification of complex high-risk tasks
    c. Avoidance of risk through education and process change
    d. All of the above

25. What is identifying, analyzing, assessing, and controlling risk?
    a. CQI
    b. PSO
    c. Risk management
    d. Productivity

26. Which strategy can help prevent eye fatigue while working?
    a. Dim the lights
    b. Move closer to the computer screen
    c. Focus on areas close to you and far away at frequent intervals
    d. All of the above

27. What type of recall would be a situation in which use or exposure to a product is not likely to cause adverse health consequences?
    a. Class I
    b. Class II
    c. Class III
    d. Class IV

28. Which segment of the NDC code represents the product code?
    a. The first 4 or 5 digits
    b. The second 3 or 4 digits
    c. The third 1 or 2 digits
    d. a and c

29. What is a sentinel event?
    a. Minor medication filling error
    b. Minor medication adverse drug event
    c. Unexpected death due to a medication error
    d. Class IV medication recall

30. Which of the following strategies will help a technician efficiently choose the correct product from the stock shelves?
    a. Audible cue barcode scanner
    b. Bringing a second technician to the shelf to check the stock with you
    c. Bringing the pharmacist to the shelf to check the stock with you
    d. None of the above

31. To prevent eye fatigue your computer screen should be how far away from you?
    a. More than 3 ft
    b. Between 20 and 26 in
    c. Closer than 12 in
    d. Between 12 and 20 in

32. Which of the following may help improve customer satisfaction?
    a. New procedures
    b. Change in workflow
    c. Education of staff
    d. All of the above

33. This agency in the Department of Health and Human Services is responsible for improving quality, safety, and efficiency in the health care system.
    a. PSO
    b. CQI
    c. AHRQ
    d. DEA

34. Why is it is necessary to perform software updates on your systems?
    a. The latest drug information can be loaded into your system
    b. The latest drug interaction information is available
    c. Software glitches and bugs will be fixed
    d. All of the above

35. All errors are preventable in a pharmacy and should never occur.
    a. True
    b. False

36. What is a bar code?
    a. An optical machine-readable representation of information related to the object to which it is attached
    b. A unique, 3-segment number that identifies drug products
    c. Issued by the DEA
    d. Issued by the State Board of Pharmacy

37. Which of the following recalls is related to serious health problems from dangerous or defective products?
    a. Class I
    b. Class II
    c. Class III
    d. Market withdrawal

38. Which organization is in charge of product recalls?
    a. DEA
    b. FDA
    c. The State Board of Pharmacy
    d. TJC

39. Where should recalled medications be stored?
    a. In the refrigerator
    b. On the shelf in alphabetical order
    c. Segregated from normal stock
    d. In the narcotic cabinet

40. Which of the following quality measures improve patient safety?
    a. Computer software updates
    b. Calibrated counting trays
    c. Barcode scanners
    d. All of the above

41. After an error has occurred, what type of analysis may be performed?
    a. FMEA
    b. Productivity report
    c. RCA
    d. Efficiency report

42. When a sentinel event occurs in a hospital, which organization is this information reported to?
    a. FDA
    b. DEA
    c. USP
    d. TJC

43. Which method of communication is best for interactive discussion?
    a. E-mail
    b. Written memo
    c. Face-to-face discussion
    d. Broadcast media

44. Which of the agency ensures safe and healthful working conditions?
    a. OSHA
    b. FDA
    c. DEA
    d. TJC

45. Which organization creates a culture of safety throughout the Veterans Health Administration?
    a. OSHA
    b. FDA
    c. NCPS
    d. USP

46. Which organization is in charge of licensing pharmacists?
    a. DEA
    b. FDA
    c. BOP
    d. TJC

47. Which of the following methods is preferred for prescription generation?
    a. Telephone
    b. E-prescribing
    c. Handwritten
    d. Faxed copy

48. What method helps decrease errors in a retail pharmacy setting?
    a. Pick the NDC for the medication based on which it is listed first
    b. Use the NDC from the medication stock bottle during data entry
    c. Choose the NDC based on memory
    d. There is no need to verify NDC during data entry

49. In what order should medications be stored in a retail pharmacy?
    a. A to Z regardless of type of medication
    b. A to Z separating fast movers
    c. Separated by type of medication
    d. A to Z separated by brand and generic medication

50. Which organization requires material safety data sheets be available?
    a. FDA
    b. OSHA
    c. P&T
    d. DEA

Medication Order Entry and Fill Process

CHAPTER
6

PTCB KNOWLEDGE AREAS

6.1 Order entry process

6.2 Intake, interpretation, and data entry

6.3 Calculate doses required

6.4 Fill process (eg, select appropriate product, apply special handling requirements, measure, and prepare product for final check)

6.5 Labeling requirements (eg, auxiliary and warning labels, expiration date, and patient-specific information)

6.6 Packaging requirements (eg, type of bags, syringes, glass, pvc, child resistant, and light resistant)

6.7 Dispensing process (eg, validation, documentation, and distribution)

KEY TERMS

Admitting order: Type of medication order written upon admission into a facility which contains previous medications being taken, new medications being ordered, any laboratory or diagnostic tests desired by the physician, and a suspected diagnosis

Automated dispensing cabinets (ADCs): A storage cabinet containing medications needed for patients in specific nursing units in which nurses can retrieve mediations in an efficient manner

Auxiliary labels: Brightly colored labels designed to provide additional warnings to patients

Blended unit dose: A unit dose system which packages all the patient's medications to be taken at the same time together

Computerized physician order entry (CPOE): Prescription orders entered by the prescriber into the pharmacy computer system directly

Counting tray: Device used to count solid oral dosage forms such as tablets or capsules

Days supply: The number of days a medication should last if used correctly

Discharge orders: Type of order given upon being discharged from the hospital

Expiration date: The date indicating when the effectiveness of a medication will diminish

Inscription: Part of the prescription that contains the name and strength of the medication and the amount prescribed

Legend drug: A drug which requires a prescription to be dispensed

Medication administration record (MAR): A record of each time a medication is administered to a patient (used in an inpatient setting); shows what time the dose was given and who administered the dose

Medication order: An order for a patient written for the inpatient setting

Modified unit dose: Also known as a blister or bingo card, a unit dose system which provides a month's supply of a medication into one card

Over-the-counter (OTC) drug: A drug which does not require a prescription to be dispensed

Patient profile: Record of information of a patient, including basic demographics, prescription filling history, allergy, and insurance information

Prescription: An order for a patient in the outpatient setting, written by a qualified health care professional and filled by a registered pharmacist

PRN orders: Type of medication order given only as needed

Scored: Tablets which have a line or crevice through the center which makes dividing the tablet in half easier and more accurate

Sig codes: Certain abbreviations for directions written on prescriptions, designed to help simplify and speed up the order entry process

Signa: Also known as sig, the part of the prescription that contains directions to the patient

STAT order: Type of medication order written for a drug that is needed immediately

Subscription: Part of the prescription that contains directions to the pharmacist such as refills or dispense as written (DAW) requirements

Superscription: Part of the prescription that is the Rx symbol

Tablet splitter: Device used to split tablets for patients taking half-tablet dosages

Unit dose: A medication that has been prepackaged for a single-dose administration

Unit dose cart: The cart filled by the pharmacy for usually a 24-hour supply of medication, and used by the nurses to pull medications from the drawers for each patient

Unit dose drug distribution system: A system which utilizes a cart of drawers containing unit doses specific for each patient in a hospital unit

Unit-of-use: A method of packaging of medications in a fixed number of units that is the most commonly prescribed amount, that is, prepacking a bottle of 30 for a medication taken daily

CASE STUDY

A patient brings a prescription into the pharmacy. You attempt to read the directions as appear in Figure 6-1.

FIGURE 6-1 Handwritten prescription.

Self-Assessment Questions
- What is this drug written for?
- What is the strength?
- What are the directions?
- How many should be dispensed and are refills permitted?

After completing this chapter, you should be able to answer the case study assessment questions presented for the illegible prescription of Figure 6-1.

INTRODUCTION

There are many processes involved in medication order entry and the filling process. This chapter focuses on all the necessary steps in prescription processing, including dosage calculations, abbreviations, packaging, and labeling requirements. After completing this chapter, you should be confident with the process of filling prescriptions and entering medication orders.

ORDER ENTRY PROCESS

A pharmacy technician plays an essential role in entering prescriptions properly into the computer, updating all patient information while ensuring the **patient profile** is accurate, and providing excellent customer service. By properly completing these and other delegated tasks, the pharmacy technician can successfully free up time for the pharmacist to spend counseling patients about medication-related questions.

As a technician, you will encounter 2 different types of orders in the pharmacy setting. In the outpatient setting, a patient will present a **prescription** written by a licensed medical practitioner; whereas, inpatient requests for medications are known as **medication orders.** Prescriptions in the outpatient setting are required for any **legend drug.** A legend drug is a drug which requires a prescription to be dispensed. Only nonprescription drugs or **over-the-counter (OTC)** medications are dispensed legally without a prescription.

Parts of the Prescription

A pharmacy technician provides the first look at the accuracy and completeness of a prescription.

The necessary components of a prescription are listed in Table 6-1:

Figure 6-2 shows an example prescription from a medical doctor. The technician reviews the prescription for completeness and then enters the information into the computer. The figure shows each important component to a prescription which is necessary for processing:

1. Prescriber information includes the address of the physician, office phone number, and a fax number.
2. Prescriber's DEA number for this prescription is not required because Topamax is not a controlled substance. A DEA number is issued by the Drug Enforcement

★ TECH ALERT: Remember, as a pharmacy technician you have many responsibilities, but you must never counsel patients. Only the pharmacist is permitted to counsel patients.

TABLE 6-1. **Required Components of a Prescription**
1. Prescriber information: Name and address of office, phone number
2. Prescriber's Drug Enforcement Administration (DEA) number (for controlled prescriptions)
3. Date
4. Patient information: Name, address, telephone number, and date of birth
5. Inscription: Medication prescribed, name, quantity, strength, and amount
6. Superscription: Rx symbol
7. Subscription: Directions to the pharmacist, refills or special labels
8. Signa (sig): Directions to the patient
9. DAW: Dispense as written
10. Prescriber's signature

Administration to a prescriber. This allows the physician to prescribe controlled substances. The DEA number is usually not preprinted on a prescription to prevent forgeries.

3. The date the prescription was written needs to be recorded. If no date is written on the prescription, the patient should be questioned as to when the physician was seen. If the prescription is for a controlled substance, the date is especially important, as schedules III to V medications can only be filled a maximum of 5 times within 6 months.

4. It is important to have a patient's full name and address updated in the pharmacy system. If this is not written on the prescription, the technician should ask the patient to verify the address. If the birthdate is not written on the prescription, the technician must request this information from the patient. This is essential for billing and insurance purposes, but also allows the pharmacist to verify the proper dosage of a medication.

5. The **inscription** is the part of the prescription that contains the name and strength of the medication and the amount prescribed.

6. The **superscription** is the Rx symbol located on every prescription.

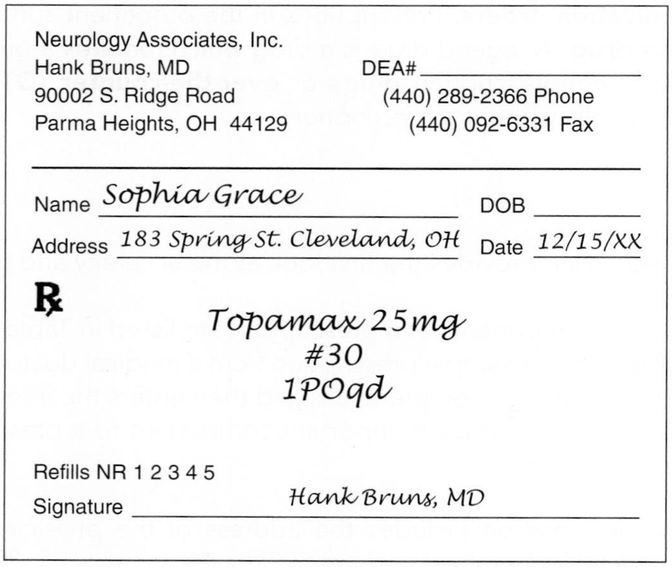

```
┌─────────────────────────────────────────────────┐
│  Neurology Associates, Inc.                       │
│  Hank Bruns, MD              DEA#_____   │
│  90002 S. Ridge Road           (440) 289-2366 Phone│
│  Parma Heights, OH  44129      (440) 092-6331 Fax │
│  _____ │
│  Name  Sophia Grace              DOB _____       │
│  Address 183 Spring St. Cleveland, OH  Date 12/15/XX│
│  ℞                                                 │
│              Topamax 25 mg                         │
│                  #30                               │
│                1 PO qd                             │
│                                                    │
│  Refills NR 1 2 3 4 5                              │
│  Signature _____ Hank Bruns, MD _____ │
└─────────────────────────────────────────────────┘
```

This figure is for educational and illustrative purposes only and is not intended to promote or endorse any specific product or organization.

FIGURE 6-2 Patient's prescription.

7. The **subscription** is the part of the prescription which lists directions to the pharmacist. These could include specific labeling requirements or instructions or refill information.

8. Directions to the patient are known as the **signa** or more commonly **sig** for short. This is the code that is translated from the prescription to the label into a more easily read format for the patient.

9. DAW is dispense as written. A prescriber will indicate this if they specifically want the brand name product to be dispensed. Patients may also request the brand name product be dispensed even when a generic is available, (and acceptable by the physician). These situations are discussed more in Chapter 9 discussing insurance billing.

10. Each prescriber must sign the prescription legibly not just able to be recognized. If a prescription is faxed, the signature may be electronic for all medications except controlled substances.

Intake, Interpretation, and Data Entry

In the outpatient setting, technicians are responsible for completing the steps to ensure proper prescription processing. This begins with receipt of a prescription from the patient or patient's representative. It is important for a technician to gather as much information during this step as possible.

A pharmacy technician is also responsible for updating and maintaining the patient profile. There are many important pieces of information that should be gathered from the patient, and maintained as the patient continues to fill medications. Some typical information on the patient profile includes the following:

- Patient's name (including middle initial and Jr./Sr. for verification purposes)
- Date of birth
- Home address and working phone number where patient can be reached
- Insurance and billing information
- Allergies
- Diagnoses
- Any OTC medications currently being taken by the patient
- Preferences for easy-off caps

After a technician has updated the profile, he or she will then enter the prescription information into the computer system. The technician should verify the correct drug, strength, and dose was entered into the system, carefully double-checking against the original prescription.

When entering prescription information into the system, most pharmacy software programs will recognize certain abbreviations for directions, to help simplify and speed up the order entry process. These are referred to as **sig codes,** and although the exact abbreviation may differ depending on the pharmacy, most follow a similar format (Tables 6-2, 6-3, 6-4 and 6-5).

Error-Prone Abbreviations

As discussed in Chapter 5, although you may still encounter these abbreviations, the Institute for Safe Medication Practices considers the following abbreviations as being frequently misinterpreted and involved in medication errors. A pharmacy

* *TECH ALERT: It is important to ask for help when reading an order that is difficult to interpret. You should never **assume** when reading prescriptions. The pharmacist relies on your knowledge to help keep patients safe. Always ask "What do you see" rather than "Do you see this?"*

TABLE 6-2. Medication Administration Abbreviations	
Abbreviation	*Meaning*
qd	Once daily
bid	Twice daily
tid	Three times daily
qid	Four times daily
ac	Before meals
pc	After meals
qam	Every morning
qpm	Every evening
qhs	Every night at bedtime (hs = hour of sleep)
q4h	Every 4 hours (can be substituted with any hour amount)
STAT	Immediately
qod	Every other day
a	Before
c	With
h, hr	Hour
PRN	As needed
qs	Sufficient quantity
Dx	Diagnosis
Tx	Treatment
Sx	Symptoms

technician should take great care when reading prescriptions that use any dangerous abbreviations. Table 6-6 lists a few examples of commonly used dangerous abbreviations.

QUICK QUIZ 6-1

1. Which part of the prescription contains the medication name and strength?

2. What is the abbreviation for twice daily?

3. What is a prescription called in the hospital setting?

4. What does the abbreviation gtt mean?

5. What part of the prescription contains the directions to the patient?

TABLE 6-3.	Dosage Forms and Route of Administration Abbreviations
Abbreviation	Meaning
AD	Right ear
Amp	Ampule
AS	Left ear
AU	Both ears
Cap	Capsule
Cmpd	Compound
cr	Cream
gtt	Drop
ID	Intradermally
IM	Intramuscularly
IV	Intravenously
liq	Liquid
lot	Lotion
MDI	Metered dose inhaler
NPO	Nothing by mouth
OD	Right eye
OS	Left eye
OU	Both eyes
PO	By mouth
PR, rec	Per rectum, rectally
PV, vag	Per vagina, vaginally
SL	Sublingual (dissolve under the tongue)
supp	Suppository
Syr	Syrup
Tab	Tablet
ung	Ointment

PHARMACY DOSAGE CALCULATIONS

When entering the prescription information into the pharmacy system, a technician must often perform certain calculations to determine proper dosages, amount to dispense, or days supply. Often, the prescriber will indicate the amount to dispense in Roman numerals. Or possibly the prescriber could specify the number of days a medication is to be given and the dosage taken, but the pharmacy must determine the quantity to dispense based on this information. A technician must perform these calculations carefully and swiftly to provide excellent and safe customer service to our patients.

★ *TECH ALERT: Remember, if a prescription is written for a controlled substance, the numerical number and written quantity must **both** be written on the prescription, for example, #20 (twenty).*

TABLE 6-4. **Measuring Quantities**	
Abbreviation	*Meaning*
tsp	Teaspoon
tbsp	Tablespoon
mL	Milliliter
L	Liter
g	Gram
mg	Milligram
kg	Kilogram
μg	Microgram
mEq	Milliequivalent
lb	Pound
gr	Grain
oz	Ounce
fl oz	Fluid ounce

TABLE 6-5. **Medication Abbreviatons**	
Abbreviation	*Meaning*
NS	Normal saline
DW	Distilled water
D5W	Dextrose 5% in water
LR	Lactated Ringer
NaCl	Sodium chloride
PCN	Penicillin
MOM	Milk of magnesia
ASA	Aspirin
EC	Enteric coated
MVI	Multivitamin
NTG	Nitroglycerin
$FeSO_4$	Ferrous sulfate
SMZ-TMP	Sulfamethoxazole and trimethoprim

A prescription is brought into the pharmacy with the directions take 2 tablets bid × 7 days. In order to calculate how many tablets the patient will need, we first need to calculate how many tablets the patient will be taking in 1 day. We can do this by multiplying the dose by the frequency of administration.

TABLE 6-6. **Dangerous Abbreviations**		
Abbreviation	Intended Meaning	Misinterpretation
AD	Right ear	Right eye
AS	Left ear	Left eye
AU	Both ears	Both eyes
OD	Right eye	Right ear
OS	Left eye	Left ear
OU	Both eyes	Both ears
qd	Every day	qid
qhs	Every night at bedtime	qhr (every hour)
qod	Every other day	qd or qid
SC, SQ	Subcutaneous	SC = SL (sublingual), SQ = 5 every
HCTZ	Hydrochlorothiazide	Hydrocortisone
$MgSO_4$	Magnesium sulfate	Morphine sulfate
MSO_4	Morphine sulfate	Magnesium sulfate

> Dose = 2 tablets
> Frequency = bid (twice daily)
> 2 tablets × 2 daily = **4 tablets daily**

To determine the total quantity needed for this prescription, we will multiply our daily quantity by the number of days of therapy.

> Daily amount = 4 tablets
> Days of therapy = 7 days
> 4 tablets × 7 days = **28 total tablets needed**

We can also calculate the **days supply** of a medication, which is the number of days a medication should last if it is used correctly. This is an important quantity to determine for insurance and third party payers that have limits to how much they will cover in a specified period.

A prescription is written for ampicillin 500 mg 1 cap qid #28. What is the days supply of this medication? Another way to look at this would be, how long will this medication last if the patient takes each dose properly? To find the days supply, first determine how many units will be taken in 1 day.

> Dose = 1 capsule
> Frequency = qid (4 times daily)
> 1 capsule × 4 times daily = **4 capsules daily**

Next to determine the amount of days this medication will last, divide the total quantity dispensed by the daily quantity taken.

> Daily amount = 4 capsules
> Amount of medication to dispense = 28 capsules
> 28 capsules ÷ 4 capsules = **7 days supply**

The same calculations can be done for liquid dosages as well. Remember the conversions for household volumes:

1 teaspoonful	5 mL
1 tablespoonful	15 mL

If a prescription calls for a suspension to be given 1 tsp tid × 10 days and the prescriber writes QS on the prescription, the pharmacy must determine the total volume to dispense for a quantity sufficient (QS) for the entire therapy. The same process is done as with any solid dosage form. First find the quantity taken in 1 day and then multiply this by the total days to determine the total volume needed.

Dosage = 1 tsp = 5 mL

Frequency = tid = 3 times daily

5 mL × 3 times daily = 15 mL daily

15 mL daily × 10 total days = 150 mL

150 mL needed for 10 days of therapy

The same can be done for days supply. If a prescription calls for a medication to be taken 2 tbsp bid, dispense 300 mL, how long will this order last the patient?

Dosage = 2 tbsp = 30 mL

Frequency = bid = twice daily

30 mL × twice daily = 60 mL daily

300 mL ÷ 60 mL = **5 days supply**

Additionally, technicians may need to calculate days supply and dosages with calculations involving insulin. The standard concentration for most insulin **100 units per every 1 mL.** Insulin vials are usually 10 mL (1,000 units) while insulin pens are usually 3 mL (300 units). Therefore, for example, if a patient is taking 20 units of insulin daily, and the pharmacy needs to calculate the days supply when dispensing 1 insulin vial, we can utilize the same concepts as before to determine this amount.

Dosage = 20 units

Frequency = daily

20 units per day

Total units per insulin vial = 100 units/1 mL × 10 mL vial = 1000 total units

1000 units/20 units per day = **50 days supply**

Technicians may also encounter days supply issues when dispensing eye- and eardrops. To solve days supply for these medications, it is essential to know how many drops are in 1 mL. This number varies based on the medication and physical properties of the solution or suspension. Therefore, for most insurance claims, pharmacies use the conversion **1 mL = 20 drops.** However, this is an estimation only so it should not be used for any dosage calculations, but merely an approximation of how long the medication will last the patient.

If a prescription is written for an eyedrop to be given 1 gtt OU qd, dispense 5 mL, what is the days supply?

Dosage = 1 gtt = 1 drop

Frequency = OU = both eyes = 2 drops daily

2 drops daily

$$\text{Total drops per bottle} = \frac{20 \text{ drops}}{1 \text{ mL}} = \frac{X \text{ drops}}{5 \text{ mL}}$$

100 drops total in 5 mL

100 drops/2 drops daily = **50 days supply**

QUICK QUIZ 6-2

1. If a prescription is written for amoxicillin 1 cap tid × 10 days, how many capsules should be dispensed?

2. A prescription is written for Omnicef suspension to be given 1 tsp qd, dispense 50 mL. What is the days supply for this medication?

3. An order is written for Bactrim suspension 3 tsp bid × 10 days QS. How much should be dispensed to this patient?

4. If a patient is given a prescription for an eyedrop to be given 1 gtt OU qid, dispense 10 mL, what is the days supply for this bottle?

5. If a patient is getting 25 units bid of insulin, is 1 vial enough to last them 30 days?

LABELING REQUIREMENTS

After the order has been entered into the pharmacy system, a label will be generated with the key information from the prescription. There are legal requirements for components of the prescription label (Figure 6-3). The required label information includes the following:

- Pharmacy's name and address
- Pharmacy's phone number
- Computer-generated prescription number (Rx number)
- Date when the prescription was filled
- Patient's name
- Directions for use of medication
- Name and strength of medication
- Quantity of medication dispensed
- If generic is filled, name of the drug manufacturer
- Refill information
- Name of the prescribing physician
- Initials of the pharmacist verifying the prescription

In addition to the prescription label, **auxiliary labels** can be used to provide additional warnings to patients. These labels can help communicate directions on administration, storage information, or special instructions that a patient may be unaware of. Auxiliary labels are brightly colored to stand out on the prescription bottle (Figures 6-4 and 6-5).

Neurology Associates, Inc.
Hank Bruns, MD   DEA#_____
90002 S. Ridge Road   (440) 289-2366 Phone
Parma Heights, OH 44129   (440) 092-6331 Fax

_____

Name *Sophia Grace*_____ DOB_____

Address *183 Spring St. Cleveland, OH* Date *12/15/XX*

℞   *Topamax 25 mg*
                      #30
                    1 PO qd

Refills NR 1 ②3 4 5

Signature _____*Dr. Hank Bruns, MD*_____

This figure is for educational and illustrative purposes only and is not intended
to promote or endorse any specific product or organization.

FIGURE 6-3 Prescription.

The Drug Store   **KAM**
330-339-4563 ~ 4249 Engle Dr.~ Cleveland, OH 44125

Rx # 6492182   **Date:** 12/20/20XX
Name: Sophia Grace
183 Spring St. Cleveland, OH 44125

TAKE ONE TABLET BY MOUTH EVERY DAY

Topiramate 25 mg (Teva) generic for Topamax 25 mg tablet
Quantity 30
Dr. Hank Bruns   2 refills remain before March 20XX

This figure is for educational and illustrative purposes only and is not intended to promote or endorse
any specific product or organization.

FIGURE 6-4 Prescription bottle label.

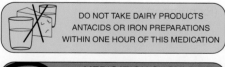
DO NOT TAKE DAIRY PRODUCTS ANTACIDS OR IRON PREPARATIONS WITHIN ONE HOUR OF THIS MEDICATION

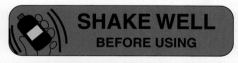
SHAKE WELL BEFORE USING

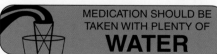
MEDICATION SHOULD BE TAKEN WITH PLENTY OF WATER

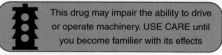
This drug may impair the ability to drive or operate machinery. USE CARE until you become familier with its effects

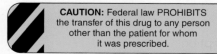
CAUTION: Federal law PROHIBITS the transfer of this drug to any person other than the patient for whom it was prescribed.

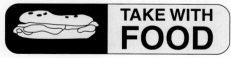
TAKE WITH FOOD

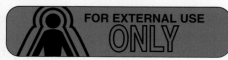
FOR EXTERNAL USE ONLY

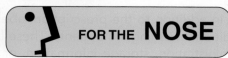
FOR THE NOSE

FIGURE 6-5 Auxiliary labels.

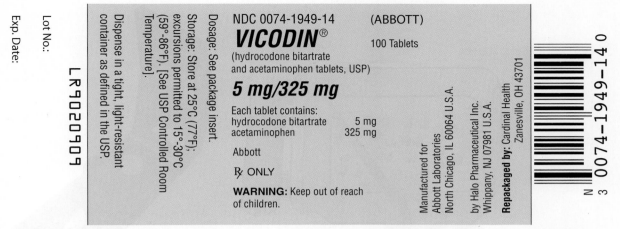

This figure is for educational and illustrative purposes only and is not intended to promote or endorse any specific product or organization.

FIGURE 6-6 Stock bottle label.

FILL PROCESS

The fill process is a multi-step process that requires attention to detail to ensure accuracy. After the label has printed, it should be verified against the original prescription to check for any discrepancies. The technician then pulls the appropriate medication from the shelf and, using the National Drug Code (NDC) number from the stock bottle, verifies that the correct medication was selected. A technician should never assume the correct stock bottle was chosen, and compare only the drug name and strength with the label (Figure 6-6).

The stock label on the bottle will give pertinent information that is essential for technicians in many situations.

1. NDC number
2. Brand name, generic name in parentheses
3. Manufacturer
4. Dosage form
5. Lot number
6. Expiration date
7. Strength per unit
8. Bar code
9. Rx only label
10. Storage requirements

If the medication is a solid dosage form, such as a tablet or capsule, a **counting tray** will be used to transfer the drug from its stock bottle to the prescription container (Figure 6-7). Medications are generally counted in multiples of 5. A counting tray and spatula should be cleaned with 70% isopropyl alcohol to prevent cross contamination of medications, especially those which leave a powder residue. Because of the severity and frequency of patient allergies, it should always be cleaned after counting sulfa or penicillin drugs.

Occasionally, patients may be prescribed half-tablets. In this case, the pharmacy may direct the patient to purchase a **tablet splitter** (also referred to as a pill cutter) to cleanly split the tablets, especially those which are **scored** (Figure 6-8).

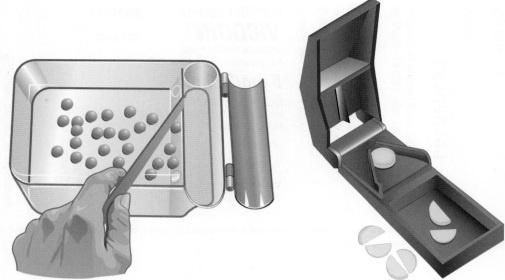

FIGURE 6-7 Counting tray.   FIGURE 6-8 Tablet splitter.

A scored tablet is one which has a line through the center, allowing the tablet to be easily split in 2 (Figure 6-9).

Pharmacy vials (Figure 6-10) come in several different sizes, and the vial chosen for each prescription should be the smallest size which can hold the medication without overfilling. The vials are arranged based on quantity held using the apothecary dram system. They range in size from 6 to 60 drams and are generally amber in color. The amber vials are light resistant which protects medications from contamination due to excessive light transmission.

A technician will fill the pharmacy vial with the medication and then select the appropriate lid. If a patient or physician has requested easy-off caps, the prescription will not be child resistant. Patients will receive child-resistant caps unless they have requested otherwise by signing a waiver. This document is kept on file within the pharmacy, as well as listed on the patient profile for future prescription filling. Certain medications are permitted to be dispensed with a nonchildproof lid, such as oral contraceptives, inhalation aerosols, and sublingual nitroglycerin.

For liquid medications, pharmacy bottles are measured in fluid ounces, and generally range in size from 2 to 16 oz (Figure 6-11). These bottles are also amber colored to protect liquid medications from exposure to ultraviolet (UV) light.

Medications can also come in **unit-of-use** packaging, which is provided by the manufacturer in the most commonly dispensed unit (Figure 6-12). The package is simply labeled with the pharmacy label, without any further modifications, eliminating the need to do any counting and thus minimizing the risk of human error. Examples of

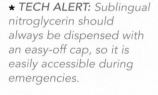

★ *TECH ALERT: Sublingual nitroglycerin should always be dispensed with an easy-off cap, so it is easily accessible during emergencies.*

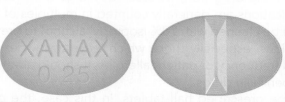

This figure is for educational and illustrative purposes only and is not intended to promote or endorse any specific product or organization.
FIGURE 6-9 Scored tablet.

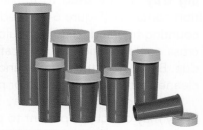

FIGURE 6-10 Pharmacy vials.

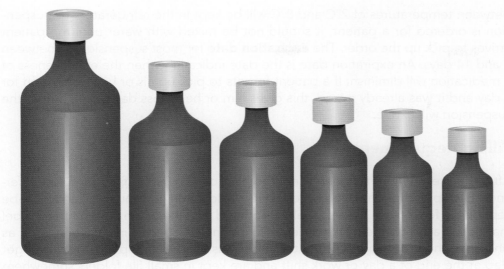

FIGURE 6-11 Pharmacy bottles.

unit-of-use packaging include manufactured bottles of 30 for a medication taken daily, oral contraceptives, or monthly packs of osteoporosis or antidepressant medications.

After the medication has been counted carefully and properly filled into the appropriately sized container, the label is applied to the vial and the prescription is sent to the pharmacist for final verification. Each prescription must be checked by a pharmacist before being dispensed to the patient. A technician should always ask the patient if they would like counseling from the pharmacist, or have any questions in regards to their prescription. In every pharmacy, there is a special consultation area which is a secluded space for the pharmacist to have a private conversation with a patient.

When an order is being prepared, a patient may decide to wait for the prescription or return later for pickup. It is important that regardless of who picks up the order, the correct patient is verified to ensure the right medication is delivered to the right person. Additionally, most insurance providers will request a signature of the person receiving the medication and depending on the coverage of the patient, a co-payment may be due.

A technician should also be mindful of where a prescription is stored while waiting to be picked up. Prescriptions stored at room temperature are generally alphabetized by last name in a specific holding area. Drugs that require storage

★ *TECH ALERT: Some examples of common drugs that are stored in the refrigerator include insulin, NuvaRing, Xalatan, and certain suppositories and vaccines.*

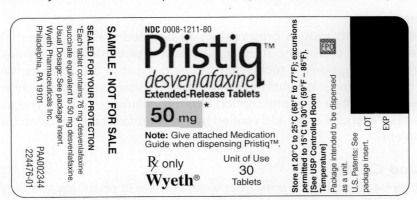

This figure is for educational and illustrative purposes only and is not intended to promote or endorse any specific product or organization.

FIGURE 6-12 Unit-of-use packaging.

between temperatures of 2°C and 8°C will be kept in the refrigerator. If a suspension is ordered for a patient, it should not be mixed with water until the patient arrives to pick up the order. The **expiration date** for most suspensions is between 7 and 14 days. An expiration date is the date indicating when the effectiveness of a medication will diminish. If a patient forgets to pick up his or her suspension for a day and it was already mixed, this gives him or her 1 less day of use before the suspension will expire.

Filling Requirements

After the prescription has been filled, the hard copy must be filed for future reference. Each prescription is filed based on its prescription or Rx number, and must be kept on file for at least 3 years. A label is printed with the original prescription label that gets placed on the back of the prescription with specific information, such as who filled the order and the date the order was filled. Prescriptions generally get filed at the end of a day or work shift and are kept in small file folders somewhere within the pharmacy grounds. If the prescription is a schedule-II controlled substance, it must be filed separately. Additionally, some states require schedule-III to -V medications to be filed separately, or the prescription to be stamped with a red "C" if filed within the other noncontrolled prescriptions.

Other Types of Orders

In the outpatient setting, a technician may be responsible for filling prescriptions other than those received directly from a patient or prescriptions that may require special handling.

Refills
A pharmacy technician may take refill requests over the phone or in person from a patient or patient's representative. In order to process the refill, a technician must have the prescription (Rx) number or patient's name and name and strength of medication. Refills are issued on the original prescription by the prescriber. If a patient has no refills remaining at the time of ordering, the pharmacy may contact the prescriber for additional refills. Sometimes the patient is out of refills because he/she is required to return to the physician for a follow-up appointment before continuing on the treatment regimen. If this is the case, the pharmacy would notify the patient to make an appointment before dispensing any refill orders.

Transfers
Many times patients require prescriptions to be filled that have been filled previously at another pharmacy. Although by law, a pharmacist is responsible for transferring prescriptions, a technician can help assist in this process. When the transfer has been received and transcribed by the pharmacist, the technician can enter the order in as a new prescription into the pharmacy system. The transfer is then filled like a regular order and verified by the pharmacist before being dispensed to the patient.

Faxes and Call-Ins
Orders may be faxed from a prescriber to an outpatient pharmacy, although this is more common in the inpatient setting. A faxed order is treated like a new prescription, and a technician may enter the order into the pharmacy system as long as they have all the patient information updated on the patient profile.

If a prescriber or nurse calls in a prescription, the order must be taken over the phone by a registered pharmacist only (some states also allow a pharmacy intern to record phoned-in prescriptions). Similar to a transfer, after the pharmacist has transcribed the order over the phone, the technician can then enter the order into the system as a new prescription to be filled.

Controlled Substances

The Controlled Substance Act permits the refilling of schedule-III to -V controlled substances a maximum amount of 5 times within 6 months. For schedule-II drugs, no refills are permitted, and a patient is required to bring a new prescription in for every C-II order. If a patient brings in a new prescription for a controlled substance, the pharmacy technician must help verify that the prescription is legal. A valid DEA number must be written on the prescription and if any forgeries are suspected, the technician should discretely bring these to the attention of the pharmacist for further inspection.

INPATIENT ORDER ENTRY PROCESS

Pharmacy technicians are also utilized in inpatient pharmacy systems, such as long-term care or hospital pharmacies. In these settings, medication orders are used in place of a prescription to communicate which medications and/or services are required for the patient. Although duties will vary by institution, most hospital pharmacists will enter medication orders to be filled by pharmacy technicians. Alternatively, some orders can be entered by the prescriber into the computer system directly. This is known as **computer physician order entry (CPOE).** This process helps assist in patient care and medication safety.

Parts of the Medication Order

More information is required on a medication order than on a prescription. The order should contain the following information:

- Date and time of order
- Patient's name
- Patient's date of birth
- Room number and bed number
- Medical or hospital record number
- Name and dose of drug
- Specific directions for use
- Route of administration and dosage form
- Frequency of administration
- Prescriber's name and signature or signature of person writing the order

Patient health information is also available. While this information will not be available on every medication order, it will be easily accessible during medication order processing.

- Allergies
- Height and weight
- Diagnosis or medical condition

> ★ *TECH ALERT: Remember the following methods for checking DEA numbers:*
>
> 1. *Add together the first, third, and fifth digits.*
> 2. *Add together the second, fourth, and sixth digits. Double this amount.*
> 3. *Add the totals from step 1 and 2 together.*
> 4. *The last digit in that total should match the last digit in the DEA number.*

There are different types of orders that may be encountered within the inpatient setting. When a patient is first admitted to the hospital, an **admitting order** is written which contains previous medications being taken, new medications being ordered, any laboratory or diagnostic tests desired by the physician, and a suspected diagnosis. A **STAT order** is written for a medication that is needed immediately for an emergency or serious medical condition. Some orders are given as **scheduled orders** or at the same time every day, based on the directions from the physician. Other orders are **PRN orders,** which are given only as needed or in response to a defined condition or parameter. Additional orders may be given upon leaving the hospital. These are known as **discharge orders,** and include any prescribed medicines the patient should continue taking until they are able to follow up with their primary care physician.

Inpatient Fill Process

After the order has been entered and verified by a pharmacist, a label is printed to be filled for the patient. In the hospital pharmacy, there are several possible methods of filling an order for a patient.

Unit Dose Distribution System

A **unit dose** is a medication that has been prepackaged for a single-dose administration. Most tablets and capsules are repackaged into unit doses, and some liquids are available as well. The **unit dose drug distribution system** is a way for patients to receive their medication from the pharmacy. In this system, the pharmacy utilizes a **unit dose cart** with drawers for each patient. The pharmacy receives the orders, and usually stocks a 24-hour supply of medication in each drawer. The nurses can then retrieve medications from the drawers prior to administration. When a medication is administered by a nurse, it is indicated on the patient's **medication administration record, or MAR.** Every time a patient receives a medication, the MAR is updated to reflect what time the medication was given and who administered the dose.

An additional type of unit dose system is known as a **modified unit dose.** Also known as bingo or blister cards, this system packages one medication into a card with a month's supply of a medication instead of 1 dose. Another unit dose system, known as the **blended unit dose,** packages all of the patient's medications that will be taken at the same time for easy dispensing.

Some medications are not always prepared in unit dose form and this may require the pharmacy staff to repackage medications. The packaging of unit doses must ensure stability of the drug and provide an airtight and light-resistant environment. In addition, proper labeling of repackaged medications is essential for patient safety. Unit doses that have been repackaged in the hospital pharmacy should include the following:

- Drug's name
- Drug's strength
- Dosage form
- Name of the manufacturer
- Lot number
- Expiration date
- Bar code for identification purposes

Automated Dispensing Cabinets

Automation is instrumental to hospital pharmacies in helping to reduce errors while also improving medication turnaround time. **Automated dispensing cabinets or ADCs** are present in many hospitals to help facilitate patient medication administration. In these systems, a storage cabinet contains medications needed for patients in specific nursing units. The system is connected through the pharmacy software, and an order can be sent to the automated machine so a nurse knows exactly which medication to retrieve for each patient. The cabinets contain additional measures and safety procedures to ensure the correct drug is selected for the correct patient. This is essential for medication and patient safety. Some examples of ADCs in hospital pharmacies are Pyxis, Omnicell, Medselect, and RxStation. Although each offers its own advantages, the main advantage lies in the safety of the patients and the ability to offer efficient and safe practices for the nursing staff.

CASE STUDY REVIEW

A patient brings a prescription into the pharmacy. You attempt to read the directions as appear in Figure 6-1.

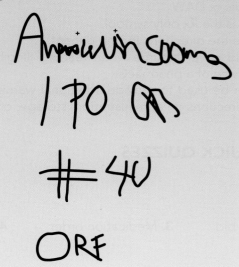

Self-Assessment Questions

- What is this drug written for and what is the strength?
  - You can tell this drug is 500 mg, but is it amoxicillin or ampicillin?
- What are the directions?
  - Do the directions say to dispense 1 PO qid or qd? Four times a day and once daily are 2 very different dosages!
- How many should be dispensed and are refills permitted?
  - Does this say #40 or #4 U as in 4 units? If a dosage is being taken by mouth, it will not be dispensed in units so we can conclude this is a quantity of 40. We can also conclude that there are no refills.

At this point, we would need to consult with the pharmacist and possibly call the physician for confirmation. This prescription is written for an antibiotic, so we can assume we are not taking it once a day, as this would have the patient taking an antibiotic for 40 days, which is highly unlikely. Instead, having a patient taking an antibiotic

4 times daily with a quantity of 40 would give an exactly days supply of 10—a much more likely scenario, but we should check with the pharmacist to make sure.

Is this drug amoxicillin or ampicillin? Although it is hard to tell, ampicillin is usually dosed 4 times daily, whereas amoxicillin is generally given just 3 times a day. After confirmation with the pharmacist and the prescriber's office, it is indeed ampicillin 500 mg, 4 times daily, dispense #40, and no refills.

CHAPTER SUMMARY

- An important task of pharmacy technicians is maintaining the patient profile and ensuring all patient information is current and accurate including insurance information, allergies, and current medications.
- A prescription is the order for a patient in the outpatient setting and a medication order is written for the inpatient setting.
- The inscription is the part of the prescription that contains the name and strength of the medication and the amount prescribed.
- The subscription is the part of the prescription with the directions to the pharmacist, such as refills or DAW.
- The superscription is the Rx only symbol.
- The signa or sig are the directions for the patient.
- A technician should never assume when reading illegible prescriptions and always seek the advice of a pharmacist.
- Auxiliary labels can be used to provide additional warnings or information to patients, such as directions on administration, storage, or special instructions.

ANSWERS TO QUICK QUIZZES

Quick Quiz 6-1

1. Inscription   **2.** bid   **3.** Medication order   **4.** Drop   **5.** Signa

Quick Quiz 6-2

1. 30 capsules   **2.** 10 days   **3.** 300 mL   **4.** 25 days   **5.** No, it will last them 20 days

CHAPTER QUESTIONS

1. Which of the following may a technician be responsible for in the retail pharmacy setting?
a. Entering prescriptions into the computer
b. Updating the patient profile
c. Counting medications on a counting tray
d. All of the above

2. Which of the following may a technician *never* do?
a. Enter prescriptions into the computer
b. Counsel patients
c. Update insurance information
d. Take a refill over the phone

40/50 = 80   39/50 = 78   10 wrong

3. Which of the following is the abbreviation for grain?
   a. g
   b. gr
   c. kg
   d. mg

4. A patient is ordered 25 mg of hydroxyzine to be taken tid for 20 days. How many capsules should be dispensed for this order, if the pharmacy stocks 25 mg capsules?
   a. 30 capsules
   b. 40 capsules
   c. 50 capsules
   d. 60 capsules

5. If a prescriber orders an MDI, this would be for which of the following?
   a. Multivitamin
   b. Metered-dose inhaler
   c. Multidrug inspection
   d. Multidrug inhalation

6. Calculate the days supply if a patient is taking ciprofloxacin PO bid #14.
   a. 7 days
   b. 10 days
   c. 14 days
   d. 20 days

7. What is an order written for a medication in the outpatient setting?
   a. Prescription
   b. Medication order
   c. Admission order
   d. Legend drug

8. Medications that can be legally dispensed without a prescription are known as which of the following?
   a. Legend drugs
   b. Over-the-counter (OTC) drugs
   c. Controlled substances
   d. None of the above

9. When is the prescriber's DEA number required on prescriptions?
   a. All the time
   b. Never
   c. On prescriptions for all controlled medications only
   d. On prescriptions for C-II medications only

10. What is the part of the prescription that contains the inscription?
    a. Directions to the pharmacist
    b. Directions to the patient
    c. The Rx symbol
    d. The amount of medication prescribed, quantity, and strength

11. What is the abbreviation for symptoms?
    a. supp
    b. Sx
    c. STAT
    d. ac

12. How would a prescriber indicate if a medication was not to be substituted with generic?
    a. No refills
    b. DAW
    c. Superscription
    d. Inscription

13. When can a medication that is scheduled III–IV be refilled?
    a. Never
    b. As many times as the patient needs
    c. Up to 5 times within 6 months
    d. Up to 6 times within a year

14. Which of the following information may be found on a patient profile?
    a. Allergy information
    b. Checking account number
    c. Credit score
    d. Social security number

15. What are abbreviations for directions written on a prescription?
    a. Diagnosis codes
    b. Sig codes
    c. Patient profile
    d. Inscriptions

16. If a prescription states to take 1 tablet QAM, then how should the medication be given?
    a. Every day in the evening
    b. Every day in the afternoon
    c. Every day at bedtime
    d. Every day in the morning

17. When a patient is taking a medication PRN, how is the patient taking the medication?
    a. Rectally
    b. As needed
    c. Every 6 hours
    d. None of the above

18. When a prescriber writes an order for a liquid medication, and specifies a quantity of QS. How much liquid should be dispensed?
    a. Quantity sufficient
    b. Dispense as written
    c. Quality standards
    d. Quinapril suspension

19. What is the abbreviation amp stands for?
    a. Drop
    b. Ointment
    c. Ampule
    d. Lotion

20. If an IV solution is to be compounded in D5W it should be made in which of the following?
    a. Dextrose 5% in sodium chloride
    b. Dextrose 5% in water
    c. Dextrose in normal saline
    d. Lactated Ringer

21. Solid dosage forms, such as tablets and capsules, are transferred from the stock bottle to the prescription container using which of the following?
    a. Oral syringe
    b. Counting tray
    c. Ointment slab
    d. Gloved hand

22. Which of the following medications is permitted to be dispensed in nonchildproof containers?
    a. Ibuprofen
    b. Oxycodone
    c. Atenolol
    d. Sublingual nitroglycerin

23. Who is responsible for final verification of the prescription?
    a. A pharmacy technician
    b. A pharmacist only
    c. The insurance company
    d. The prescriber

24. What is an expiration date?
    a. The date which indicates when the drug was dispensed
    b. The date which indicates when the drug was manufactured
    c. The date which indicates when the drug will no longer be effective
    d. None of the above

25. What is the abbreviation for teaspoon?
    a. tbsp
    b. Tx
    c. tp
    d. tsp

26. Which of the following medications would be stored in the refrigerator?
    a. Lantus
    b. Metoprolol tablets
    c. Amoxicillin capsules
    d. Nexium capsules

27. What is a medication that is prepackaged for a single-dose administration?
    a. Unit-of-use
    b. Stat order
    c. Unit dose
    d. ADC

28. What is a device used to halve tablets for patients taking half-tablet doses?
    a. Counting tray
    b. Tablet splitter
    c. Auxiliary label
    d. Inscription

29. Calculate the days supply if a patient is taking Zantac 300 mg #60 1 PO bid.
    a. 15 days
    b. 30 days
    c. 60 days
    d. 90 days

30. When should the following medication be taken: Lunesta 1 PO qhs?
    a. Every morning
    b. At bedtime
    c. Every day at lunch
    d. Every day at breakfast

31. What is the abbreviation for liter?
    a. mL
    b. L
    c. gr
    d. Liq

32. Which of the following parts of the prescription would contain the refill information?
    a. Inscription
    b. Superscription
    c. Subscription
    d. Signa

33. How many tablets should be dispensed for the following prescription: Plavix 1 PO qd #XXX
    a. 15 tablets
    b. 30 tablets
    c. 45 tablets
    d. 60 tablets

34. What is an order written for a medication in the hospital setting?
    a. Prescription
    b. Controlled substance
    c. Medication order
    d. Inscription

35. If a patient was taking a medication q8h, how many times per day would this medication be taken?
    a. 2
    b. 3
    c. 4
    d. 5

36. You receive an order for a prescription for a cough medicine that is to be given 1 tsp qid × 10 days QS. How much should be dispensed?
    a. 100 mL
    b. 150 mL
    c. 200 mL
    d. 250 mL

37. A patient has a prescription with the abbreviation ung. What route should this medication be administered?
    a. Orally
    b. Intravenously
    c. Rectally
    d. Topically

38. Which of the following is the abbreviation for sodium chloride?
    a. KCl
    b. PCN
    c. NaCl
    d. NS

39. If a patient is taking 25 units of insulin in the morning and 35 units in the evening, how long will 1 vial of Lantus last?
    a. 10 days
    b. 16 days
    c. 20 days
    d. 30 days

40. Which of the following is correct about superscription?
    a. Rx symbol
    b. Refill(s) amount
    c. Directions given to the patient
    d. Medication prescribed, quantity, and strength

41. What is the abbreviation for capsule?
    a. tab
    b. PO
    c. syr
    d. cap

42. What is a fl oz?
    a. Ounce
    b. Fluid ounce
    c. Dram
    d. Grain

43. If a patient receives 10 fl oz of medication, and is taking 1 tbsp bid, how long will the medication last?
    a. 5 days
    b. 7 days
    c. 10 days
    d. 15 days

44. What is the abbreviation for the word before?
    a. c
    b. a
    c. qs
    d. pc

45. Which type of medication order would be issued for a medication needed immediately?
    a. STAT order
    b. Discharge order
    c. PRN order
    d. Admitting order

46. A patient presents the following order, how many prednisone 10 mg tablets are needed?

    Take 60 mg × 2 days
    Take 50 mg × 1 day
    Take 40 mg × 2 days
    Take 30 mg × 1 day
    Take 20 mg × 2 days
    Take 10 mg × 1 day
    Take 5 mg × 2 days

    a. 28 tablets
    b. 32 tablets
    c. 34 tablets
    d. 36 tablets

47. What is a medication that requires a prescription?
    a. Legend drug
    b. Over-the-counter drug
    c. Behind-the-counter drug
    d. None of the above

48. If a prescription is written for ASA 325 mg, what should the pharmacy dispense?
    a. Acetaminophen 325 mg
    b. Advil 325 mg
    c. Aspirin 325 mg
    d. Allegra 325 mg

49. What are directions to the patient?
    a. Inscription
    b. Subscription
    c. Sig
    d. Superscription

50. OS is the abbreviation for which of the following?
    a. Right ear
    b. Left eye
    c. Both ears
    d. Left ear

Pharmacy Inventory Management

CHAPTER
7

PTCB KNOWLEDGE AREAS

7.1 Function and application of National Drug Code (NDC), lot numbers, and expiration dates

7.2 Formulary or approved/preferred product lists

7.3 Ordering and receiving processes (eg, maintaining par levels and rotating stock)

7.4 Storage requirements (eg, frozen, refrigerated, and room temperature)

7.5 Removal (eg, recalls, returns, outdates, and reverse distribution)

KEY TERMS

Average wholesale price (AWP): A suggested price assigned to each drug listed in various published pricing guides. Insurance companies reimburse pharmacies based on the AWP of the medication dispensed.

Discount: A percentage at which the selling price of an item is reduced. Discounts are usually taken on non-prescription merchandise or over-the-counter (OTC) products.

Dispensing fee: A charge for the services provided by the pharmacy, including overhead expenses, salaries, equipment cost, and a selected profit margin.

Expiration date: The length of time in which the medication retains optimal potency and stability.

Formulary: A list of preferred medications.

Inventory turnover rate: A method for measuring the overall effectiveness of purchasing and inventory control processes, equals total annual inventory purchases divided by cost of inventory on hand.

Invoice: A bill of sale for products ordered.

Lot numbers: A unique identifier assigned to each batch of medication produced at a given time.

Markup: The difference in price between the cost at which a business purchases a product and the price at which they sell it.

National Drug Code (NDC): A 10-digit product identifying code used for all drugs marketed in the United States.

New Drug Application (NDA): The process by which new drugs are proposed to the Food and Drug Administration (FDA) for approval to market and sell in the United States.

Periodic automatic replacement (PAR): The optimal amount of each item that should be stocked at any given time.

Prime vendor: The wholesaler from whom the pharmacy has committed to purchase the majority of its inventory.

Profit: Generating more revenue than expenses in business operations.

Purchase order (PO): A document used to purchase inventory containing information about the pharmacy, the vendor, and details about each of the products ordered.

Rotating stock: Moving the products with the shortest expiration date to the front of the shelf when stocking.

Usual and customary price (U&C): Cash price charged for a prescription if there is no insurance coverage.

Wholesaler (distributor): Company that carries a selection of medications, medical devices, and supplies.

CASE STUDY

You are working as a pharmacy technician in a retail pharmacy. You are in the process of filling the prescription of Figure 7-1.

Patient: Melanie Williams
Address: 24 Eastwood Lane Springfield, OH 43215

DOB: 3/3/1974

Lipitor 20mg
Sig i qhs
Disp #90

Refills: 3

Carla Black MD
Dr. Carla Black, MD

This figure is for educational and illustrative purposes only and is not intended to promote or endorse any specific product or organization.

FIGURE 7-1 Sample prescription.

Self-Assessment Questions
- How do you know which NDC of atorvastatin (Lipitor) to choose?
- Where will you find Lipitor stocked in the pharmacy?
- How do you handle the situation if there is not enough Lipitor in stock to fill the entire prescription?

INTRODUCTION

It takes an average of 12 years of research and over $300 million before a new drug reaches pharmacy shelves. Once on the shelf, pharmacy technicians can utilize certain required tools to ensure proper drug selection, inventory measures, and ordering and receiving processes. This chapter will discuss the process of drug creation and approval and continue the path of the drug to ordering from a wholesaler and receipt within the pharmacy. Additionally, general pharmacy business calculations will be discussed.

DRUG-APPROVAL PROCESS

A new drug faces over 3 years of laboratory testing before it can even be submitted to the FDA for approval to begin trials in humans. Once the FDA approves the

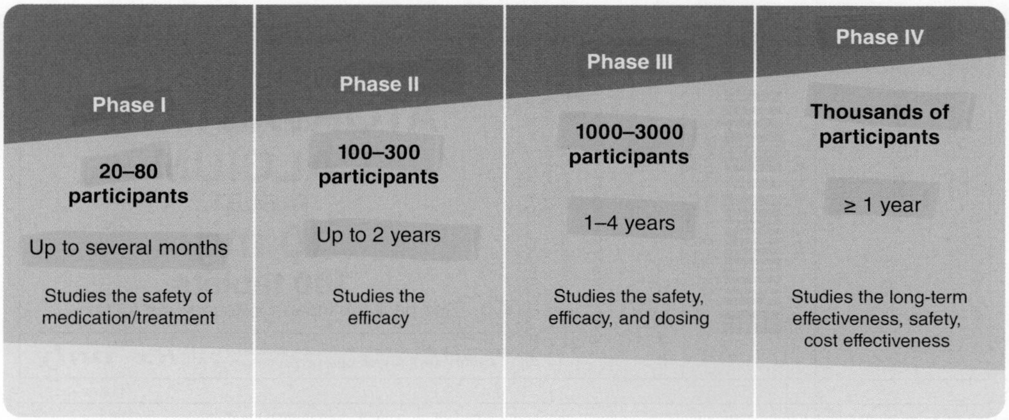

FIGURE 7-2 Phases of clinical trials.

investigational new drug, clinical trials can begin. Clinical trials include the 4 phases as given in Figure 7-2.

After the first 3 phases of clinical trials are complete, the pharmaceutical company submits an NDA to the FDA for final approval. The NDA contains all of the findings of the clinical trials in extensive detail. It can take several years for the NDA to be approved. Once the FDA approves the drug, it then becomes available for marketing and sale in the United States. But the work of a pharmaceutical company is still not done, as they must continue to monitor reports of adverse effects and other clinical data. This postmarketing surveillance for safety, efficacy, and cost-effectiveness is considered phase 4 of clinical trials.

Identifying Characteristics on Manufacturer Labels

The **National Drug Code (NDC)** is a product identifying code used for all drugs marketed in the United States. Every drug has a unique 11 digit NDC in a 5-4-2 format. The NDC is divided into 3 sections identifying the manufacturer, the product, and the package size. The first set of numbers is the labeler code. This is a unique code assigned by the FDA to all companies that manufacture or distribute medications. The second set of numbers, the product code, identifies the strength, dosage form, and formulation of the medication. The third set of numbers, the package code, identifies the package type and size.

The NDC is an important way of identifying medications. When dispensing a medication, one should always ensure that the NDC on the stock bottle matches the NDC on the prescription label. If the NDC does not match, it may indicate that the wrong product, strength, dosage form, or package size has been selected. Figure 7-3 illustrates how the NDC is displayed on a manufacturer's label.

During manufacturing, each medication is assigned a lot number for identification. **Lot numbers** are unique to each batch of medication produced at a given time. Lot numbers make it possible to identify when a particular tablet, capsule, or injectable was produced. This allows for easy tracking in the event that a problem occurs with a given batch, necessitating a product recall. Without lot numbers, a problem with one batch of medication would mean that every lot of that medication would need to be recalled, leaving the drug completely unavailable to patients. Lot numbers allow manufacturers to remove specific bottles that might be affected by a recall while keeping safe, effective products available to consumers.

★ *TECH ALERT: When converting from a 10 digit to an 11 digit NDC, add a zero in the section that is missing a number.*
For example:
9999-9999-99 = 0̲9999-9999-99
99999-999-99 = 99999-0̲999-99
99999-9999-9 = 99999-9999-0̲9

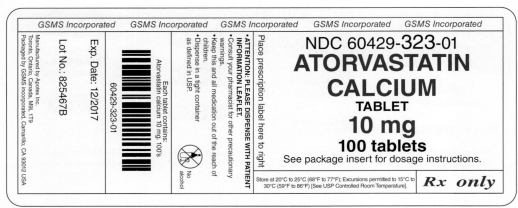

FIGURE 7-3 Identifying characteristics on a manufacturer's label.

Lot numbers are always included in the documentation of sterile or nonsterile compounding. This ensures that any affected compounded products can be isolated in the event of a recall. Lot numbers can be a range of lengths and may contain both letters and numbers. Figure 7-3 demonstrates how a lot number is displayed on a manufacturer's label.

Every medication is assigned an expiration date during the manufacturing process. The **expiration date** defines the length of time in which the medication retains the intended potency and stability. Medications typically expire 1 to 5 years after manufacturing. Medications should not be dispensed or consumed after the expiration date.

However, to ensure safety, most patient-specific pharmacy labels list the expiration date of the medication as one year after it was dispensed or the actual expiration date if it is shorter than one year.

Some expiration dates are expressed with month, date, and year of expiration. Others define only the month and year of expiration. When an expiration date lists only a month and year, the medication can be safely used through the last day of that month. For example, a drug with an expiration date of 8/15 should not be used after August 31, 2015. Figure 7-3 illustrates a manufacturer's label with an expiration date containing only the month and year.

INVENTORY MANAGEMENT

One of the primary responsibilities of a pharmacy technician is to maintain an appropriate inventory of medications in the pharmacy. This helps to ensure that there is an adequate supply of medications to dispense all prescriptions. Some pharmacies order stock manually, but most utilize electronic ordering systems. Either way, the pharmacy technician must be aware of the ordering and receiving process. Additionally, many pharmacies may utilize a perpetual inventory system, which reflects exactly what is on hand at that particular time. This system helps with the ordering process.

Each pharmacy has a master inventory list of all drugs, equipment, supplies, and specialty items on hand in the pharmacy. A complete or detailed pharmacy inventory should be conducted annually, although state law may specify otherwise. Additionally, an inventory must be conducted of all controlled substances when a new pharmacy opens or there is a change in the pharmacy director. A biennial inventory is required for controlled substances. Schedule II drugs must be counted, while schedule III through V drugs may be estimated.

Inventory turnover rate is a method for measuring the overall effectiveness of purchasing and inventory control processes. The inventory turnover rate represents the number of times the total pharmacy inventory is sold, or turned over, throughout the year. The inventory turnover rate is calculated by dividing the total cost of stock purchased in a year by the actual value of stock on the pharmacy shelves at any point in time. If the pharmacy spends $8,000,000 on drugs over 1 year, and the inventory on hand at the current time is $727,000, then the pharmacy's inventory turnover rate is approximately 11. This means the stock turns over 11 times over 1 year. Most pharmacies aim for a turn rate of approximately 15. A lower inventory turnover rate indicates that stock is sitting on the shelves for longer than desired, and tying up a larger amount of money than necessary. An inventory turnover rate higher than 15 might indicate that not enough stock is being ordered, leading to inefficient ordering processes and pharmacy stock-outs.

Ordering Processes

Medications may be obtained from several different sources. Pharmacies generally obtain most of their medications from a distributor, or **wholesaler.** Wholesalers carry a selection of medications, medical devices, and supplies. This makes it more efficient for the pharmacy because most of their products can be ordered from one location, limiting the amount of paperwork and number of deliveries required. Often wholesalers offer discounts in exchange for a pharmacy committing to order the majority of its stock (generally 80%-85%) from them. In this case, the wholesaler is referred to as the **prime vendor** for the pharmacy. Pharmacies might also order some medications directly from the manufacturer. This usually occurs when a medication is used in limited quantities or under special circumstances.

Additionally, pharmacies may pay to participate in a group purchasing organization (GPO). This is a company which helps negotiate discounts from wholesalers and other pharmacy suppliers. For example, a pharmacy may need to purchase a medication from a wholesaler, and pays $100 for this drug. But the same medication purchased by a pharmacy contracted with a GPO, may only cost the pharmacy $65.

The type of ordering completed by a pharmacy generally depends on the volume of prescriptions the pharmacy fills. Smaller pharmacies may utilize just-in-time ordering, which is a process that helps to minimize costs associated with having excessive inventory or product on the shelves. This method must be monitored continuously, to help prevent overlooking of a needed medication which may not get ordered. It also requires attention to drug shortages, as other larger organizations may be stockpiling shorted drugs.

Regardless of the ordering process, a **purchase order (PO)** is required when ordering medications, medical devices, or supplies. A purchase order contains identifying information about the pharmacy purchasing the products, the vendor selling the products, and details about each of the products ordered. The purchase order is usually assigned a number for tracking.

Once the purchase order is transmitted to the vendor, an invoice is generated. An **invoice** is a bill of sale for the products ordered. The information on the invoice should be carefully checked against the purchase order prior to submitting payment. Also, once the shipment is received in by the pharmacy, the order should be checked against the invoice to ensure the correct products were received.

Every pharmacy has an established amount of each medication to be kept on hand. This is referred to as the **periodic automatic replacement (PAR)** level. The PAR level is the optimal amount of a product that should be stocked at any time. When creating or revising PAR levels it is important to carefully consider the usage patterns of each individual medication. Medications that are used frequently, sometimes referred to as "fast movers," will have a high PAR level to ensure that the medication does not run out. Medications that are used infrequently, or "slow movers," will generally have a small PAR level to minimize the amount of stock kept on hand. If PAR levels are too low, the pharmacy will run out of stock frequently and may have to submit costly special orders to restock medications. If PAR levels are too high, there will be a large number of medications that expire on the shelves and the pharmacy will incur associated excessive inventory costs.

Similar to PAR levels, minimum and maximum (min/max) levels are determined for each medication for manual ordering; the minimum and maximum amount that should be on the shelf is known, so for ordering purposes, it is easy to determine how much of a product needs to be replenished.

Automated ordering systems utilize PAR levels and predetermined reorder points to create a purchase list. The benefits of electronic ordering systems include automated reports, product turnover rates, and maintenance of a perpetual inventory. However, electronic ordering systems are not flawless and the purchase list should be checked and verified by a pharmacy technician prior to submission.

Close attention should be paid to medications that run out of stock throughout the day. The ordering technician or purchaser must be sure that these medications are included in the subsequent order. Keeping medications in stock is crucial to pharmacy operations. Occasionally medications will run out of stock in the middle of filling a patient's prescription. When this occurs, the pharmacy fills a portion of the prescription and informs the patient of the date that he or she can come back to obtain the remainder of the prescription when the medication is back in stock.

When a medication runs out of stock, it is important to consider the nature of that medication. Is it an urgent medication that must be dispensed immediately when a patient presents a prescription? Is it a chronic medication in which the course of therapy should not be interrupted? Is it a "fast mover" medication that is dispensed to many patients? In these cases, it may be appropriate to ration the medication in the dispensing process. That is, fill just enough of the prescription to get each patient through until the medication is restocked and the remainder of their prescriptions can be filled. This helps ensure that each patient who presents a prescription can obtain the urgently required doses of the medication.

★ TECH ALERT: PAR levels must account for ordering, shipping, and receiving time from a pharmacy's prime vendor.

★ TECH ALERT: Medication stock-outs are a source of patient dissatisfaction, and keeping common medications in stock must be a priority.

★ TECH ALERT: "Partial fill" is a term used when a prescription cannot be completely filled due to lack of stock.

QUICK QUIZ 7-1

1. What is the inventory turnover rate if a pharmacy purchases $5,000,000 in inventory annually and has $400,000 worth of inventory currently on their shelves?

2. What is the inventory turnover rate if a pharmacy purchases $12,500,000 in inventory annually and has $920,000 worth of inventory currently on their shelves?

3. A retail pharmacy opened 1 year ago. So far, they have purchased $2,125,000 worth of inventory. There is currently $375,000 in inventory on their shelves. What was their inventory turnover rate in the first year?

4. What does the inventory turnover rate in question #3 say about the new pharmacy's inventory management?

5. What should the pharmacy do to help increase its turnover rate?

~~~~~~

Controlled Substance Ordering

There are special requirements for ordering and recording the purchase of controlled medications. Please review Chapter 2 for full details.

Receiving Processes

Proper receiving and stocking of medications is essential in maintaining pharmacy operations. During the receiving process, it is important to double check the items received against the invoice to be sure that all items were shipped correctly and in the appropriate quantities. Discrepancies in the items or quantities shipped should be verified against the purchase order and corrected as necessary. It is also important to inspect all received items for damage, defect, and expiration date. Generally, medications with short expiration dates are not accepted because it is unlikely they will be dispensed prior to outdating.

It is important to stock all medications in the appropriate location throughout the pharmacy. Some pharmacies are arranged alphabetically by medication brand name, some by generic name, and others by fast or slow movers. No matter which system a pharmacy uses, stocking medications in their proper positions helps to ensure that patients receive the correct medication in a timely manner.

Rotating stock, or moving the products with the shortest expiration date to the front of the shelf, is an important component to pharmacy stocking. Rotating stock helps decrease the number of items that outdate on the shelf prior to dispensing. When stocking a medication, it is important to compare the expiration dates of the newly received items with those currently on the shelf and move the one with the shortest expiration date to the front. Many pharmacies also utilize a system in which items with short expiration dates (usually products that will expire within the next 3 to 6 months) are stickered to alert all staff.

> ★ *TECH ALERT: Medications that require refrigeration or freezing should be stocked first to minimize the time spent at room temperature.*

> ★ *TECH ALERT: An important role of the pharmacy technician is monitoring outdates. Hospital pharmacy technicians must inspect medications in all units of the hospital, not just the pharmacy.*

Storage Requirements for Pharmacy Stock

It is important to follow manufacturer's requirements for storage of medications. Failure to store medications according to these guidelines can render the medications adulterated and unusable. Manufacturers clearly label the storage requirements for medications on the product label and in the package insert. Medical equipment, devices, and supplies stocked in a pharmacy must also be stored according to manufacturer's requirements. Common storage conditions and their corresponding temperature requirements are listed in Table 7-1.

Some medications must be protected from light. Medications that must be PFL should be stored in the original container until use. Some medications must also be packaged in light-protective bags or syringes when dispensed to protect the product from exposure to light.

TABLE 7-1. Storage Condition Temperature Requirements	
Storage Condition	Temperature
Frozen	−20°C to −10°C
Refrigerated	2°C to 8°C
Room temperature	15°C to 30°C
Warm	30°C to 40°C

Many medications, including all sterile powders for injection and powders for reconstitution, must be protected from humidity. The addition of water greatly decreases the stability of these medications and can rapidly degrade the efficacy. Storing medications in their original containers in a climate-controlled environment is the most appropriate way to ensure the medication is not compromised.

Controlled medications in schedules III-V may be stored on the shelves with other medications, dispersed throughout the pharmacy. Schedule-II medications must be kept in a secure area accessible only to authorized personnel. Many pharmacies choose to store all controlled substances in a secure location to limit accessibility and risk of diversion.

Formularies and Preferred Product Lists

Many hospitals, clinics, long-term care facilities, and insurance companies have drug formularies. A **formulary** is a list of preferred medications. In the inpatient setting, a formulary represents the medications that are carried by the pharmacy. In the outpatient or retail setting, a formulary is the list of preferred medications on a patient's insurance plan. Because there are many different insurance companies, retail pharmacies typically carry a wide variety of medications to accommodate all insurance company formularies.

Inpatient formularies are set by the Pharmacy and Therapeutics (P&T) Committee. Some health systems have an open formulary. An open formulary means that most medications prescribed by physicians are stocked in the pharmacy, or able to be ordered if requested. Other health systems have a closed formulary. A closed, or restricted, formulary is a specific list of medications stocked in the pharmacy and available for prescribing. In a closed formulary, only certain medications in each pharmacologic class are available. Health systems with closed formularies generally have therapeutic interchange protocols. This means when a physician prescribes a nonformulary medication for a patient, it is automatically interchanged with a therapeutically equivalent formulary medication.

In retail pharmacy, the term formulary most often refers to the preferred medication list for an insurance plan. The medications included in an insurance plan's formulary are identified by the NDC. The NDC of a medication from one manufacturer might be covered, while the NDC of the same medication from another manufacturer is not. Nonformulary medications might also be covered at a higher co-pay, require prior authorization, or not be covered at all. These will be discussed in greater detail in Chapter 8.

Inventory Returns

Unwanted pharmacy stock, including medications, medical equipment, devices, and supplies, can be returned to the wholesaler or manufacturer. The primary reasons for returns are manufacturer recalls, product outdates, and damaged or adulterated goods. Some pharmacies handle return processes on their own, and others utilize licensed return companies to sort, package, and maintain records of the returned inventory.

Recalled Products

Medications, medical equipment, devices, and medical supplies are regulated by the FDA. If the FDA determines that there is a problem with a product, it requests a recall from the manufacturer. Although this request is considered voluntary, the FDA does have the jurisdiction to mandate the recall if necessary. Manufacturers are also required to monitor their products and submit recalls if defects are identified. The most common reasons for product recalls are inappropriate manufacturing practices, contamination or mislabeling in the manufacturing and distribution processes, or serious unexpected adverse effects.

As discussed in Chapter 2, recalls are categorized into 3 classes based on the relative health risk. Table 7-2 reviews the classifications of recalls. Regardless of the class of recall, all recalled products must be removed from inventory and returned to the manufacturer. Most frequently, only specific lot numbers of a given product are recalled. The cost of the medications returned by a pharmacy during a recall is reimbursed by the manufacturer.

★ *TECH ALERT: Some manufacturers offer full refunds or replacement of unopened packages of medication returned more than 3 months prior to expiration.*

The FDA obtains information about medications and medical products from the public and health care providers, including pharmacists and pharmacy technicians. The FDA utilizes a program called MedWatch to gather information about medications. Pharmacists and pharmacy technicians are important reporters of adverse effects or unexpected reactions. Pharmacy technicians should be comfortable reporting potential problems with medications to the FDA. The MedWatch form is available at www.fda.gov/medwatch.

Outdated Products

★ *TECH ALERT: Always have another authorized person witness when wasting controlled substances. This protects you, your coworkers, and your pharmacy in the event of a discrepancy.*

Outdated, or expired, products must be removed from pharmacy inventory and kept in a separate area until disposal. Most pharmacies remove stock from inventory not less than 3 months prior to expiration. Vigilant inventory monitoring and rotating stock helps ensure that expired products do not stay on the shelves. Outdated products are considered adulterated and cannot be dispensed.

TABLE 7-2. **Recall Classifications**	
Recall Class	*Description*
Class 1	• The most serious recall • Recalled product may cause serious injury or death • Includes mislabeled products that do not list possible allergy-causing ingredients
Class 2	• Recalled product may cause temporary adverse effects, small probability of causing serious harm • Includes medications that contain less active ingredient than intended
Class 3	• Least severe recall • Recalled products have minor defects without the probability of causing harm • Includes products with minor discrepancies in labeling and container defects

Special Considerations

Some medications require additional considerations in ordering, receiving, storage, and documenting. Investigational drugs, or drugs used in a study protocol, generally have strict documentation requirements. These medications are typically ordered and received directly from the pharmaceutical company or the sponsor of the study, and should be stored separately from general pharmacy stock. Any medication left over after the completion of the study or course of therapy should be returned to the manufacturer or study sponsor.

Business Math

Another important aspect of inventory management is understanding basic business practices and business math. Just like any other business, a retail pharmacy must make a profit in order to stay in business. A **profit** means generating more revenue than expenses in operating the business. Although revenue and expenses are calculated in the inpatient setting also, the inpatient pharmacy is a necessary component of the health system and its revenue is linked directly with overall health system profitability.

Technicians help ensure profitability of the pharmacy by assisting with product markup and discounts. A **markup** is the difference of the price the pharmacy paid for a product and the price at which they sell it. The amount of markup on medications will vary between each pharmacy, based on store revenue and operating costs. Markup can be calculated by subtracting the original purchase price from the pharmacy selling price.

> Markup = pharmacy selling price – pharmacy purchase price

For example, if a pharmacy purchased one 30-count bottle of Lexapro at a cost of $89 and sold it for $126, the markup would be calculated as below:

> Pharmacy selling price = $126
> Pharmacy purchase price = $89
> $126 – $89 = $37
> **Markup = $37**

The markup rate can also be determined as a percentage. To find the markup rate, take the amount of markup, and divide it by the original purchase price. Then multiply by 100 to convert the decimal into a percentage.

> Markup rate = (amount of markup/pharmacy purchase price) × 100

Using the same example from above, determine the markup rate from the bottle of Lexapro the pharmacy sold.

> Markup = $37
> Pharmacy purchase price = $89
> ($37/$89) × 100 = 41.57
> **Markup rate = 41.57%**

Other situations may warrant a pharmacy to **discount** a product. Discounts are usually taken on nonprescription merchandise or OTC products. A discount is calculated in the same way as a markup, only the price sold will be *less* than the

259

original price. For example, a pharmacy is selling a lip balm at 40% off the original price. If the original price was $1, the discount is determined by multiplying the price by the discount rate.

> Discount = list price × discount percentage rate

When determining the discount, the discount rate is given as a percent, and must be converted to a decimal before multiplying by the list price. To convert a percentage to a decimal, divide the percentage by 100. For example, 40% as a decimal is 0.4.

> Discount rate = 40% = 0.4
> List price = $1
> Discount = $1 × 0.4 = 0.4
> **Discount = 0.4**

Now the new selling price of the product can be calculated by subtracting the discount from the original list price.

> Discount = 0.4
> List price = $1
> New price = $1 − 0.4 = $0.60
> **The new selling price is $0.60**

QUICK QUIZ 7-2

1. If a drug costs a pharmacy $24, and the pharmacy sells it for $52, what is the markup and markup rate?

2. If a pharmacy sells an antibiotic for $4, and it costs the pharmacy $2.34 for this medication, what is the markup and markup rate?

3. If the markup of a medication is $15, and the pharmacy sold it for $35, what was the pharmacy purchase price of this medication?

4. If a pharmacy is discounting a knee brace 25% and the list price is $38, what is the discount and what is the new selling price?

5. If a pharmacy is discounting canes for 75% and the list price is $19, how much is the discount and what is the new selling price?

When calculating cost of medications, retail pharmacies may charge a **dispensing fee.** This is the charge for the services provided by the pharmacy, including overhead expenses, salaries, equipment cost, and a selected profit margin. Most insurance companies use this method for payment of pharmacy prescriptions. Dispensing fees do not include any cost of the drug being dispensed.

Along with dispensing fees, retail pharmacy costs are reimbursed using the **average wholesale price (AWP)** of drugs. This is a suggested price assigned to each drug listed in various published pricing guides, such as the *Red Book*. The AWP is the average price pharmacies pay for medications; however, most pharmacies earn discounts or rebates from the wholesalers and pay less than AWP. If a patient does not have insurance or if a medication is not covered by a patient's insurance plan, the patient is charged the **usual and customary price (U&C)** for the prescription. This amount is generally determined at a corporate level by the pharmacy.

To determine the reimbursement amount based on AWP, the following formula is generally followed:

> Reimbursement = AWP ± percentage + dispensing fee

For example, a pharmacy has a dispensing fee of $5. AWP of a drug is $50, but the wholesaler gives the pharmacy a 10% discount on their purchase price. The insurance company will pay the pharmacy AWP plus 2%. The profit can be determined using the formula above.

AWP = $50
Dispensing fee = $5
Wholesaler discount = 10%
Reimbursement markup = 2%

1. **Determine the pharmacy's cost of drug.**

   First find the discount.
   $50 × 0.1 = $5 = discount
   Next find the pharmacy purchase price.
   $50 − $5 = $45

2. **Calculate pharmacy reimbursement rate from the insurance company.**

   AWP × reimbursement markup
   ($50) × (0.02) = $1

3. **Compute the reimbursement total.**

   AWP + reimbursement markup + dispensing fee
   $50 + $1 + $5 = $56

4. **Find the profit of the pharmacy.**

   Reimbursement total − pharmacy drug cost
   $56 − $45 = $11

For this prescription, the pharmacy made **$11 profit.**

QUICK QUIZ 7-3

1. If the AWP for a medication is $15 and the dispensing fee is $4, how much will the pharmacy be reimbursed if the insurance company will reimburse at plus 3%?

2. If the AWP for a medication is $10 and the dispensing fee is $3.50, how much will the pharmacy be reimbursed if the insurance company will reimburse at plus 2%?

3. If the AWP for a medication is $15 and the dispensing fee is $4, how much will the pharmacy profit if the wholesaler gives the pharmacy a 5% discount and they are being reimbursed at plus 2%?

4. If the AWP for a medication is $50 and the dispensing fee is $5.50, how much will the pharmacy profit if the wholesaler gives the pharmacy a 15% discount and they are being reimbursed at plus 3%?

5. What is the term for the cash price of a medication?

CASE STUDY REVIEW

You are working as a pharmacy technician in a retail pharmacy. You are in the process of filling the prescription of Figure 7-1.

Patient: *Melanie Williams*
Address: *24 Eastwood Lane   Springfield, OH 43215*

DOB: *3/3/1974*

Lipitor 20mg
Sig i qhs
Disp #90

Refills: 3

Carla Black MD
Dr. Carla Black, MD

This figure is for educational and illustrative purposes only and is not intended to promote or endorse any specific product or organization.

Self-Assessment Questions
- How do you know which NDC of atorvastatin (Lipitor) to choose?
  - The NDC of atorvastatin dispensed depends on the formulary for the patient's insurance plan.
- Where will you find atorvastatin stocked in the pharmacy?
  - Atorvastatin is stocked at room temperature, and is a fast mover in many retail pharmacies.
- How do you handle the situation if there is not enough atorvastatin in stock to fill the entire prescription?
  - There are 2 ways to handle this situation. If the atorvastatin is due back in stock shortly, all of the medication on hand could be dispensed to the patient. The patient would purchase the entire prescription at this time and pick up the remainder when it is back in stock. If there will likely be additional patients who need some of the atorvastatin before the medication is restocked, Ms. Williams should be dispensed only enough to cover the doses until the atorvastatin will be restocked. In this case, the patient might pay for the medication when the remainder (the majority) of the prescription is dispensed.

CHAPTER SUMMARY

- The NDC is a unique 11-digit product identifying code used for all drugs marketed in the United States.
- Lot numbers are unique to each batch of medication produced at a given time. Lot numbers make it possible to identify when a particular tablet, capsule, or injectable was produced.
- Every medication is assigned an expiration date during the manufacturing process. The expiration date defines the length of time in which the medication retains optimum potency and stability.
- Ordering and receiving processes are essential pharmacy technician duties in maintaining an efficient, productive pharmacy.
- Just-in-time ordering is a process of ordering a medication as it is needed, to avoid excess inventory and abundance of outdates.
- Medical equipment, devices, and supplies stored in a pharmacy must also be stored according to manufacturer's requirements. Failure to storage medications and medical products according to these guidelines can render the items adulterated and unusable.
- A formulary is a list of preferred medications. In hospitals, clinics, and long-term care facilities, the formulary represents the medications that are carried by the pharmacy. With respect to insurance companies, a formulary is the list of preferred medications on a patient's insurance plan.
- Sometimes pharmacy stock, including medications, medical equipment, devices, and supplies, must be returned to the wholesaler or manufacturer. The primary reasons for returns are manufacturer recalls, product outdates, and damaged or adulterated goods. Records for returns, recalls, and outdated products must be completed and retained by the pharmacy as specified by the DEA, FDA, and State Boards of Pharmacy.
- Basic understanding of business management is an important skill for pharmacy technicians. Inventory management and business math including profitability calculations, markups and discounts, and AWP are essential in pharmacy management.

ANSWERS TO QUICK QUIZZES

Quick Quiz 7-1

1. 12.5

2. 13.6

3. 5.6

4. They are not turning over inventory frequently enough and probably have too many products expiring before use.

5. Decrease the PAR levels on its slow-moving inventory.

Quick Quiz 7-2

1. Markup = $28, markup % = 116.7%

2. Markup = $1.66, markup % = 70.9%

3. $20

4. Discount = $9.50, new selling price = $28.50

5. Discount = $14.25, new selling price = $4.75

Quick Quiz 7-3

1. $19.45

2. $13.70

3. $5.05

4. $14.50

5. Usual and customary price (U&C)

CHAPTER QUESTIONS

1. A(n) _____ formulary is a system in which therapeutic interchange protocols are utilized to convert prescribed nonformulary medications to formulary alternatives.
   a. Open
   b. Closed
   c. Retail
   d. Inventory

2. A bottle of Xalatan eyedrop has been stored in the pharmacy at approximately 24°C for the past 7 days. Xalatan requires refrigeration. Is this product safe to dispense?
   a. Yes
   b. No

3. What is the DEA electronic program used for ordering C-II medications?
   a. FDAS
   b. DEAS
   c. CSOS
   d. CMOS

4. If the AWP for a medication is $180 and the dispensing fee is $4, how much will the pharmacy be reimbursed if the insurance company will reimburse at minus 4%?
   a. $172.80
   b. $176.64
   c. $184
   d. $191.20

5. Which DEA form is used for the purchase and sale of C-II medications?
   a. Form 41
   b. Form 106
   c. Form 222
   d. Form 224

6. Which calculation is used to measure the overall effectiveness of purchasing and inventory control processes?
   a. Lot numbers
   b. Inventory turnover rate
   c. AWP
   d. Rotating stock

7. A lot number is a unique identifying code assigned to each _____ of medication produced at a given time.
   a. Unit
   b. Brand
   c. Batch
   d. Strength

8. Which of the following is a required information sheet that instructs proper storage, handling, and containment procedures for hazardous substances?
   a. Formulary
   b. NDC
   c. MSDS
   d. PAR

9. The optimal amount of each item that should be stocked at any given time is called the _____ level.
   a. Minimum
   b. Maximum
   c. Average
   d. PAR

10. Which term is used to describe the wholesaler from whom a pharmacy has committed to purchase the majority of its inventory?
    a. Prime vendor
    b. Manufacturer
    c. Formulary
    d. Distributor

11. Which of the following medications can become toxic after its expiration date?
    a. Aspirin
    b. Vicodin
    c. Tetracycline
    d. Lorazepam

12. What is the term for a company that carries a selection of medications, medical devices, and supplies from which a pharmacy may order?
    a. Wholesaler
    b. Manufacturer
    c. Reverse distributor
    d. AWP

13. What is the second section of the NDC code?
    a. The labeler code, identifying the manufacturer
    b. The product code, identifying the product
    c. The package code, identifying the package
    d. It varies

14. Rotating stock is a process in which products with the _____ expiration dates are moved to the front of the shelf when stocking.
    a. Shortest
    b. Longest
    c. Same
    d. Outdated

15. When is the last day that a medication can be safely used if it has an expiration date of 9/16/2017?
    a. 9/1/2017
    b. 9/15/2017
    c. 9/16/2017
    d. 9/17/2017

16. Why is ordering from a wholesaler more efficient for a pharmacy than ordering from each individual manufacturer?
    a. Most of the products come from one place, limiting the amount of paperwork and number of deliveries
    b. Wholesalers are always less expensive than manufacturers
    c. Most of the products come from different places, creating additional purchase orders and increasing the number of deliveries
    d. Ordering from wholesalers is not more efficient than ordering from manufacturers

17. How much of its total inventory does a pharmacy need to purchase from a single wholesaler before that wholesaler is considered its prime vendor?
    a. 30% to 35%
    b. 50% to 55%
    c. 80% to 85%
    d. 100%

18. What is the benefit of having a prime vendor for a pharmacy?
    a. Discounts are offered
    b. Markups are offered
    c. Reverse distributor status
    d. Use of CSOS is allowed

19. Which of the following is correct regarding purchasing?
    a. Once a purchase order is transmitted to a vendor, an invoice is generated
    b. Once an invoice is generated, the purchase order is transmitted to a vendor
    c. A purchase order is also known as a bill of sale
    d. Once the shipment is received, it does not need to be checked against the invoice or purchase order for accuracy

20. Recalls classified as class 2 or 3 are optional, and products do not need to be removed from inventory.
    a. True
    b. False

21. Medications that are used frequently ("fast movers") should have _____ PAR levels.
    a. Small
    b. Large
    c. Varying
    d. None of the above

22. If a pharmacy's inventory turnover rate is 13 and the annual purchases are $16,000,000, what is the value of the inventory on hand?
    a. $1,230,800
    b. $2,080,000
    c. $13,920,000
    d. $14,960,000

23. Which of the following are not benefits of electronic ordering systems?
    a. Technicians do not need to check or verify the orders
    b. Automated inventory turnover rate calculations
    c. Perpetual inventory counts
    d. All of the above are benefits

24. The bottom (blue) copy of a DEA form 222 is retained by which of the following?
    a. Supplier
    b. Manufacturer
    c. DEA
    d. Pharmacy

25. The top (tan) copy of a DEA form 222 is retained by which of the following?
    a. Supplier
    b. Manufacturer
    c. DEA
    d. Pharmacy

26. Per the DEA, how long must the form 222 and record of receipt for C-II medications be kept on file?
    a. 1 year
    b. 2 years
    c. 5 years
    d. 7 years

27. Which medication should be processed first when a shipment is received?
    a. A package of NuvaRing which requires refrigeration
    b. A bottle of expensive Plavix tablets
    c. A bottle of metformin with short expiration dates
    d. A box of OTC insulin needles

28. Where are storage requirements for medications listed?
    a. Manufacturer's label
    b. Package insert
    c. Neither a or b, storage is at the discretion of the pharmacist
    d. Both a and b

29. Manufacturer's guidelines for storage are suggestions and products are still usable if not stored accordingly.
    a. True
    b. False

30. What is the temperature range for storage of frozen products?
    a. −20°C to −10°C
    b. 2°C to 8°C
    c. −20°F to −10°F
    d. 2°F to 8°F

31. A(n) _____ formulary is a system in which most medications are stocked in the pharmacy, or able to be ordered if prescribed.
    a. Open
    b. Closed
    c. Retail
    d. Inventory

32. The medications included in an insurance plan's formulary are identified by which of the following?
    a. AWP
    b. NDC
    c. Lot number
    d. Medication name

33. Which of the following are common reasons for a pharmacy to return inventory?
    a. Manufacturer recalls
    b. Product outdates
    c. Damaged or adulterated good
    d. All of the above

34. What is the third section of the NDC code?
    a. The labeler code, identifying the manufacturer
    b. The product code, identifying the product
    c. The package code, identifying the package
    d. It varies

35. The FDA only has the authority to request a recall from a manufacturer if it deems there is a problem with a medication, it cannot mandate the recall.
    a. True
    b. False

36. How many classes of drug recalls are there?
    a. 2
    b. 3
    c. 5
    d. 7

37. Which recall class is defined by the following statement: recalled products in this class may cause temporary adverse effects but have a very small probability of causing serious harm.
    a. Class 1
    b. Class 2
    c. Class 3
    d. None of the above

38. Which recall class is the least severe?
    a. Class 1
    b. Class 2
    c. Class 3
    d. All are equally as severe

39. Which program does the FDA use to collect data about medications, including adverse effects and unexpected reactions?
    a. CSOS
    b. MedAlert
    c. DEA
    d. MedWatch

40. Which of the following is an identifying code used for all drugs marketed in the United States?
    a. Lot
    b. PAR
    c. NDC
    d. CSOS

41. What is the term used to describe a bill of sale of products ordered?
    a. Invoice
    b. Purchase order
    c. MSDS
    d. Formulary

42. Per the DEA, how long must records of controlled substance destruction be kept on file?
    a. 1 year
    b. 2 years
    c. 5 years
    d. 7 years

43. Which DEA form is used to document the destruction of controlled substances?
    a. Form 41
    b. Form 106
    c. Form 222
    d. Form 224

44. The DEA form 222 is a(n) _____ form designed specifically for the sale of C-II medications.
    a. Duplicate
    b. Triplicate
    c. Electronic
    d. Optional

45. How do insurance companies handle medications that are not in the plan formulary?
    a. Cover them at a higher co-pay
    b. Require prior authorization
    c. Not cover them at all
    d. Any of the above are possible

46. The label on a blood pressure monitor indicates the product must be stored at controlled room temperature. What is the appropriate temperature range?
    a. 15°C to 30°C
    b. 30°C to 40°C
    c. 15°F to 30°F
    d. 30°F to 40°F

47. A lot of Tylenol has been determined to contain only 160 mg per tablet rather than the labeled 325 mg. In which class would this product be recalled?
    a. Class 1
    b. Class 2
    c. Class 3
    d. This product would not be recalled

48. The middle (green) copy of a DEA form 222 is retained by which of the following?
    a. Supplier
    b. Manufacturer
    c. DEA
    d. Pharmacy

49. What is the first section of the NDC code?
    a. The labeler code, identifying the manufacturer
    b. The product code, identifying the product
    c. The package code, identifying the package
    d. It varies

50. An insulin vial has been stored at 6°C for the past 2 months. Insulin vials require refrigeration. Is this product safe to dispense?
    a. Yes
    b. No

Pharmacy Billing and Reimbursement

CHAPTER

PTCB KNOWLEDGE AREAS

8.1 Reimbursement policies and plans (eg, HMOs, PPO, CMS, and private plans)

8.2 Third party resolution (eg, prior authorization, rejected claims, and plan limitations)

8.3 Third party reimbursement systems (eg, PBM, medication assistance programs, coupons, and self-pay)

8.4 Health care reimbursement systems (eg, home health, long-term care, and home infusion)

8.5 Coordination of benefits (COB)

KEY TERMS

Adjudication: The process of determining whether or not the drug will be covered under the patient's insurance plan

Centers for Medicare and Medicaid Services (CMS): Federal organization that oversees Medicare and Medicaid

CHAMPVA: Government program that helps pay medical expenses for the families of veterans who have been disabled because of injuries related to military service

Coinsurance: An out-of-pocket expense similar to a co-payment except a patient pays a percentage of the costs of the service as determined by the insurance provider

Coordination of benefits (COB): If a patient has multiple insurance providers, one is selected as primary and is billed first. The second insurance company is not billed unless there are still unpaid claims remaining, and then they are billed only the remainder of the costs, so there is not a duplication of payment

Co-payment: An out-of-pocket expense a patient must pay at the time services are rendered

Deductible: The amount a patient must pay each year before the insurance policy will cover remaining costs

Dependent: Usually a spouse, same-sex partner or child(ren) of the subscriber

Formulary: A list of approved medications

Health maintenance organizations (HMOs): A managed care organization in which a patient must select a primary care physician (PCP) from a network and must first see or get a referral from their physician to obtain any covered services

Medicaid: State-run benefits program for patients with low incomes or certain disabilities

Medicare: Federal health insurance program that offers benefits to those who are 65 and older and younger citizens with long-term disabilities

Medicare Part A: Provides coverage for patients eligible for Medicare for inpatient hospital stays, nursing facilities, home health care services, and hospice care

Medicare Part B: Provides coverage for patients eligible for Medicare for durable medical equipment (DME), outpatient services from hospitals, and physician services

Medicare Part C: Known as Medicare Advantage plan; patients must be enrolled in both Medicare Parts A and B to receive Part C benefits through a separate provider

Medicare Part D: Voluntary prescription drug coverage program for Medicare

Out-of-pocket expenses: All expenses a member is responsible for and pays directly

Pharmacy benefit manager (PBM): A third party administrator of prescription drug programs, processes and pays for the drug claims and maintains the formulary for each plan

Point-of-service (POS): A type of managed care plan that combines the benefits of an HMO and PPO; typically members do not make a choice about service until the point at which it is needed

Preferred provider organizations (PPOs): A managed care organization in which a patient can obtain services from any physician as long as it is within network, without a prior referral

Premium: Cost of the insurance coverage that a patient must pay to be eligible for services

Prior authorization (PA): A special approval needed before an insurance company will cover a specific medication for a patient, generally an expensive brand name drug that is not present on the formulary

Refill-too-soon (RTS): A patient's attempt to get their prescription refilled before the insurance company permits a scheduled fill

Subscriber: Cardholder of the insurance plan

Third Party: Insurance company paying for a patient's medical or prescription claim

TRICARE: Health benefits program for military personnel and retirees, also includes dependents of active-duty service members

Workers' compensation insurance: Medical coverage for a person who is injured on the job or becomes ill due to a work-related environment

CASE STUDY

You are working as a pharmacy technician when a patient brings you in a prescription for a very expensive brand name medication. When you submit the claim to the insurance, it is rejected with a rejection code saying "prior authorization required."

Self-Assessment Questions
- What does "prior authorization required" mean?
- How do you explain to the patient what a prior authorization is?
- How long does the prior authorization submission and approval process take?

After completing this chapter, you should be able to answer the case study assessment questions on prior authorization.

INTRODUCTION

In order for a pharmacy to be profitable it must be reimbursed for the cost of filling and processing prescriptions. This chapter will focus on understanding third party and private insurance plans, insurance billing or claims submission, claim rejections, and reimbursement procedures used in pharmacy practice.

REIMBURSEMENT POLICIES AND PLANS

As a pharmacy technician, you will be responsible for processing many different types of insurance plans. It is essential to have an understanding of common terms dealing with health insurance, as well as an understanding of insurance policies and the meaning behind rejected claims and other third party issues.

Third-Party and Private Plans

The term **third party** refers to the insurance company representing the first party (patient) who is receiving the medication from the pharmacy (second party). Third party plans can include HMOs, PPOs, government, and private insurance plans.

Health maintenance organizations (HMOs) were developed as a way to control rising health care costs. They are a type of managed care organization which contracts with employers to provide health services to their employees. A member of an HMO must select a PCP from a network of physicians contracted within the HMO. To see any specialist or obtain other services, the patient must first see their PCP and get a referral, or expenses are not covered unless it is an emergency.

Preferred provider organizations (PPOs) are another type of managed care plan that differs slightly from HMOs. In this plan, patients need not select a PCP but can obtain services from any physician contracted within the PPO network. The advantage to this system is that patients may see specialists within their network without first getting a referral from a PCP. Some services obtained outside of the network may even be partially reimbursed under this plan.

A combination of HMO and PPO is an option called **point-of-service (POS)**. This plan operates similar to an HMO in that the patient picks a PCP, but if the patient decides to go outside of the network, they will pay more for service. It is known as point-of-service because at the time services are needed, the patient has the option to stay in network and allow the PCP to manage care, or leave the network and seek other care without a referral.

Most HMO and PPO plans are provided through private health care companies. Patients generally enroll in private plans through group contracts offered by employers. Some examples of private plans include the Blue Cross–Blue Shield Association (BCBS), Humana, Aetna, and The Kaiser Foundation. There are many others you will encounter as a technician, and although each policy and plan may be unique, the basic structure for each patient will be similar.

There are some drug manufacturers who may offer discounts or coupons for drug products. These are generally given to the physician who passes the savings on to his or her patients when prescribing. These coupons are generally processed similar as insurance, but are usually only good on a one time basis.

Each patient will pay a **premium,** which is the cost of the coverage of the insurance policy. This amount is usually deducted from the patient's paycheck or paid in a monthly fee. The patient who is the cardholder of the insurance plan is also known as the **subscriber** or member. The member may have **dependent**(s) that are also included on the policy. An example of a dependent may be the subscriber's spouse, same-sex partner, or child(ren).

When a patient picks up a prescription in the pharmacy, he or she may be responsible for an out-of-pocket expense known as a **co-payment.** This amount will vary based on the type of insurance plan the patient has, as well as the medication the patient is receiving. Most insurance companies offer less expensive co-pay for generic medications and a higher charge for brand name drugs. The co-pay may also fluctuate based on the subscriber's **deductible.** This is the amount that is paid each year by the member before the policy benefits begin. Generally, the higher a patient pays for a premium, the lower the deductible will be. A patient may also have **coinsurance** which tends to differ from co-pay in that with coinsurance the patient is responsible for a percentage of the cost of services covered by the insurer. Any costs that a member pays are referred to as **out-of-pocket expenses.** Some insurance plans limit a subscriber's out-of-pocket expenses to a certain dollar amount each year.

TECH ALERT: If a patient has 80% coinsurance and has a prescription for $100, the insurance company will cover $80 and they will be responsible for the remaining $20.

A more popular trend growing with some employers is to offer the option of a Health Savings Account (HSA). These accounts are established by the employee and are used to pay only for medical expenses, which includes prescriptions. The patient can contribute funds into the HSA tax free, automatically deducted from their paycheck within a set limit. These insurance plans have a high deductible, and regulations are established by the US government.

QUICK QUIZ 8-1

1. What must a patient pay each year before insurance benefits begin?

2. In which type of plan does a patient select a PCP and have to obtain referral for any outside specialist seen?

3. What is a child or spouse on a member's plan is known as?

4. What is it known as when a patient pays a percentage of the costs and the insurance company pays the remaining percent?

5. Generic medications will generally have a cheaper co-pay than name brand.
   a. True
   b. False

Government Insurance Plans

Medicare is the federal health insurance program that offers benefits to those who are 65 and older and younger citizens with long-term disabilities. It has 4 areas of coverage as described below:

In **Medicare Part A,** patients have coverage for inpatient hospital stays, nursing facilities, home health care services, and hospice care. If a patient is eligible for social security benefits, they are automatically enrolled in part A.

Any patient eligible for Part A has the option of enrolling in **Medicare Part B.** This coverage requires a monthly premium and a deductible must be met before benefits begin. Medicare Part B covers DME, outpatient services from hospitals, and physician services.

The Medicare insurance card, shown in Figure 8-1, is given to each patient showing dates effective for Parts A and B coverage. Each member will also have a Medicare claim number, which is the patient's social security number.

Originally known as Medicare + Choice plan, **Medicare Part C** became an option to individuals eligible for Parts A and B. Under this plan, private companies can offer Medicare benefits through their own policies. This is now known as the Medicare Advantage plan and these provide all coverage included in Parts A and B, as well as additional benefits.

The latest addition to Medicare is Part D. **Medicare Part D** was created to cover the costs of medications for Medicare patients. This is a voluntary program, and patients must enroll during a designated period to be eligible for benefits. As a pharmacy technician, Part D will be a very important component of insurance processing to be familiar with, as there are many plans and difference costs and formularies associated with each policy.

Medicaid is a program designed for patients with low incomes. It is a state-run program that varies in structure for co-pays, coverage, and services based on location. Other patients that may be covered are those who are blind or have permanent disabilities. Each state determines the income level required for eligibility, within federal guidelines.

Both Medicaid and Medicare are overseen by a federal organization known as the **Centers for Medicare and Medicaid Services (CMS).** In order for any facility to receive reimbursements for patients covered by Medicaid or Medicare, they must receive approval by CMS and the facility must also be inspected and approved to provide care to eligible patients.

TRICARE is a benefits program for military personnel and retirees. It also covers dependents of active-duty service members, and some former spouses and survivors of deceased military members. There are 3 options of TRICARE coverage: standard, extra, or prime.

The Civilian Health and Medical Program of the Veterans Administration **(CHAMPVA)** is a government program that helps pay medical expenses for the

★ *TECH ALERT: A Medicaid Spend Down is a minimum paid by patient before being eligible for full benefits. This is similar to a deductible, but must be met monthly not yearly.*

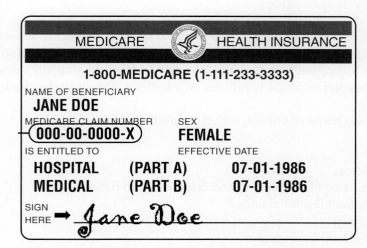

FIGURE 8-1 Sample Medicare insurance card (red, white, and blue).

families of veterans who have been disabled because of injuries related to military service. This coverage also extends to spouses and children of veterans who may have died from a service-related incident.

In the event a person is injured on the job or becomes ill due to a work-related environment, medical costs are covered by a state or federal plan known as **workers' compensation insurance.** Under this plan, the patient provides the pharmacy or other provider with the workers' compensation information, including the date of injury, and the patient is not billed any fees for services.

QUICK QUIZ 8-2

1. Which type of benefits program is offered for military personnel?

2. Which type of Medicare plan would be used to cover prescription drugs?

3. Is Medicare a federal or state-run program?

4. Which Medicare plan is responsible for DME?

5. If a person is injured on the job, what insurance program may they be eligible for?

* TECH ALERT: Government insurance plans include Medicare, Medicaid, TRICARE, CHAMPVA, and workers' compensation.

Coordination of Benefits

There are situations when patients may be covered under multiple insurance plans. It is essential that the benefits of each policy are coordinated so that the maximum benefits are paid, but not duplicated. This is known as **coordination of benefits.** This process occurs when one insurance company is designated as the primary insurer and claims are sent to this company first. Then if the primary insurer does not pay the entire claim in full, the secondary insurer may be billed for any remaining charges.

Third Party Resolution

An important role of a pharmacy technician is helping to resolve issues related to rejected third party claims. Each insurance company requires specific information, and it is up to the technician to gather this information from the patient. Some necessary information needed to properly process an insurance claim includes the following:

- First and last name of patient, including middle initial
- Gender
- Birthdate
- Home address
- Member's name (if not patient) and relationship to patient
- Member's identification number
- Group number
- Insurance carrier or processor
- Medication prescribed, dose, and quantity
- Drug allergy information

THIRD PARTY REIMBURSEMENT SYSTEMS

A third party administrator of prescription drug programs is known as a **pharmacy benefit manager (PBM).** A PBM processes and pays for the drug claims and maintains the formulary for each plan. In addition, because a PBM represents a large group of employers, they can negotiate better discounts and prices with drug manufacturers.

Below is a sample insurance card from Health Rx PBM (Figures 8-2a and 8-2b). This company will process any claims for prescription medications for patients whose employers utilize insurance providers that work with Health Rx. Health Rx is an example of a PBM because it processes the claims of not just one insurance provider, but many. This helps to negotiate better discounts for this company's prescription drug coverage program.

When you receive a prescription insurance card for a patient, you will first notice the name of the member on the card. This will be the subscriber, also known as the cardholder. You may also be filling a prescription for the cardholder's spouse or child—otherwise known as a dependent. The person number affiliated with the cardholder will be 1 or 01. For the spouse or first dependent, the person number will be 2 or 02, and for each dependent following, the number will proceed in succession, depending on birthdate. It is a good practice to always ask the patient what their relationship is to the cardholder to expedite this process.

After you determine the ID number and person number, the biller identification number (BIN) and group numbers should be entered into your pharmacy software system. The BIN is unique to each third party and identifies where the claim is being sent. The BIN number is usually listed on the insurance card and consists of 6 numbers. Unlike the BIN number, the group number may consist of numbers and letters. The processor control number (PCN) helps direct the electronic claim to the proper location. Like the group number, the PCN does not have a consistent format, and can contain letters and numbers in varying quantities.

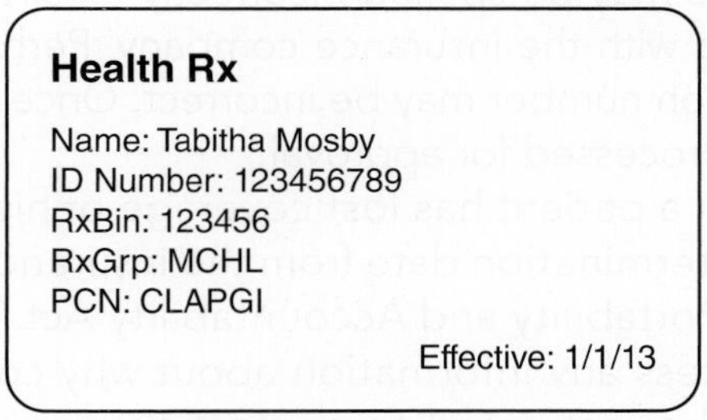

Health Rx

Name: Tabitha Mosby
ID Number: 123456789
RxBin: 123456
RxGrp: MCHL
PCN: CLAPGI

Effective: 1/1/13

FIGURE 8-2a Front of Health Rx PBM card.

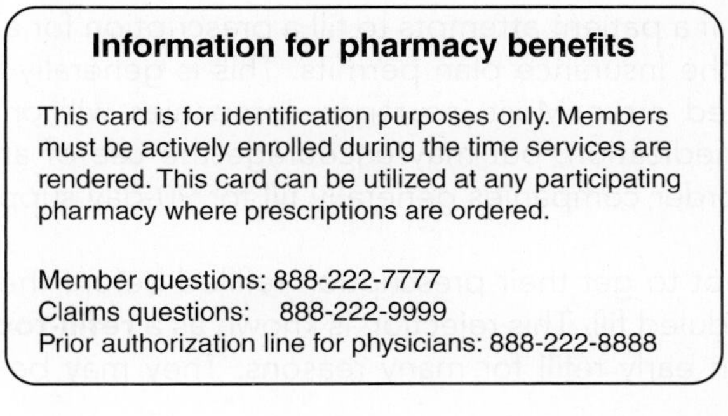

Information for pharmacy benefits

This card is for identification purposes only. Members must be actively enrolled during the time services are rendered. This card can be utilized at any participating pharmacy where prescriptions are ordered.

Member questions: 888-222-7777
Claims questions: 888-222-9999
Prior authorization line for physicians: 888-222-8888

FIGURE 8-2b Back of Health Rx PBM card.

* TECH ALERT: The RxBin number is a 6-digit number on insurance cards and the RxGroup and PCN number can be combinations of numbers and letters.

QUICK QUIZ 8-3

1. What BIN number would you enter for this patient?

2. What ID number would you enter?

3. If you were filling a prescription for Tabitha's husband, what person code would you enter?

4. If the doctor's office called and asked about what number to call for a prior authorization, where would you direct them?

5. The insurance rejects the claim, and we realize we forgot to submit the group number. What would you need to enter into the system to make sure the claim was approved?

Insurance Processing

After the prescription has been entered into the system, the claim can be transmitted electronically where it undergoes **adjudication.** This is the process of determining whether or not the drug will be covered under the patient's insurance plan. If the information is correct and the medication is indeed covered under the patient's policy, the claim will be processed. The pharmacy will receive an electronic transmission of what the patient's insurance company will pay and the patient's remaining co-pay.

There are many reasons why a prescription may not be covered by an insurance company. Some are basic issues that require a simple change within the pharmacy computer system. A patient's name may be spelled incorrectly or birthdate could be different from what is on record with the insurance company. Perhaps a group number is missing or an identification number may be incorrect. Once these issues are corrected, the claim can be reprocessed for approval.

A claim can also be rejected if a patient has lost coverage of his or her policy. The pharmacy will be given a termination date from the insurance company, but due to the Health Insurance Portability and Accountability Act (HIPAA), the pharmacy is not permitted to access any information about why coverage was terminated. The patient should be instructed to contact the insurance company and will have to pay full price for any medications until the issue can be resolved.

A rejection can also occur if a patient attempts to fill a prescription for a quantity that is in excess of what the insurance plan permits. This is generally known as a plan limitations exceeded error. Most insurance companies will only pay for a thirty-day supply of a medication, but may encourage the use of an affiliated mail-order facility. Mail-order companies generally fill for 90-day supplies of medications.

Some patients may attempt to get their prescription refilled before the insurance company permits a scheduled fill. This rejection is known as a **refill-too-soon** error. Patients may request an early refill for many reasons. They may be going on vacation out of the country and they need to ensure they will have a sufficient quantity to last their entire trip. A technician must call the insurance company to explain the situation and be given the directions for how to proceed. The patient may have to pay cash for the vacation quantity or be given an override for a certain amount that will be covered under their plan. Another scenario could be that a patient's physician has increased their dosage and they are now taking the medication more often and therefore ran out before the scheduled time. The patient will be required to obtain a new prescription from the doctor, but again, the technician will need to call the insurance company to receive proper instructions on how to process this claim.

Sometimes patients are prescribed a medication that is not covered under the insurance company's **formulary,** or list of approved medications within the member's plan. If a drug is not covered, the patient may be required to receive a **prior authorization (PA)** for this medication. To obtain prior authorization, the pharmacy calls the prescriber and notifies them of the patient's insurance rejection. The prescriber is then responsible for either changing the medication, or explaining to the patient's insurance company why the patient must have this specific medication.

When the pharmacy submits a claim, the **dispense as written (DAW)** code is used for third parties to determine if the proper brand or generic medication was used to fill the prescription. These codes are a type of National Council for Prescription Drug Programs' (NCPDP) code. The NCPDP is responsible for providing each pharmacy with a provider ID and then maintaining the database of all pharmacies. The DAW codes for submitting claims are shown in Table 8-1.

After the claim has been submitted, it undergoes a **drug utilization review (DUR).** This process consists of an evaluation of the prescribed medication against specific criteria that helps to ensure drug safety, and help reduce unnecessary costs. In the event a claim is rejected, the pharmacy will be notified immediately that there is a problem. Examples of DUR rejections are shown Table 8-2.

TABLE 8-1. **DAW Codes**	
DAW 0	Default code used when dispensing a generic drug or when dispensing a brand name product that does not have a generic available
DAW 1	Prescriber indicates dispense as written
DAW 2	Prescriber indicates generic is permitted, but patient requests brand name product
DAW 3	Prescriber indicates generic is permitted, but pharmacist requests brand name product be dispensed
DAW 4	Prescriber indicates generic is permitted, but the generic is not in stock so the brand name product must be dispensed
DAW 5	Brand name drug dispensed but priced as generic
DAW 6	Override—brand name is necessary—usually for prior authorization cases
DAW 7	Substitution not allowed, brand mandated by law
DAW 8	Generic is not currently available, not being manufactured or distributed
DAW 9	Other

TABLE 8-2. DUR Rejections and Examples	
DUR Rejection	*Example*
Drug–drug interaction	A patient is prescribed an antacid while on a tetracycline antibiotic which interact
Therapeutic duplication	A patient has a prescription for both meloxicam (Mobic) and ibuprofen (Motrin) and both are nonsteroidal anti-inflammatory drugs (NSAIDs)
Allergy	A patient has an allergy to penicillin and is prescribed amoxicillin (Amoxil)
Low/high dose	A patient is prescribed a dose that is either below therapeutic level or too high and potentially toxic
Contraindicated	A patient who is pregnant is given a medication not to be taken during pregnancy, an elderly or pediatric patient is given a medication that may be inappropriately dosed for their age group

CASE STUDY REVIEW

You are working as a pharmacy technician when a patient brings you in a prescription for a very expensive brand name medication. When you submit the claim to the insurance, it is rejected with a rejection code saying "prior authorization required."

Self-Assessment Questions
- What does this mean?
  - A prior authorization is required by the insurance company for brand name medications that are usually expensive and not on the formulary.
- How do you explain to the patient what a prior authorization is?
  - The patient should be informed that the prescriber will be notified and will need to decide if he or she wants the patient on the medication or wants to switch to another drug. If the prescriber does want the patient on the rejected medication, the prescriber must call the insurance company explaining why the patient should specifically have this medication.
- How long does the prior authorization submission and approval process take?
  - The patient will likely have to wait a few days for this process to be completed; it will definitely take more than a few minutes for the approval to be processed at the insurance company.

CHAPTER SUMMARY

It is important as a pharmacy technician to be familiar with insurance in many different ways. Knowing the different plans and co-pay structures will be helpful when communicating prices to patients, as well as being familiar with rejections and DUR issues that may arise. Being knowledgeable in these and other areas pertaining to insurance can make a technician a great asset in a pharmacy and a dependable member of the pharmacy team.

ANSWERS TO QUICK QUIZZES

Quick Quiz 8-1

1. Premium

2. HMO

3. Dependent

4. Coinsurance

5. True

Quick Quiz 8-2

1. TRICARE

2. Part D

3. Federal

4. Part B

5. Workers' compensation

Quick Quiz 8-3

1. 610455

2. 106395135

3. 2

4. 888-222-8888

5. MCHL

CHAPTER QUESTIONS

1. Which government insurance plans offered 4 different parts or areas of different coverage?
   a. Medicare
   b. Medicaid
   c. TRICARE
   d. CHAMPVA

2. DAW stands for which of the following?
   a. Dispense as written
   b. Distribute and work
   c. Distribution and working
   d. Dispense as well

3. Which of the following third party plans requires the patient to designate a primary care physician (PCP)?
   a. Health maintenance organization (HMO)
   b. Preferred provider organization (PPO)
   c. Medicare Part D
   d. TRICARE

4. The cost of the coverage of an insurance policy is known as which of the following?
   a. Deductible
   b. Co-payment
   c. Coinsurance
   d. Premium

5. Which of the following is another name for the cardholder of the insurance policy?
   a. Subscriber
   b. Dependent
   c. Patient
   d. Third party

6. When a patient picks up a prescription in the pharmacy, he or she may be responsible for an out-of-pocket expense known as which of the following?
   a. Co-payment
   b. Premium
   c. Deductible
   d. Third party

7. The part of Medicare that covers the costs of prescriptions for Medicare patients is known as which of the following?
   a. Part A
   b. Part B
   c. Part C
   d. Part D

8. Which organization oversees Medicaid and Medicare?
   a. Food and Drug Administration (FDA)
   b. Drug Enforcement Administration (DEA)
   c. Centers for Medicare and Medicaid Services (CMS)
   d. United States Pharmacopeia (USP)

9. Which of the following is a formulary?
   a. List of insurance companies that offer pharmacy benefits
   b. List of providers that are included in an HMO
   c. List of approved medications in a member's plan
   d. Recipe for how to make specific medications

10. If a drug is not covered under a patient's prescription plan, but the prescriber specifically wants the patient to have this medication, the insurance company may require which of the following?
    a. Formulary
    b. Prior authorization
    c. Adjudication
    d. Coordination of benefits

11. Which code is used for the third party to determine if the proper brand or generic medication was used to fill the prescription?
    a. USAN
    b. DAW
    c. Adjudication
    d. Trade

12. Which of the following DAW code is submitted when a generic drug is dispensed or a brand name product that does not have a generic available?
    a. DAW 0
    b. DAW 1
    c. DAW 2
    d. DAW 3

13. After a claim has been submitted, what is the process of evaluating a medication for specific drug safety and cost-effectiveness measures known as?
    a. Coordination of benefits
    b. Drug utilization review
    c. Prior authorization
    d. Coinsurance

14. The deductible is the amount that must be paid when?
    a. Each time when a prescription is picked up
    b. Each year before the policy kicks in
    c. Monthly to cover the insurance plan
    d. As a percentage of the cost of services

15. If a patient has coinsurance that pays 90% of services, and their prescription costs $50, how much will they owe the pharmacy?
    a. $5
    b. $10
    c. $15
    d. $25

16. Which of the following is an example of a third party plan?
    a. HMO
    b. Prior authorization
    c. Adjudication
    d. Premium

17. Which of the following is an example of a private insurance company?
    a. Medicare
    b. Medicaid
    c. TRICARE
    d. Aetna

18. A patient pays a $500 deductible and a total of $100 in co-pays for the year. The total $600 is called which of the following?
    a. Premium
    b. Out-of-pocket expenses
    c. Coinsurance
    d. Point-of-service

19. CMS represents which organizations?
    a. TRICARE and Medicare
    b. Medicare and Medicaid
    c. TRICARE and CHAMPVA
    d. CHAMPVA and Medicare

20. To ensure that the maximum benefits are paid, but not duplicated, patients covered under multiple insurance plans will undergo which of the following?
    a. Adjudication
    b. PCN
    c. PBM
    d. Coordination of benefits

21. Which of the following DAW code is submitted when the patient requests a brand name product, although the prescriber says generic substitution is permitted?
    a. DAW 1
    b. DAW 2

c. DAW 3
d. DAW 5

22. Which of the following information must be gathered from the patient to process an insurance claim?
    a. First and last name
    b. Birthdate
    c. Drug allergy information
    d. All of the above

23. Which of the following might have a person number of 3?
    a. Member
    b. Spouse of member
    c. Child of member
    d. None of the above

24. PCN stands for which of the following?
    a. Patient-controlled narcotics
    b. Processor control number
    c. Pharmacy control number
    d. Patient-centered number

25. Which of the following is required to submit an insurance claim?
    a. Rx Bin number
    b. Rx Group number
    c. Patient ID number
    d. All of the above

26. What type of pharmacy would pay for a 90-day supply of a medication?
    a. Retail
    b. Mail-order
    c. Nuclear
    d. Long-term care

27. When is a prior authorization required?
    a. A patient is going on vacation
    b. A patient has a change in dosage
    c. A patient has a prescription for an expensive medication or one not on the formulary
    d. A patient only wants a generic drug

28. Which of the following might cause a refill-too-soon rejection?
    a. A patient attempts to refill their prescription before the insurance company permits a scheduled fill
    b. A patient is going on vacation, and attempts to get a larger quantity than normal
    c. A patient had an increased dosage by their physician, and is taking a larger quantity than before so they run out before the scheduled refill date
    d. All of the above

29. If a DAW 0 was used, what does this mean?
    a. The prescriber wants a name brand dispensed
    b. The generic is dispensed or brand name only if there is no generic available
    c. The pharmacist wants the patient to have the brand name
    d. There is no generic available due to manufacturing or distribution issues

30. A patient is taking an antacid while also on a tetracycline antibiotic. The antacid will cause the antibiotic to cease working. This is an example of which type of DUR rejection?
    a. Drug–drug interaction
    b. Therapeutic duplication
    c. Allergy
    d. Contraindication

31. In a PPO, if a patient wants to see a specialist, they must do which of the following?
    a. Get a referral from their primary care physician
    b. Get approval from the pharmacy
    c. See any provider as long as they are in network
    d. None of the above

32. Coinsurance is similar to a co-payment, except patients do not pay a flat fee for prescriptions but a _____.
    a. Premium
    b. Cheaper cost
    c. Variable rate
    d. Percentage of the cost

33. Which of the following would *not* be covered under Medicare Part A?
    a. Inpatient hospital stays
    b. Prescription drugs
    c. Hospice care
    d. Home health care services

34. In order to be enrolled in Medicare Part C, a patient must be enrolled in which of the following Medicare parts?
    a. Parts A and B
    b. Parts A and D
    c. Parts B and D
    d. None of the above

35. Which of the following would Medicare Part D *not* cover?
    a. DME
    b. Lipitor
    c. Lisinipril
    d. Zetia

36. A patient learns that a medication the doctor has prescribed is not on the approved list of drugs covered by her insurance company. What is this list of drugs called?
    a. Adjudication
    b. Coordination of benefits
    c. Pharmacy benefit manager
    d. Formulary

37. Most patients enroll in private health care plans through contracts offered by which of he following?
    a. The pharmacy
    b. The insurance company
    c. Their employer
    d. None of the above

38. If a patient's services cost a total of $100, and they are responsible for 20% of the costs, this is known as which of the following?
    a. A co-payment
    b. A deductible
    c. A premium
    d. Coinsurance

39. Which part of Medicare covers DME and physician services or outpatient hospital visits?
    a. Part A
    b. Part B

c. Part C

d. Part D

40. A pharmacy benefit manager processes and pays for drug claims for which of the following?
    a. One insurance provider
    b. Multiple insurance providers
    c. Multiple pharmacies
    d. One pharmacy

41. How many numbers is the BIN number on each insurance card?
    a. 3
    b. 4
    c. 5
    d. 6

42. If a patient has had his or her coverage terminated, what restricts the pharmacy from accessing information about why the patient no longer has coverage?
    a. DEA
    b. HIPAA
    c. FDA
    d. State laws

43. When does a refill-too-soon error occurs?
    a. A patient attempts to get a 90-day supply of a medication
    b. A patient attempts to get a name brand of a medication
    c. A patient attempts to get their prescription filled before the insurance company permits a scheduled fill
    d. A prior authorization is needed

44. You are filling a prescription for a patient who insists on getting the brand name medication. What DAW code would this be?
    a. DAW 0
    b. DAW 1
    c. DAW 2
    d. DAW 3

45. DUR stands for which of the following?
    a. Drug utilization remission
    b. Drug utility recess
    c. Drug utilization review
    d. Director utilization review

46. A PA is also known as which of the following?
    a. Prior authorization
    b. Part A
    c. Premium assistance
    d. Pharmacy assistance

47. Which part of Medicare supplies patients with coverage for inpatient hospital stays and nursing facilities?
    a. Part A
    b. Part B
    c. Part C
    d. Part D

48. Which of the following is the Part D plan for Medicare?
    a. Is a voluntary program for Medicare patients
    b. Must be enrolled in during a designated period
    c. Is very important for pharmacy technicians to be familiar with
    d. All of the above

49. If a patient is pregnant, and given a medication that is a pregnancy class D, this would be considered what type of DUR rejection?
    a. Drug–drug interaction
    b. Therapeutic duplication
    c. Allergy
    d. Contraindication

50. Which of the DAW code is submitted when the prescriber indicates he or she wants the brand name dispensed?
    a. DAW 0
    b. DAW 1
    c. DAW 2
    d. DAW 3

Pharmacy Information System Usage and Applications

PTCB KNOWLEDGE AREAS

9.1 Pharmacy-related computer applications for documenting the dispensing of prescriptions or medication orders (eg, maintaining the electronic medical record, patient adherence, risk factors, alcohol drug use, drug allergies, and side effects)

9.2 Databases, pharmacy computer applications, and document management (eg, user access, drug database, interface, inventory report, usage reports, override reports, and diversion reports)

KEY TERMS

Biometrics: Identification of a person by their characteristics (ie, fingerprint, face recognition, DNA, palm print, iris recognition, and voice)

Clinical information system (CIS): An integrated system to store, manipulate, and retrieve electronic orders, medication administration records, evidence-based medicine, point-of-care applications, and nonclinical and administrative information

Drug information: Any written or electronic resource used to find answers to questions from patients, prescribers, or other pharmacists as related to the practice of dispensing or using medication for the treatment or prevention of illness and disease

Left click: A basic computer mouse has 2 buttons. When you press the left one, it is called a left click. This is typically the main button on the

mouse and is used for the most common tasks such as selecting or double clicking

Medication administration record (MAR): A computer-generated schedule for administering medications to a patient for a defined period of time

Multifunction printers (MFP): Office machine which incorporates the functionality of multiple devices in one. Provides centralized document management

Patient profile: A record of patient's medical information. Generally, used to identify valuable information necessary to aid the pharmacist in the practice of dispensing medication

Right click: A basic computer mouse has 2 buttons. When you press the right one, it is called a right click. This is typically used to open menus depending on where you click

CASE STUDY

The phone rings in at your workstation. Upon answering the phone a patient asks several questions regarding her medication therapy. First, she asks for the date her furosemide was last dispensed. Next, she wants to know if her physician's office has faxed over a new prescription for a β blocker. Lastly, she is wondering what some of the common side effects of this new medication may be.

Self-Assessment Questions
- Where should you begin when you investigate her questions?
- How many different pieces of equipment do you need to know how to operate in order to assist the patient?
- Which question should be passed to the pharmacist and how do you accomplish a successful transfer of the phone call?

INTRODUCTION

Pharmacists and technicians rely on well-organized, easily retrievable patient information to help them fill prescriptions and educate and counsel patients. With information coming into the pharmacy through different sources it is imperative for the pharmacy to have a robust information system to document and retrieve information about a patient's medication therapy. Pharmacy information systems have been around as long as there are pharmacies. This chapter will investigate the basics of these systems, and how the pharmacy technician interacts with them in order to provide assistance to the pharmacist.

BASIC PHARMACY HARDWARE

Pharmacy technicians must be familiar with the basic pieces of equipment in the pharmacy and understand how to use each of these in order to have a sufficiently operating pharmacy.

Phone

Mastering the telephone system in the pharmacy is essential. Many phone systems also include wireless devices, hands-free headsets, or earpieces to make working within the pharmacy easier and more efficient. There may even a required log-on to the phone similar to a computer log-on.

Proper phone training includes how to correctly answer a ringing line, how to place someone on hold, and how to transfer a call. More advanced skills include conferencing calls, overhead paging another person using the phone, and retrieving voicemails or refill requests. Confidence with the phone system will improve your ability to serve patients.

★ TECH ALERT: *Keep a list of frequently used commands or functions near the phone to quickly care for a customer and provide excellent customer service.*

Printing and Faxing Devices

In many pharmacies, single-use machines are now being replaced with multifunction devices (MFD) that can copy, print, and fax. There are many essential skills needed to properly use this hardware and each device is unique. Two important tasks include knowing where and how to load more paper and how to change the toner. Being able to perform this type of maintenance will keep the pharmacy workflow moving.

Computers

Computer skills are required to function effectively as a pharmacy technician. Familiarity with both hardware and software will help you navigate through pharmacy programs and patient profiles. For optimal computer performance, regular software updates and virus protection are required.

There are multiple types of computers as below:

- Mainframe: Large, powerful computers used to house and process large amounts of information
- Minicomputer: Smaller version of the mainframe
- Dumb terminal: Allows multiple users to access patient information
- Personal computer (PC): Any stand-alone computer system (ie, desktop, laptop, and tablet)
  - Desktop computer: PC used at a single location; contains a tower that houses the hardware and software, monitor, keyboard, and mouse
  - Laptop computer: Portable PC that can be used in any location; contains the same components as a desktop computer, but connected together
  - Tablet computer: Portable computer with a touch screen display; may or may not contain a keyboard; all components house in the tablet; size varies

Computers contain many different components depending on the type of machine (Table 9-1). It is important to understand the vocabulary in order to speak with information technology specialists, especially when a computer is not working.

★ *TECH ALERT: It is important to know your pharmacy's down-time procedure in case of computer system failure.*

TABLE 9-1. **Computer Components**	
Hardware	Physical components of a computer which are controlled by software
Monitor	Output device; display device that looks like a television
Mouse	Input device; computer pointing device, usually contains a trackball and 2 or more buttons
Hard disk drive	Data storage device within the computer
Keyboard	Input device; contains letters and numbers; however, may have other function keys needed for prescription processing
Printer	Output device; allows for a hard copy of information instead of on computer monitor
Light pen	Input device; used to scan in information (ie, medication bar code)
Disk drive	Input/output device; devices that uses light to read or write onto a disk (ie, compact disk); temporary storage
Scanner	Input device; scans an image or bar code to convert it to a digital image (ie, handheld scanner)
Modem	Device that allows a computer to communicate over a network
Universal Serial Bus (USB) drive	Input/output device; device that is similar to a compact disk, but much smaller in size and can hold a significant amount of data; also know as a flash or jump drive
Software	Machine-readable instructions that directs a computer to perform functions
Memory	Space available on a computer to save information, also known as random access memory (RAM)

PHARMACY-RELATED COMPUTER APPLICATIONS

Health systems are moving toward a fully integrated **clinical information system (CIS)** that houses all of the information necessary to successfully and efficiently treat a patient. The CIS is a robust combination of all the information related to the medical treatment of a patient. Pharmacy information is a large part of the CIS and it is important to know what information may be found there and how it can assist with the medication management of a patient.

Electronic Health Record

The electronic health record (EHR) is a digital record of a patient's health information that can be shared among different health care settings (ie, hospital, doctor's office, and pharmacy). The features of an EHR vary between systems. There are many advantages of using an EHR:

- Enables the tracking of patient care (ie, prescriptions and laboratory/radiology orders)
- Follows up with outcomes (ie, laboratory/radiology results and vitals)
- Prompt warnings (ie, drug interactions and allergies)
- Triggers patient reminders (ie, vaccines and mammograms)
- Sends and receives orders, reports, and results
- Improves care coordination
- Improves the work flow of health care workers (i.e physician, pharmacist, etc) with all results in one location

★ TECH ALERT: "Meaningful use" is the term used by Medicare and Medicaid for providing financial incentives. Providers have to show that they are "meaningfully using" their EHRs to obtain payment.

While EHRs have advantages, there are several known problems with their use. Implementing an EHR system is very costly. There are also many systems available, which make it difficult for the provider to choose a system and that system may not interact well with other systems. There is also the concern of privacy and confidentiality of the EHR system. Even though there are concerns with use, the EHR is utilized throughout the country and improves patient care on a daily basis.

Computerized Physician Order Entry

Computerized physician order entry (CPOE) is a way of entering orders for medications, laboratories, radiology, and nursing directly into the computer. The CPOE system sends the order to the appropriate department so that it may be fulfilled. This method of ordering is utilized in an inpatient setting (ie, hospital and nursing home). CPOE allows for real-time transmission of orders, so in the pharmacy, prescriptions can be verified immediately, and patients receive medications when needed.

Medication Administration Record

A **medication administration record (MAR)** is the document that is the record for the medications administered to a patient at a health care facility (ie, hospital and nursing home). The MAR is a permanent and legal record in the patient's medical record. An electronic record of a MAR is often called e-MAR.

The contents of a MAR vary based on setting; however, they typically contain the following:

- Patient information
  - Name
  - Medical record
  - Bed number
  - Admitting physician
  - Allergies, height, or weight
- Medication information
  - Drug name
  - Drug strength and formulation
  - Route of administration
  - Frequency
  - Medication indication
  - Prescribing physician
  - Time of actual administration
  - Signature or initials of the nurse administering medication

E-Prescribing

E-prescribing is a computer-based method that allows a prescriber to send a prescription directly to a pharmacy from the point of care. E-prescribing takes the place of a paper or faxed prescription. There are several advantages to e-prescribing: improved patient safety through a written order instead of illegible handwriting, increased quality of care, decrease time calling to pharmacy and call-backs to physician offices, improved formulary compliance, and increased patient convenience. Even though e-prescribing streamlines workflow, it does have some limitations. The disadvantages of e-prescribing are increased initial cost by the implementation of an e-prescribing system as well as switch fees the pharmacy may incur, system downtime, security risks, and choosing the right software. The use of e-prescribing has significantly increased due to payment incentives by insurance companies.

★ *TECH ALERT:*
E-prescribing and CPOE software often require 2 passwords or identifiers prior to allowing a prescriber to order a medication.

Telepharmacy

Telepharmacy is the delivery of pharmaceutical services via the computer when a pharmacy is unable to provide patients with direct contact to a pharmacist. Videoconferencing allows for patient counseling and interactions with other health care providers. This method is utilized in many smaller hospitals, where the cost of staying open during the night, greatly exceeds the cost of a telepharmacy service.

QUICK QUIZ 9-1

1. Which of the following types of computers may be utilized in a pharmacy setting?
   a. Laptop computer
   b. Desktop computer
   c. Tablet computer
   d. All of the above

2. Which of the following is a paperless transmission of a prescription from a prescriber directly to a pharmacy?

   a. CPOE

   b. Telepharmacy

   c. E-prescribing

   d. E-MAR

3. Which of the following is a computerized order entry method for prescribers?

   a. CPOE

   b. Telepharmacy

   c. E-prescribing

   d. MAR

4. All medications given to a patient must be documented on which of the following?

   a. CPOE

   b. MAR

   c. USB

   d. Hardware

5. Which of the following is an advantage to electronic medical records?

   a. Streamlines physician workflow

   b. Improvement in the coordination of care between practitioners

   c. Immediate alerting of potential issues

   d. All of the above

HIPAA AND PHARMACY TECHNOLOGY

The Health Insurance Portability and Accountability Act (HIPAA) sets minimum standards for privacy and security of protected health information (PHI). Various records kept in the pharmacy are examples of PHI, including prescription records, billing records, and patient profiles. The HIPAA privacy rule states that all PHI must be kept private and only the minimum information should be discussed for health care operations. HIPAA also discusses the security of PHI. Some examples of how to keep PHI secure include the following:

- Transmit PHI with encryption software
- Secure passwords with 2 factor identification
  - Something you know (ie, password)
  - Something you are (ie, biometric characteristic such as fingerprint or retina scan)
  - Something you have (ie, hard token that generates a one-time number and badge with imbedded identification)
- Role-based access that only allows providers to access certain data and function (ie, pharmacists and technicians have access to different sets of data and functions)

Clinical Decision Support System

The clinical decision support system (CDSS) is an interactive computer system that allows for the pharmacist to monitor the patient. The CDSS allows the pharmacist to be compliant with OBRA'90 and perform a prospective drug review. Some functions performed by a CDSS include the following:

- Over- or underutilization: Evaluates the day supply of the previous prescription and compares it to the current prescription. This allows for evaluation of patient adherence.
- Therapeutic duplication: Identifies medications in the same pharmacologic category.
- Drug–disease interaction: Detect medications that should not be taken with certain disease states.
- Drug–drug interaction: Triggers alerts for medications that should not be taken together.
- Incorrect dosage or duration of treatment: Warns for doses or duration of treatment that are outside of the appropriate range.
- Drug–allergy interaction: Notifies of medications that should not be taken based on allergic reaction.
- Drug–laboratory interaction: Alerts for medications that may need to be adjusted based on specific laboratory parameters.
- Pharmacokinetic monitoring: Evaluates medications that may need special monitoring due to narrow therapeutic ranges.
- Intravenous compatibility: Detects medications that are incompatible with each other.

Patient Profiles

The **patient profile** (Figure 9-1) is a legal record of medication dispensing where the necessary information for accurate dispensing is stored. It is also a reference for the pharmacist to refer when filling new medications for a patient, helping to prevent patient harm. It is important as a technician to gather as much information as possible when a patient is filling a prescription for the first time, and to inquire about any new changes, each time following. Listed below are important sections in a patient profile.

Demographics
Patient's demographic information includes patient's name, address, telephone number, and date of birth.

Allergies
Drug allergies are generally required to be input on a patient profile even before any medication orders can be entered. In a hospital setting, during an emergency, this system can be overridden to allow for the care of the patient during an emergency code. Documenting allergy information allows the pharmacist to properly evaluate any new prescription products for potentially dangerous reactions that may occur. But allergies to medications may not be the only issue, as even food allergies such as eggs, peanuts and gluten may all be real problems for patients when taking prescription products. Therefore, the allergy section of the patient profile should be filled out in its entirety to keep the patient safe from unnecessary harm.

★ *TECH ALERT: The allergic reaction to the medication should also be documented. This allows the pharmacist to evaluate potential cross-reactivity with other medications.*

```
Patient: Art Dealer_____
Address: 321 Lost Drive, Wherever, NV _____
Phone Number: 555-600-0006 _____
DOB: 05/30/1976_____
Gender: Male_____

Allergy information:
Penicillin – Rash_____
Peanuts – Throat swells, SOB_____

Other medication:
Daily multivitamin, acetaminophen 325-mg tablets as needed, omeprazole 40-mg tablet daily

Medical history:
GERD (2012), family history of HTN, family history of stroke _____

Insurance:
BIN: 456789, ID #: 123567891, Rx GRP: THB3ST_____
```

Rx#	DATE	Medication	QTY	Dose	Refills	Prescriber
856794	1/6/13	Epinephrine	2 autojects	0.3 mg PRN	2	Shaw, D.
856795	1/6/13	Albuterol HFA	1 inhaler	1 puff q4h PRN SOB	4	Shaw, D.

FIGURE 9-1 Patient profile example.

Concurrent Medications

Of equal importance for patient safety is documentation of all the other medications taken, including both prescription and **over-the-counter (OTC)** medication. It is important to update this information continually, as a patient's medication regimen may change frequently.

Medical History

A patient's medical history may include important family history facts as well as the patient's own medical history, such as a diagnosis, alcohol or drug use, and even past history of surgeries. In an inpatient setting, this information is readily available for the pharmacist to review prior to dispensing medications.

Special Considerations

Special considerations for patients are also documented in the patient profile. For example, some patients may have limited vision and require special labeling in order to use the product correctly. Some pharmacies provide services to patients that require labels or instructions to be printed in a foreign language. In any case, these notes are essential to provide a positive patient experience and safe medication use.

Insurance Information

★ **TECH ALERT:** *"Self-pay" is the term used when a patient does not have insurance and is responsible for the entire amount out-of-pocket.*

Pharmacy technicians and pharmacists are responsible for keeping insurance information up to date in order to ensure proper billing for each patient. Insurance information will include the details regarding a patient's third party insurance such as the member's ID number or group number. It should also be documented if the patient does not have any insurance.

Medication Order

The patient profile will show current medication status. Details such as the date of dispensing, amount dispensed, refills remaining, and date of next refill are all fields that could be available for a quick overview of the patient's various prescriptions. Keep in mind that hard copies of the original prescriptions must be kept in a readily retrievable form (such as printed files) as required by the State Board of Pharmacy. The patient profile should serve as a quick reference tool for the hard copies of those prescriptions.

PHARMACY REPORTING SYSTEMS

Pharmacy computer applications allow for many types of reports to be completed. Reports are essential to improving patient care, managing inventory, and detecting diversion. Some reports that are commonly evaluated include the following:

- Medication usage patterns including nonformulary drug use
- Monthly drug costs
- Productivity and workload
- Clinical interventions performed and documented by pharmacists
- Controlled substance use and waste report to evaluate for diversion
- Financial reports to evaluate reimbursement
- Override reports
- Recall reports

Automation

Today, there are many ways the pharmacy team is assisted with new and even some old automation. Dispensing cabinets, barcode scanners, tablet and capsule counting machines, and robots are creating a more efficient and safer pharmacy for patients.

Automated Dispensing Cabinets

Automated dispensing cabinets (ADCs) (ie, Pyxis, AcuDose, Omnicell, etc.) are systems that are used daily in hundreds of hospitals and other direct patient care organizations. These cabinets make it easier for a caregiver to retrieve a single dose of medication to be immediately administered to a patient. Pharmacy technicians play a role in keeping cabinets stocked and secure. These cabinets are able to store, dispense, track inventory, and even create charges for the medication being administered to the patient. The cabinets have the capability to directly interface with the patient profile and allow nursing staff to obtain medication specific for the patient after the order has been reviewed by a pharmacist.

Barcode Scanners

Barcode scanners allow patient caregivers to identify medication correctly by scanning the bar code found on the medication packaging. A retail pharmacy uses this technology to speed up the medication identification and checking process and a health care system uses this technology to verify the correct medication has been selected, medication administration times, and the correct patient (wrist band bar code). The challenges with using a barcode scanning system for medication administration include the following:

- Products with unreadable or missing bar codes
- Scanners that only read a specific barcode label (there are a variety in use)
- False sense of security and safety when administering medications

These issues with bar codes tend to be barriers to proper implementation. The cost of implementing a barcode scanning system can also be very high and therefore seem unappealing to a pharmacy. However, any step toward reducing error potential should be considered as a viable quality improvement project and investigated thoroughly before being dismissed as too costly.

Other Automation Examples

Tabletop tablet counters can be used in place of the typical tray and spatula to count tablets for dispensing. This may increase productivity and improve accuracy. Many of the robots found in retail and health system settings are larger scale versions of the tablet and capsule counters capable of interfacing with the dispensing software to generate the final medication product that is ready to be checked by the pharmacist. The introduction of miniature cameras, positive identification upon logging in to a system, and the scalability of the robots create an efficient workflow system for the pharmacy that allows the pharmacist more time to provide care to the patient and reduce the time spent on checking medication.

Drug Information

TECH ALERT: The number of the poison control center throughout the United States is 1-800-222-1222.

Required references in a pharmacy vary by state, and the drug information resources needed in each pharmacy location vary by setting (Table 9-2). For example, the desired drug information books would be different in an inpatient pediatric hospital when compared to an outpatient adult-only compounding pharmacy.

QUICK QUIZ 9-2

1. Which of the following would not be necessary in a patient profile?
- **a.** Name
- **b.** Address
- **c.** Mother's maiden name
- **d.** Date of birth

2. Which of the following information is checked against the patient profile?
- **a.** Drug–allergy risk
- **b.** Drug–drug interaction risk
- **c.** Drug–indication risk
- **d.** All of the above may be checked against a patient profile

TABLE 9-2. **Examples of Drug Information Resources**	
Federal and state law reference	Available online or hard copy for each individual state
Pharmacotherapy	*Applied Therapeutics: The Clinical Use of Drugs* *Conn's Current Therapy* *Goodman and Gilman's The Pharmacological Basis of Therapeutics* *Pharmacotherapy: A Pathophysiological Approach*
Dosage and toxicology	*American Drug Index* *American Hospital Formulary Service Drug Information* *Drug Information Handbook* *Drug Facts and Comparisons* *Handbook on Injectable Drugs* *Lexi-Comp: Drug Information Handbook* *Merck Manual* *Physician's Desk Reference* *The Red Book* *USP Dispensing Information*
Equivalency	*The Orange Book: Approved Drug Products with Therapeutic Equivalence Equations*
Natural and herbal	*Lexi-Comp: Natural Products Index* *Natural Medicines Comprehensive Database* *Natural Standard* *Review of Natural Products*
Nonprescription	*Handbook of Nonprescription Drugs* *PDR for Nonprescription Drugs, Dietary Supplements, and Herbs*
Pediatrics	*Harriet Lane Handbook* *NeoFax* *Pediatric Dosage Handbook*
Pregnancy	*American Academy of Pediatrics: Transfer of Drugs and Other Chemicals into Human Milk* *Brigg's Drugs in Pregnancy and Lactation*

3. Which of the following is an example of automation in the pharmacy?

   a. ADC

   b. Bar coding

   c. Robots

   d. All of the above

4. Which reference text may be utilized if a patient has a question about an OTC vitamin?

   a. FDA's the *Orange Book*

   b. *Brigg's Drugs in Pregnancy and Lactation*

   c. *Lexi-Comp: Natural Products Index*

   d. *Goodman and Gilman's The Pharmacological Basis of Therapeutics*

5. Biometric screening could include the positive identification of which of the following?

    a. Fingerprint

    b. Retina scan

    c. Password set at computer log in

    d. a and b only

~~~~~~

Today, many pharmacies are able to meet the set requirements by subscribing to online and electronic versions of texts and drug information. These virtual libraries may even be integrated into the dispensing software. They are available for reference at the point of order entry and at the point of any final checking of the finished product being dispensed.

New drug information is emerging every day, thus an electronic medium is more likely to be current (Table 9-3). The convenience of electronic systems is evident, but they also present a challenge for every pharmacy team member. The proper use of these systems should be evaluated and the content updated as required by the vendor in order to maintain the integrity of the information. Managing and maintaining a quality drug information library is a necessity for each pharmacy.

TABLE 9-3. **Web-Based Drug Information Resources**	
Clinical Pharmacology	www.clinicalpharmacology-ip.com
Facts and Comparisons e-Answers	www.factsandcomparisons.com
Lexi-Comp Online	www.lexi.com
Medline Plus	www.nlm.nih.gov/medlineplus
Micromedex	www.micromedex.com
ToxNet	www.toxnet.nlm.nih.gov
Up To Date	www.uptodate.com

CASE STUDY REVIEW

The phone rings at your workstation. Upon answering the phone, a patient asks several questions regarding her medication therapy. First, she asks for the date her furosemide was last dispensed. Next, she wants to know if her physician's office has faxed over a new prescription for a β blocker. Lastly, she is wondering what some of the common side effects of this new medication may be.

Self-Assessment Questions

- Where should you begin when you investigate her questions?
  - You will begin to help the patient on the phone by answering the call in a timely manner and making sure you positively identify the patient according to the pharmacy policies. At this point, you would access the patient profile.

The patient profile is likely to be accessed on a computer terminal by opening the dispensing software and searching for the patient by name, birthday, telephone number, or other form of identification.

- How many different pieces of equipment do you need to know how to operate in order to assist the patient?
  - Throughout your interaction with this patient you will need to use the phone system, computer, and fax machine.
- Which question should be passed to the pharmacist and how do you accomplish a successful transfer of the phone call?
  - When the patient asks a particular question regarding the adverse effects of the new medication, you will have to transfer the phone call to the pharmacist and at that point the pharmacist may begin using a drug information system to find answers to the patient's questions.

CHAPTER SUMMARY

- Understanding the functions and how to troubleshoot the phone, fax, printer, and computer are part of the pharmacy operations and workflow.
- The patient profile is used to document and retrieve information about a patient's medication use, medical history, and allergy information.
- Drug information resources aid the pharmacist and technician when answering difficult questions or when researching basic medication facts and dosing.
- Clinical information systems provide all of the patient information in one spot to aid all prescribers and clinicians when caring for a patient.
- Reporting software and systems are used to easily read and evaluate specific information about a patient.

ANSWERS TO QUICK QUIZZES

Quick Quiz 9-1

1. All of the above
2. E-prescribing
3. CPOE
4. USB
5. All of the above

Quick Quiz 9-2

1. Mother's maiden name
2. All of the above may be checked against a patient profile
3. All of the above
4. *Lexi-Comp: Natural Products Index*
5. Fingerprint and retina scan

CHAPTER QUESTIONS

1. Which of the following is *not* a type of pharmacy automation?
   a. Robot
   b. Ointment slab and spatula
   c. Barcode scanner
   d. Tabletop tablet counter

2. In which reference book would you find detailed patient counseling information?
   a. State Law Book
   b. Federal Law Book
   c. Natural Product Reference
   d. Patient Handout Information Reference

3. A computer mouse is used for which of the following commands?
   a. Double click
   b. Tap the screen
   c. Type a password
   d. Press the function key

4. Which of the following are drug information resources?
   a. Written references used to find answers to questions
   b. Electronic references used to find answers to questions
   c. Available for patients and pharmacists to read and review
   d. All of the above

5. Which CDSS function helps identify patient adherence?
   a. Therapeutic duplication
   b. Drug-allergy
   c. Drug-laboratory
   d. Over- or underutilization

6. What pharmacy system allows a pharmacist to counsel a patient in a different location?
   a. CPOE
   b. E-prescribing
   c. Telepharmacy
   d. EHR

7. A clinical information system may contain which of the following information?
   a. Electronic orders
   b. Medication administration records

   c. Patient information
   d. All of the above

8. The MAR stands for which of the following?
   a. Medication administration record
   b. Multiple admission record
   c. Memory amplified recording
   d. None of the above

9. In which reference book would you find information regarding the storage requirements of a medication?
   a. *Drug Facts and Comparisons*
   b. *Natural Standard*
   c. *Federal Law Book*
   d. *NeoFax*

10. What basic information is *not* contained in the patient profile?
    a. Patient's name
    b. Medication allergies
    c. Social security number
    d. Insurance information

11. Which of the following technology is used frequently in the pharmacy?
    a. Computer
    b. Automated tablet counters
    c. Barcode scanner
    d. All of the above

12. Which of the following is *not* used to input information into a computer?
    a. Mouse
    b. Monitor
    c. USB
    d. Light pen

13. When are down-time procedures used in a pharmacy?
    a. Power outage
    b. Fax machines run out of paper
    c. The label printer is switched off
    d. 1 of 4 computers is not working

14. A patient profile may be updated using any of the following *except* which one?
    a. A keyboard
    b. A mouse

c. A touch screen monitor
d. A speaker

15. Which of the following is correct about patient allergy information?
    a. Is not necessary
    b. Should be reviewed frequently with patients
    c. Should include *only* drug allergy information
    d. May not be collected by technicians

16. Which of the following reports is most useful to identify a product's availability?
    a. Inventory report
    b. Usage report
    c. Override report
    d. Diversion report

17. Medication doses given to patients are recorded on which of the following?
    a. CIS
    b. Monitor
    c. MAR
    d. Barcode scanner

18. Which of the following is correct about the bar-code scanner?
    a. Prevents all medication errors
    b. May not be able to read some bar codes
    c. Is used only for medication
    d. Should only be used "sometimes"

19. The list of a patient's current medications should *not* include which of the following?
    a. Over-the-counter medications
    b. Other prescription medications
    c. Nutritional supplements
    d. All of the above should be included

20. If a patient has limited vision which of the following is correct?
    a. That information should be on the patient profile
    b. It is best to ask each and every time the patient needs care
    c. No special considerations should be taken
    d. The patient must remember to ask for bold print labeling

21. In which reference book would you find information regarding dosage forms available for a specific medication?

    a. *Natural Product Reference*
    b. *Federal Law Book*
    c. *General Drug Information Reference*
    d. *Patient Handout Information Reference*

22. A patient's insurance card is likely to include all of the following except which one?
    a. Member's ID number
    b. Member's group number
    c. Billing identification number (BIN)
    d. Contracted pricing structure

23. In which reference book would you find information regarding record keeping requirements for prescriptions?
    a. *State Law Book*
    b. *Natural Product Reference*
    c. *Drug Information Reference*
    d. *Patient Handout Information Reference*

24. What allows a computer to communicate over a network?
    a. Modem
    b. Light pen
    c. Universal Serial Bus
    d. Disk drive

25. In which reference book would you find information regarding recommended doses of ginkgo?
    a. *State Law book*
    b. *Natural Standard*
    c. *Harriet Lane Handbook*
    d. *Brigg's Drug in Pregnancy and Lactation*

26. What is the number for the poison control center?
    a. 1-800-222-1222
    b. 1-888-111-2111
    c. 1-800-111-2111
    d. 1-800-POISONC

27. To improve efficiency, health systems may use an ADM stocked with medication. What is an ADM?
    a. Accurate dose meter
    b. Automated dispensing machine
    c. Administration drug monitor
    d. Actual dispensing monitor

28. Allergy information collected on a patient profile should include which of the following?
    a. Food allergies
    b. Medication allergies
    c. Environmental allergies
    d. All of the above

29. In which reference book would you find information regarding whether or not a medication should be taken with food?
    a. General Drug information Reference
    b. Federal Law Book
    c. Patient Handout Information Reference
    d. Both a and c

30. Which of the following is not an important part of a patient profile?
    a. Address
    b. Phone number
    c. Allergies
    d. All are important in a patient profile

31. Which is an example of a drug–allergy interaction?
    a. Amoxicillin prescribed for a penicillin allergic patient
    b. Amoxicillin prescribed for a patient on Augmentin
    c. Amoxicillin prescribed for a patient with a bacterial infection
    d. Amoxicillin prescribed for a patient by a dentist

32. In which reference book would you find information regarding the Drug Enforcement Administration (DEA) classification of a medication?
    a. Federal Law Book
    b. Patient Handout Information Reference
    c. General Drug Information Reference
    d. Both a and c

33. A patient's insurance card is likely to include all of the following except which one?
    a. Member's ID number
    b. Patient's height and weight
    c. Member's group number
    d. Billing identification number (BIN)

34. The MAR is useful for determining which of the following?
    a. When a dose of medication is due
    b. If the patient has had an adverse reaction
    c. How much urine output the patient has had for the past 8 hours
    d. The patient's red blood cell count

35. Which of the following is *not* a type of pharmacy automation?
    a. Robot
    b. Dispensing cabinet
    c. Barcode scanner
    d. Tray and spatula

36. In which reference book would you find information regarding the requirements of a prescription label?
    a. Natural Product Reference
    b. Patient Handout Information Reference
    c. State Law Book
    d. Drug Information Reference

37. Which of the following computers is used to house and process large amounts of data?
    a. Desktop
    b. Mainframe
    c. Laptop
    d. Tablet

38. Which of the following is an output device?
    a. Modem
    b. Keyboard
    c. Light pen
    d. Disk drive

39. Which of the following is *not* an advantage of an electronic health record (EHR)?
    a. Quickly track prescriptions
    b. Low cost
    c. Triggers patient care reminders
    d. Prompts allergy warnings

40. Which method of prescribing decreases handwriting errors?
    a. Pen or paper
    b. Faxing written order
    c. E-prescribing
    d. Verbal orders

41. Which of the following pieces of information are found on a MAR?
    a. Patient's name
    b. Patient's next of kin
    c. Medication cost
    d. Patient's insurance data

42. Which of the following is *not* an example of a secure identifier to protect PHI?
    a. Password
    b. Biometric fingerprint
    c. Hard token generator
    d. All of the above are secure identifiers

43. Which of the following may be provided by a clinical decision support system (CDSS)?
    a. Drug-allergy
    b. Therapeutic duplication
    c. Pharmacokinetic monitoring
    d. All of the above

44. Which of the following devices store medications on a nursing unit?
    a. Barcode scanners
    b. Automated dispensing cabinets
    c. Tabletop tablet counters
    d. Robots

45. Which of the following may increase the speed of prescription dispensing?
    a. Robots
    b. Tabletop tablet counters
    c. Automated dispensing cabinets
    d. All of the above

46. Which of the following books is used to obtain equivalency information?
    a. *NeoFax*
    b. *Brigg's Drugs in Pregnancy and Lactation*
    c. *The Orange Book*
    d. *Handbook for Nonprescription Drugs*

47. Which of the following reports is most useful to identify a fast-moving product?
    a. Inventory report
    b. Usage report
    c. Override report
    d. Diversion report

48. Which is an example of a drug–drug interaction?
    a. Bactrim prescribed for a penicillin allergic patient
    b. Amoxicillin prescribed for a patient on Augmentin
    c. Acyclovir prescribed for a patient with a bacterial infection
    d. Oxycodone prescribed for a patient by a dentist

49. In which reference book would you find information regarding the stability of a medication compounded in a sterile IV solution?
    a. State Law Book
    b. Federal Law Book
    c. General Drug Information Reference
    d. Natural Product Reference

50. A patient's insurance card is likely to include all of the following except which one?
    a. Member's ID number
    b. Member's group number
    c. Patient diagnosis
    d. Billing identification number (BIN)

Answers to Chapter Questions

MATH REVIEW

1. c: There are 60 mg per grain.

2. b: $\dfrac{1600\ \mu g}{mL} \times \dfrac{1\ mg}{1000\ \mu g} \times 250\ mL = 400\ mg$

3. d: There are 2.2 lb per kg.

4. b: x = 10, l = 50, v = 5. Since the x is first and smaller than the l, it is 50 − 10 + 5 = 45.

5. d: There are 3 teaspoons per tablespoon.

6. d: 30/60.

7. d: 0.5.

8. b: There are approximately 30 mL per fluid ounce.

9. c: $\dfrac{1}{100\ g} = \dfrac{X}{30\ g}$

     X = 0.3 g or 300 mg.

10. c: There are approximately 5 mL per dram.

11. c: Electrolytes are typically expressed in milliequivalent.

12. b: Each patch will last 3 days. (72 hours = 3 days); 5 patches will last 15 days (2 weeks = 14 days)

13. c: 0.5 g = 500 mg. Thus, 250 mg × 2 capsules × 4 times per day × 10 days = 80.

14. b: 120 mg divided by 4 doses is 30 mg.

15. a: There are approximately 480 mL per pint.

16. b: Apothecary is the system using grains and drams.

17. a: x = 10, v = 5; so, xxv = 25.

18. a: Injectable solutions are expressed as weight per volume or w/v.

19. b: There are approximately 30 mL per fluid ounce.

20. d: Units should not be abbreviated.

21. d: °F = °C × (9/5) + 32. Thus, 23 × (9/5) + 32 = 73.4.

22. b: x = 10, i = 1, v = 5. Since the i is smaller than the v, it is 5 − 1 = 4 + 10 = 14.

23. b: The avoirdupois system uses tablespoon and teaspoon.

24. d: 1000 μg = 1 mg, so 560/1000 μg = 0.56 mg.

25. d: $\dfrac{1\,g}{100\,mL} = \dfrac{X}{20\,mL}$

    X = 0.2 g or 200 mg.

26. b: There are 60 mg per grain.

27. c: $\dfrac{3200\,\mu g}{mL} \times \dfrac{1\,mg}{1000\,\mu g} \times 250\,mL = 800\,mg.$

28. c: There are 2.2 lb per kg.

29. a: X = 10, l = 50. Since the x is first and smaller than the l, it is 50 − 10 = 40.

30. d: There are 5 mL per tablespoon.

31. d: 20/60.

32. d: 0.3.

33. c: There are approximately 30 mL per fluid ounce.

34. b: There are approximately 5 mL per teaspoon. So, 10/5 mL = 2 teaspoons.

35. c: $\dfrac{1}{100\,g} = \dfrac{X}{60\,g}$

    X = 0.6 g or 600 mg.

36. b: Ointment is a solid in a solid, thus expressed as weight/weight or w/w.

37. d: There are approximately 5 mL per dram.

38. c: Potassium chloride is expressed in milliequivalent.

39. b: Each patch will last 3 days. (72 hours = 3 days); 3 patches will last 9 days (1 week = 7 days).

40. b: $\dfrac{1\,g}{100\,mL} = \dfrac{X}{0.1\,mL}$

    X = 0.001 g or 1 mg.

41. d: Twice daily × 2 days = 4 doses, then once daily × 7 days = 7 doses; thus 4 + 7 = 11 × 1 mg = 11 mg total treatment course.

42. c: $\dfrac{1\,dose}{0.1\,mL} = \dfrac{X\,doses}{2.5\,mL}$

    X = 25 doses.

43. a: Yes, the patient needs 11 doses and the bottle contains 25 doses.

44. b: Each drop contains 0.05 mL. So, 0.1 mL/0.05 = 2 drops.

45. d: 18/35.

46. d: 0.51.

47. b: 0.5 g = 500 mg. Thus, 250 mg × 2 caps × 3 times per day × 7 days = 42.

48. d: Insulin is expressed in units.

49. b: 180 mg divided by 4 doses = 45 mg per dose.

50. a: There are approximately 480 mL per pint.

ONE

1. a: Diflucan (fluconazole) is available as intravenous solution, suspension, and tablet.

2. d: Mobic (meloxicam) is a nonsteroidal anti-inflammatory drug (NSAID) that can increase the risk of bleeding in patients receiving aspirin and warfarin.

3. a: Diclofenac is the generic of Voltaren and is an NSAID.

4. a: NSAIDs can increase the risk of gastrointestinal bleeding.

5. a: Opioids cause constipation, sedation, and respiratory failure.

6. b: Fentanyl transdermal (Duragesic) is in DEA class II.

7. c: Sumatriptan is indicated for the acute treatment of migraines.

8. b: Grapefruit juice can increase potency of statins and make them toxic.

9. d: Rosuvastatin is the generic name of Crestor and is a statin.

10. a: Lotensin (benazepril) is a category X medication and contraindicated in pregnancy.

11. d: Ramipril is the generic name of Altace and is an angiotensin-converting enzyme inhibitor (ACEI).

12. a: Only levothyroxine is available in an injection formulation.

13. c: The most common side effects of Augmentin (amoxicillin/clavulanate) are diarrhea, allergic reaction, and rash.

14. a: Lisinopril is an ACEI.

15. c: Inderal (propranolol) can exacerbate asthma by blocking β receptors.

16. d: Toprol XL (metoprolol extended release) should not be crushed.

17. d: Statins are indicated for hypercholesterolemia.

18. c: Atenolol is indicated for hypertension.

19. a: Lasix (furosemide) should be taken early in the day to minimize nighttime diuresis.

20. d: Nitroglycerin can be used to treat anal fissures, angina, and heart failure.

21. b: Clopidogrel is the generic name of Plavix.

22. b: Metformin is contraindicated in patients with renal failure.

23. c: There is a potential cross-reaction between cephalosporins and penicillins.

24. a: Amaryl (glimepiride) should be given before the first meal of the day.

25. b: Intravenous injection directly goes into the blood stream, thus having the fastest onset of action.

26. d: Trazodone is indicated in the treatment of depression.

27. a: OD means the right eye.

28. a: Pioglitazone can exacerbate heart failure by causing edema.

29. b: Rosiglitazone is the generic name for Avandia.

30. c: Methimazole is indicated for hyperthyroidism.

31. b: A side effect of ACE inhibitors is cough.

32. d: Tylenol #4 contains 60 mg of codeine and is a C-III.

33. a: Zyban (bupropion) is indicated for smoking cessation.

34. c: Effexor XR (venlafaxine) cannot be crushed or chewed.

35. a: Ketoconazole is an antifungal.

36. c: Ativan (lorazepam) may be refilled for 6 months.

37. a: Zolpidem is indicated for insomnia.

38. a: Spiriva (tiotropium) can cause blurred vision if the contents are sprayed in the eyes.

39. a: Diuretics cause an increase in excretion of urine and electrolytes.

40. c: Guaifenesin is an expectorant.

41. d: Patients who are of age greater than 35 years or smoke are at a greater risk of cardiovascular side effects.

42. c: *The Orange Book* contains therapeutic equivalence information.

43. d: Lyrica (pregabalin) is in DEA class V.

44. c: The generic name of Crestor is rosuvastatin and the brand name of lovastatin is Mevacor.

45. c: Wellbutrin (bupropion) is indicated for depression.

46. c: Sinemet (carbidopa/levodopa) increases the levels of dopamine.

47. c: Atypical antipsychotics increase blood sugar and the risk of diabetes.

48. c: A common side effect of Zyprexa (olanzapine) is weight gain.

49. a: Ritalin (methylphenidate) can cause insomnia.

50. d: Antacids can bind with ferrous sulfate, ciprofloxacin, and doxycycline and decrease their effectiveness.

TWO

1. a: United States Pharmacopeia.

2. c: DEA form 106 is used to report document theft or loss of C-II medications.

3. d: Methadone is a C-II medication.

4. d: The Pure Food and Drug Act of 1906 required drugs not be mislabeled and set standards for strength and purity.

5. d: Drugs are intended for the use of prevention, treatment, and diagnosis of disease.

6. c: Medications with a low abuse potential and acceptable medication use are in schedule IV.

7. b: The Durham-Humphrey Amendment created 2 medication classes: OTC and prescription.

8. c: The Drug Listing Act required each drug to be assigned a NDC number.

9. d: To accurately dispense a prescription, the pharmacy should obtain the patient's name, address, and age.

10. b: The Poison Prevention Act created the standard requirement of child-resistant containers.

11. a: Anabolic steroids are in DEA schedule III.

12. b: Asking other patrons to step away from the counter during a counseling session promotes the protection of PHI.

13. d: Pseudoephedrine is the main ingredient in methamphetamine.

14. d: The pharmacy must keep track of the name and address of the purchaser, date and time of sale, and the name of the product, in order to abide by the law.

15. b: The Drug Enforcement Administration (DEA) enforces the controlled substance laws.

16. a: United States Pharmacopeia (USP) sets standards for the identity, strength, quality, and purity of medicines, food ingredients, and dietary supplements manufactured, distributed, and consumed worldwide.

17. c: $1 + 3 + 5 = 9$, $2 + 4 + 6 = 12 \times 2 = 24 + 9 = 3\underline{3}$. The letter A is a letter that is used for physicians and the physician's last name begins with the letter S.

18. c: The DEA 222 is used to order C-II medications.

19. d: Facsimile, telephone, and e-script may be used to transmit a prescription to the pharmacy.

20. d: A valid prescription requires date of issue, name and address of the practitioner, and the name of the patient.

21. d: A C-II prescription requires the quantity written in numerical and alpha form, and a physician's DEA.

22. a: The Health Insurance Portability and Accountability Act (HIPAA) protects the privacy of a patients' protected health information.

23. b: The Food and Drug Administration (FDA) protects the public by assuring safety, effectiveness and control of drugs, cosmetics, food, dietary supplements, and other medical products and devices.

24. e: Medication labels must contain the name of the pharmacy, address, phone number, and name of the patient.

25. a: When faced with different state and federal laws, the more strict law should be followed.

26. a: Over-the-counter (OTC) medications may be sold without a prescription.

27. d: The Pure Food and Drug Act of 1906 required that drugs not be mislabeled, be industry pure and of standard strength, and contain the amount stated on the label.

28. a: The Food, Drug, and Cosmetic Act of 1938 was passed to legally define a drug and establish policies to determine safety.

29. b: The Controlled Substances Act defined drug schedules.

30. c: Clonazepam is a schedule IV medication.

31. a: Medications are listed in the USP.

32. d: Natural supplements are not drugs, because they cannot claim to prevent, treat, or diagnose a disease.

33. d: The most restrictive class is C-I.

34. b: PHI stands for protected health information.

35. c: Medication schedules are defined by abuse potential and safety information.

36. a: The Durham-Humphrey Amendment created 2 medication classes: OTC and prescription.

37. c: The Health Insurance Portability and Accountability Act (HIPAA) protects the privacy of a patients' protected health information.

38. b: "Caution: Federal law prohibits dispensing without a prescription" is the federal legend.

39. d: The Omnibus Budget Reconciliation Act of 1990 (OBRA'90) required patient counseling.

40. b: HIPAA protects PHI.

41. c: The HIPAA sets standards for storing patient information.

42. d: Pseudoephedrine is the main ingredient in methamphetamine.

43. c: The Drug Enforcement Administration (DEA) enforces the controlled substance laws.

44. b: The State Board of Pharmacy licenses pharmacists.

45. d: Ketamine is a schedule III medication.

46. b: The National Formulary (NF) includes standards for excipients, botanicals, and other similar products.

47. a: The Drug Enforcement Administration (DEA) enforces the controlled substance laws.

48. d: The Food, Drug, and Cosmetic Act of 1938 officially defined drugs and established policies to determine drug safety.

49. a: Birth control pills do not require child-resistant packaging.

50. c: Inviting more than one patient at a time into the counseling area does not promote the protection of PHI.

THREE

1. b: Trituration is the act of grinding particles into fine powders with the use of a mortar and pestle.

2. b: Levigation is the process of reducing the particle size of a powder through the addition of a liquid.

3. d: A suspension is a homogeneous mixture in which the active ingredient is not completely dissolved, but rather suspended, in liquid.

4. b: Subcutaneous medications are injected directly into the fatty layer below the skin's surface.

5. b: IV piggybacks are a small volume of medication, typically less than 250 mL, which is infused through the same lines as a primary IV fluid.

6. d: The drip rate is the rate at which an IV medication is infused.

7. a: Conical graduates are best suited for viscous liquids because the sloped sides allow for more product to be emptied from the graduate.

8. c: The volume of a liquid in a graduate should be read at the bottom of the meniscus.

9. a: Powders for reconstitution are commercially available, and thus do not require extemporaneous compounding.

10. a: Horizontal flow hoods should be cleaned with isopropyl alcohol in the direction of clean air flow, from back to front.

11. b: Aseptic technique dictates compounding should occur 6 in from the front and sides of the laminar flow hood.

12. b: 5 mg—equal parts just be mixed together using the principle of geometric dilution.

13. c: Oral preparations do not need to be kept sterile.

14. c: $\dfrac{12.5 \text{ mg}}{5 \text{ mL}} \times 20 \text{ mL} = 50 \text{ mg}$

15. a: Oral preparations have a beyond-use date of 14 days.

16. b: Even if stored in the refrigerator, oral preparations have a beyond-use date of 14 days.

17. c: Reverse distribution is a process in which unused or expired medications are returned to the manufacturer.

18. a: The beyond-use date of a product prepared at a patient's bedside must be immediate use only.

19. b: TPNs are medium-risk sterile products, which have a beyond-use date of 30 hours.

20. a: A precipitant has formed in the solution and the bag should not be dispensed.

21. c: Eye preparations should always be sterile.

22. a: Filters must be used with ampules because of the risk of glass shards entering the final product.

23. a: Special PPE must be worn while compounding chemotherapy due to the potential hazards of the medications.

24. d: Amino acids, dextrose, and lipids are all found in TPNs.

25. d: Multidose vials contain preservatives and preservatives should never be given epidurally.

26. b: Shoes should remain on, but shoe covers should be worn in sterile compounding areas.

27. c: Aseptic technique limits the risk of microbial contamination.

28. a: The downward flow of air protects the user from exposure to the potentially hazardous chemotherapy medications.

29. b: Appropriate hand washing means washing for at least 30 seconds with antimicrobial soap and water.

30. a: USP Chapter 795 defines guidelines for nonsterile compounding, USP Chapter 797 defines guidelines for sterile compounding.

31. b: IV push is the rapid administration of a small volume of medication into the vein.

32. c: Total volume 60 mL – volume of powder 12.4 mL = 47.6 mL water

33. c: $\dfrac{25 \text{ mg}}{5 \text{ mL}} \times \dfrac{100 \text{ mg}}{X}$

    X = 20 mL or 4 teaspoons (1 teaspoon = 5 mL)

34. b: 20 mL × 2 doses per day × 7 days = 280 mL

35. b: $15 \text{ lb} \times \dfrac{1 \text{ lb}}{2.2 \text{ kg}} = 6.8 \text{ kg}$

    $\dfrac{2.2 \text{ mg}}{\text{kg}} \times 6.8 \text{ kg} = 15 \text{ mg}$

36. a: $\dfrac{25 \text{ mg}}{5 \text{ mL}} = \dfrac{15 \text{ mg}}{X}$

    X = 3 mL

37. b: D10W is the abbreviation for dextrose 10% in water.

38. a: 4.2 mL/h × 12 h = 50.4 mL

    $\dfrac{20 \text{ mg}}{100 \text{ mL}} = \dfrac{X}{50.4 \text{ mL}}$

    X = 10 mg

39. c: $\dfrac{0.25 \text{ mL}}{\text{min}} \times \dfrac{60 \text{ min}}{1 \text{ h}} \times 6 \text{ h} = 90 \text{ mL in 6 h}$

    $\dfrac{1 \text{ mg}}{\text{mL}} = \dfrac{X}{90 \text{ mL}}$

    X = 90 mg

40. a: Geometric dilution is a process in which ingredients are mixed together in equal proportions to ensure a homogeneous final product.

41. c: TPN is also referred to as hyperalimentation.

42. a: Rectal products do not need to be sterile, while TPNs, epidurals, and ophthalmic solutions must be sterile.

43. b: Beakers are less accurate in measuring volume than graduated cylinders.

44. d: Suspensions are heterogeneous mixtures in which the active ingredient is not completely dissolved, but rather suspended, in the liquid. Therefore, to distribute the active ingredient evenly, they must be shaken well before use.

45. b: Topical ointments contain some water, and thus have a beyond-use date of 30 days.

46. d: The vertical flow of air protects the user from exposure to hazardous chemicals.

47. a: Morphine multidose vials contain preservative which should not be used in neonates.

48. d: Needles, ampules, and broken glass vials should all be disposed in a sharps container.

49. a: Pharmaceutical waste is regulated by the EPA because intact pharmaceuticals can leach into drinking water and cause toxicity.

50. a: You should put PPE on in the anteroom or designated gowning area.

FOUR

1. d: Trailing zeros should be avoided.

2. b: Computerized physician order entry (CPOE) decreases handwriting errors.

3. a: IU should be spelled out to international unit.

4. c: qod should be spelled out to every other day.

5. c: The dispensing pharmacist is responsible for all dispensed medications.

6. d: Date of birth, height, and weight are all essential to prevent errors.

7. a: The pharmacist should discuss the clinical situation with the patient and physician.

8. a: Insulin and heparin are both high-alert medications.

9. b: The apothecary system (grain) should be avoided to minimize errors.

10. d: Many distractions can occur during a verbal order including cell phone connection issues, accent, and similar sounding medications.

11. a: Reading the verbal order back to the prescriber helps to verify the order.

12. a: Infants are at the highest risk of a calculation error due to their small size.

13. b: Tall-man lettering can help distinguish between look-alike sound alike-medications.

14. a: The ISMP is dedicated solely to medication error prevention.

15. c: Shelf dividers can help prevent look-alike packaging errors.

16. d: Insulin, heparin, and morphine are all high-alert medications.

17. d: High-alert medications have the potential to cause devastating adverse effects.

18. b: Medications should be sorted regardless of dosage form by generic name A to Z to minimize errors.

19. a: The dose will be 2 mL, thus a 2.5-mL syringe is closest in size.

20. d: Only a pharmacist can counsel a patient on medication use.

21. d: There are many factors to medication errors including poor lighting, clutter, and noise.

22. a: Adequate lighting can help decrease medication errors.

23. c: The Pharmacy and Therapeutics (P&T) Committee develops a formulary.

24. b: Redesigning systems and processes that lead to errors is the best way to decrease errors.

25. d: A pharmacy technician should always alert a pharmacist to make a clinical decision.

26. a: OBRA '90 required pharmacies to perform a prospective drug utilization review.

27. a: Trailing zeros can cause medication errors.

28. d: There are many sections to a drug utilization review.

29. c: The Pharmacy and Therapeutics (P&T) Committee develops a formulary.

30. a: Norvasc-amlodipine is the only example of a brand-generic substitution.

31. a: Protonix-Prevacid is the only example of a therapeutic substitution.

32. c: Required medication guides must be dispensed with every dispensed prescription.

33. c: Only a pharmacist can make a clinical decision for an OTC recommendation.

34. b: Pharmacy technicians may perform generic substitutions where allowed by law.

35. a: qd should be spelled out as daily or once daily.

36. d: The OBRA '90 requires a prospective drug utilization review.

37. d: FDA stands for Food and Drug Administration.

38. c: Pharmacy technicians may not counsel patients.

39. a: Pharmacy technicians may not perform drug utilization review.

40. c: A pharmacy technician should alert the pharmacist when encountering an alert during a prospective drug utilization review.

41. d: Only a pharmacist may make recommendation to a patient.

42. b: Tall-man lettering helps decrease errors from look-alike drugs.

43. c: A formulary is a list of medications that is approved by the P&T Committee.

44. c: The OBRA '90 requires a pharmacist to offer to counsel a patient.

45. d: Multiple strategies may be employed to decrease medication errors.

46. c: Redesigning processes have shown to decrease medication errors.

47. c: CPOE can help prevent illegible handwriting errors.

48. c: Warfarin is a high-alert medication.

49. c: Phenytoin has a narrow therapeutic range.

50. c: Tall-man lettering can help prevent look-alike-sound-alike errors.

FIVE

1. b: The NDC is a unique, 3-segment number which identifies drug products.

2. a: The ISMP oversees MERP.

3. b: Productivity is the quality of being productive or being able to produce.

4. d: A written memo is most efficient for a policy announcement.

5. d: DEA stands for Drug Enforcement Agency.

6. c: A failure mode and effects analysis (FMEA) is performed *prior* to a high-risk process.

7. a: Efficiency is the time, effort, or cost of producing an outcome.

8. a: A formal line of communication is employee to direct supervisor.

9. c: The USP sets standards for medications, biologics, medical devices, and compounded products.

10. b: The FDA issues a medication recall.

11. a: A class I recall is when a drug company is required to remove their medication from market due to the risk of death.

12. b: The Department of Health and Human Services created patient safety organizations.

13. c: The AHRQ is in the Department of Health and Human Services and dedicated to improve quality, safety, and efficiency of health care.

14. a: The NDC consists of the labeler code (4 or 5 digits), the product code (3 or 4 digits), and the package code (1 or 2 digits).

15. a: The FDA oversees Medwatch.

16. c: Quality control investigates a problem after completion.

17. c: Continuous quality improvement is a process to ensure programs are intentionally improving services.

18. a: Productivity is measured via amount of work accomplished during a set period of time.

19. a: PSO stands for patient safety organization.

20. b: The NDC is the unique, 3-segment number which identifies a drug product.

21. d: ISMP is dedicated solely to medication error prevention.

22. d: Continuous quality improvement ensures that programs are intentionally improving service and increasing positive outcomes.

23. a: Patient safety organizations (PSOs) are classified by the Department of Health and Human Services to improve quality and safety of health care services.

24. d: Risk management minimizes risk by analyzing workflow, identifying high-risk tasks, and avoidance of risk through education and process change.

25. d: Risk management is identifying, analyzing, assessing, and controlling risk.

26. c: Focusing on areas close to you and far away at frequent intervals can help prevent eye fatigue.

27. c: A class III recall is when exposure to a product is not likely to cause adverse health consequences.

28. b: The NDC consists of the labeler code (4 or 5 digits), the product code (3 or 4 digits), and the package code (1 or 2 digits).

29. c: A sentinel event is an unexpected death due to a medication error.

30. a: Audible cue barcode scanner will help a technician efficiently chose the right product.

31. b: A computer screen should be between 20 and 26 in away to help prevent eye fatigue.

32. d: New procedures, change in workflow, and education of the staff can help improve customer service.

33. c: The AHRQ is in the Department of Health and Human Services and dedicated to improve quality, safety, and efficiency of health care.

34. d: Software updates are needed to keep the latest drug information and drug interaction software, and help fix bugs.

35. b: All errors are not preventable.

36. a: A bar code is an optical machine-readable representation of information related to the object to which it is attached.

37. a: Class I recalls are related to a serious health problem from dangerous or defective products.

38. b: The FDA is in charge of product recalls.

39. c: Recalled medications should be stored segregated from normal stock.

40. d: Computer software updates, calibrated counting trays, and barcode scanners all improve patient safety.

41. c: Root cause analysis (RCA) occurs *after* an error has occurred.

42. d: Sentinel events are reported to The Joint Commission (TJC).

43. c: Face-to-face discussion is best for interactive discussion.

44. a: Occupational Safety and Health Administration (OSHA) ensures safe and healthful working conditions.

45. c: NCPS creates a culture of safety throughout the Veterans Health Administration.

46. c: Individual State Boards of Pharmacy (BOP) are in charge of licensing pharmacists.

47. b: E-prescribing is preferred for prescription generation.

48. b: Using the NDC from the medication bottle during data entry is preferred to decrease errors in a retail setting.

49. a: Medications should be stored A to Z regardless of type of medications.

50. b: OSHA requires material safety data sheets.

SIX

1. d: A technician may enter prescriptions into the computer, update the patient profile, and count medications on a counting tray.

2. b: A pharmacy technician may never counsel patients.

3. b: The abbreviation for grain is gr.

4. d: 1 capsule × 3 doses per day × 20 days = 60 capsules.

5. b: MDI is the abbreviation for metered-dose inhaler.

6. a: 14 doses/2 doses per day = 7 days.

7. a: A written order for a medication in the outpatient setting is a prescription.

8. b: Over-the-counter (OTC) medications can be obtained without a prescription; legend drugs require a prescription.

9. c: A DEA number is required to be present on a prescription when a physician prescribes a controlled substance.

10. d: The inscription is the part of the prescription that contains the name and strength of the medication and the amount prescribed.

11. b: The abbreviation for symptoms is Sx.

12. b: Dispense as written (DAW) is what a prescriber would indicate if they want the patient to be given the name brand medication.

13. c: A medication that is scheduled III-IV can be refilled up to 5 times within 6 months.

14. a: Allergy information may be found on a patient profile.

15. b: Sig codes are abbreviations for directions written on a prescription.

16. d: 1 tablet qAM is interpreted as the patient should take 1 table everyday in the morning.

17. b: The medication should be taken as needed (PRN).

18. a: Quantity sufficient (QS).

19. c: The abbreviation amp is for ampule.

20. b: D5W is the common abbreviation for dextrose 5% in water.

21. b: A counting tray is used to transfer solid dosage forms from a stock bottle to a prescription container.

22. d: Certain medications are permitted to be dispensed with a non-childproof lid, such as oral contraceptives, inhalation aerosols, and sublingual nitroglycerin. Nitroglycerin should always be dispensed with an easy-off cap, so it is easily accessible during emergencies.

23. b: The pharmacist is responsible for the final verification of the prescription.

24. c: An expiration date indicates when the effectiveness of the drug will diminish.

25. d: The abbreviation for teaspoon is tsp.

26. a: Lantus is an insulin and should be stored in the refrigerator in the pharmacy.

27. c: Unit doses are medication used in the hospital and have been prepackaged for a single-dose administration.

28. b: A tablet splitter easily and cleanly splits a tablet into 2 pieces.

29. b: 1 tablet 2 times per day = 2 tablets/day; 60 tablets/2 tablets = 30 days.

30. b: The abbreviation qhs means at bedtime.

31. b: Liter = L.

32. c: The subscription is the part of the prescription that contains directions to the pharmacist such as refills or DAW requirements.

33. b: X = 10, thus 10 + 10 + 10 = 30.

34. c: An order written in the hospital setting is a medication order.

35. b: 24 hours per day/8 hours = 3 times per day.

36. c: 1 tsp = 5 mL, qid = 4 times per day, thus 5 mL × 4 times per day × 10 days = 200 mL.

37. d: ung is the abbreviation for ointment, thus it should be applied topically.

38. c: Na = sodium, Cl = chloride.

39. b: 25 units + 35 units = 60 Units/day

1 vial of insulin = 100 Units/mL × 10 mL = 1000 Units/vial

1000 Units/60 = 16 days

40. a: The superscription is the Rx symbol.

41. d: cap is the abbreviation for capsule.

42. b: Fluid ounce (fl oz) = 30 mL.

43. c: 1 tbsp = 15 mL × 2 times daily = 30 mL per day

$$\frac{30\ mL}{1\ fl\ oz} = \frac{X}{10\ fl\ oz}$$

X = 300 mL

300 mL/30 mL per day = 10 days

44. b: The word before is abbreviated "a."

45. a: A STAT order would be needed immediately.

46. c: Take 60 mg (6 tablets) × 2 days = 12

Take 50 mg (5 tablets) × 1 day = 5

Take 40 mg (4 tablets) × 2 days = 8

Take 30 mg (3 tablets) × 1 day = 3

Take 20 mg (2 tablets) × 2 days = 4

Take 10 mg (1 tablet) × 1 day = 1

Take 5 mg (0.5 tablet) × 2 days = 1

12 + 5 + 8 + 3 + 4 + 1 + 1 = 34

47. a: A legend drug requires a prescription.

48. c: The pharmacy should dispense aspirin (ASA) 325 mg.

49. b: The subscription is the part of the prescription that contains directions to the pharmacist such as refills or DAW requirements.

50. b: O = abbreviation for eye, S = abbreviation for left, OS = left eye.

SEVEN

1. b: A closed formulary is a system in which therapeutic interchange protocols are utilized to convert prescribed nonformulary medications to formulary alternatives.

2. b: No, Refrigerated products require temperatures ranging from 2° to 8°C.

3. c: The Controlled Substances Ordering System (CSOS) is the DEA electronic program used to order C-II medications.

4. b: $180 + $4 = 184 × 0.04 = 7.36; 184 − 7.36 = $176.64.

5. c: Form 222 is used for the purchase and sale of C-II medications.

6. b: Inventory turnover rate is a method for measuring the overall effectiveness of purchasing and inventory control processes.

7. c: A lot number is a unique identifying code assigned to each batch of medication produced at a given time.

8. c: Material safety data sheet (MSDS) contains instructions for proper storage, handling, and containment procedures for a hazardous substance.

9. d: The optimal amount of each item that should be stocked at any given time is called the PAR level.

10. a: The prime vendor is the wholesaler from whom the pharmacy has committed to purchase the majority of its inventory.

11. c: Tetracycline can become toxic after its expiration date and cause liver failure.

12. a: A wholesaler, or distributor, is a company that carries a selection of medications, medical devices, and supplies.

13. b: The second section of the NDC code is the product code which identifies the product.

14. a: Rotating stock is a process in which products with the shortest expiration dates are moved to the front of the shelf when stocking.

15. c: When the actual date is listed, that is the actual expiration date. When it is the month and year it is till the last day of the month.

16. a: When ordering most of the products come from one place, limiting the amount of paperwork and number of deliveries.

17. c: A pharmacy usually needs to order 80% to 85% of its total inventory from a single wholesaler to be considered its prime vendor.

18. a: A prime vendor gives a pharmacy discounts on product.

19. a: Once a purchase order is transmitted to a vendor, an invoice is generated.

20. b: False. All recalls must be complied with, regardless of the recall class.

21. b: Medications that are used frequently ("fast movers") should have large PAR levels and more of the medication should be stocked.

22. a: Inventory turnover rate $= \dfrac{\text{Total annual inventory purchases}}{\text{Cost of inventory on hand}}$

$$13 = \frac{16,000,000}{X}$$

$$\frac{13X}{13} = \frac{16,000,000}{13}$$

$$X = \$1,230,800$$

23. a: Electronic ordering systems still require human thought and judgment to be sure the pharmacy is adequately stocked.

24. d: The bottom (blue) copy of a DEA form 222 is retained by the pharmacy.

25. a: The top (tan) copy of a DEA form 222 is retained by the supplier.

26. d: Per the DEA, form 222 must be kept on file for 7 years.

27. a: Refrigerated medications should be put away first so as to limit the amount of time spent at room temperature.

28. d: Storage requirements for medications are listed on the manufacturer's label and the package insert.

29. b: False. If medications are not stored correctly, they are considered adulterated and are not usable.

30. a: Frozen products are stored at −20° to −10°C.

31. a: An open formulary is a system in which most medications are stocked in the pharmacy, or able to be ordered if prescribed.

32. b: The medications included in an insurance plan's formulary are identified by the NDC.

33. d: The most common reasons that pharmacies return inventory is due to manufacturer recalls, expired products, or damaged goods.

34. c: The third section of the NDC code is the package code, identifying the package.

35. b: False. The FDA does have the authority to mandate a recall, but usually the manufacturers choose to voluntarily compile with the recall request.

36. b: There are 3 classes of drug recalls.

37. b: Class 2 recalled products may cause temporary adverse effects but have a small probability of causing serious harm.

38. c: Class 3 recall is the least severe recall class.

39. d: MedWatch collects data about medications, including adverse effects and unexpected reactions.

40. c: The NDC is a 11-digit product identifying code used for all drugs marketed in the United States.

41. a: An invoice is a bill of sale for products ordered.

42. b: The DEA states that records of controlled substance destruction must be kept on file for 2 years.

43. a: Form 41 is used to document the destruction of controlled substances.

44. b: The DEA form 222 is a triplicate form designed specifically for the sale of C-II medications.

45. d: Nonformulary medications might be covered at a higher co-pay, require prior authorization from the prescriber, or may not be covered at all.

46. a: Appropriate controlled room temperature is 15° to 30°C.

47. b: Class 2 recalls include medications that contain less active ingredient than intended.

48. c: The middle (green) copy of a DEA form 222 is retained by the DEA.

49. a: The first section of the NDC code is the labeler code, identifying the manufacturer.

50. a: Yes refrigerated products require temperatures ranging from 2° to 8°C.

EIGHT

1. a: Medicare has parts A, B, C, and D.

2. b: DAW stands for dispense as written.

3. a: Health maintenance organizations (HMOs) require the designation of a primary care physician (PCP).

4. d: Patients must pay a premium to have insurance coverage.

5. a: A subscriber is another name for the cardholder of the insurance policy.

6. a: A co-payment is a fee which is due at the time services are rendered.

7. d: Medicare Part D is the voluntary prescription drug coverage program for Medicare.

8. c: Centers for Medicare and Medicaid Services (CMS) is a federal organization that oversees Medicare and Medicaid.

9. c: A formulary is a list of approved medications in a member's plan.

10. b: A prior authorization is special approval needed before an insurance company will cover a specific medication for a patient. These are generally expensive brand name drugs that are not on the insurance formulary.

11. b: The DAW code is used for third parties to determine if the proper brand or generic medication was used to fill the prescription.

12. a: DAW 0 is the default code used when dispensing a generic drug or when dispensing a brand name product that does not have a generic available.

13. b: A drug utilization review (DUR) is a process which consists of an evaluation of the prescribed medication against specific criteria that helps to ensure drug safety and help reduce unnecessary costs.

14. b: A deductible must be met each year before the insurance policy will cover remaining costs.

15. a: The patient's insurance will pay 90% so 90% of 50 = (0.9) × (50) = 45. This is the amount the insurance will pay. To determine the amount the patient must pay, subtract this amount from the total billed: $50 − $45 = $5. The patient owes the pharmacy $5.

16. a: A health maintenance organization (HMO) is a type of third party plan which requires the designation of a primary care physician.

17. d: Medicaid, Medicare, and TRICARE are all government sponsored insurance plans, Aetna is a privately run insurance company.

18. b: Money that a patient pays from their pocket is known as out-of-pocket expense.

19. b: CMS is a federal organization that oversees Medicare and Medicaid.

20. d: Coordination of benefits occurs if a patient has multiple insurance providers, then one is selected as primary and is billed first. The second insurance company is not billed unless there are still unpaid claims remaining, then they are billed only the remainder of the costs, so there is not a duplication of payment.

21. b: DAW 2 is the code used when the prescriber indicates generic is permitted, but the patient requests a brand name product.

22. d: In order to process a claim, the pharmacy must know the patient's first and last name, birthdate, allergy information in addition to a valid prescription and insurance information.

23. c: A member would have a person code of 1, a spouse would have 2, and then a child could be 3.

24. b: The PCN, or processor control number, helps direct the electronic claim to the proper location.

25. d: The RxBin, RxGroup, and member ID number are all required to submit an insurance claim properly.

26. d: Mail-order pharmacies can supply medications for 90-day supplies.

27. c: A prior authorization is a special approval needed before an insurance company will cover a specific medication for a patient, generally an expensive brand name drug that is not present on the formulary.

28. d: If a patient attempts to get a prescription refilled before the insurance company permits a scheduled fill, the insurance company will reject the claim with a refill-too-soon error.

29. b: DAW 0 is the default code used when dispensing a generic drug or when dispensing a brand name product that does not have a generic available.

30. a: When 2 drugs interact with each other and the effectiveness of one or both is altered, this is a drug-drug interaction.

31. c: PPO patient does not require a referral from a PCP prior to seeing a specialist provided this physician is in network.

32. d: Coinsurance is an out-of-pocket expense similar to a co-payment except a patient pays a percentage of the costs of the service as determined by the insurance provider.

33. b: Medicare Part A provides coverage for patients eligible for Medicare for inpatient hospital stays, nursing facilities, home health care services, and hospice care; Medicare Part D covers prescription drugs.

34. a: Medicare Part C is a Medicare plan in which patients must be enrolled in both Medicare Parts A and B a to receive Part C benefits through a separate provider.

35. a: Medicare Part D provides coverage for prescription drugs; Medicare Part B provides coverage for durable medical equipment (DME).

36. d: Formulary is a list of approved drugs on a patient's insurance plan.

37. c: Private health insurance plans are offered through most employers, not the pharmacy.

38. d: Coinsurance is an out-of-pocket expense similar to a co-payment except a patient pays a percentage of the costs of the service as determined by the insurance provider.

39. a: Medicare Part A provides coverage for patients eligible for Medicare for inpatient hospital stays, nursing facilities, home health care services, and hospice care.

40. b: A pharmacy benefit manager is a third party administrator of prescription drug programs and processes and pays for the drug claims and maintains the formulary for each plan.

41. d: The BIN or biller identification number is unique to each third party and identifies where the claim is being sent. The BIN number is usually listed on the insurance card and consists of 6 numbers.

42. b: The pharmacy will be given a termination date from the insurance company, but due to HIPAA, the pharmacy is not permitted to access any information about why coverage was terminated. The patient should be instructed to contact the insurance company and will have to pay full price for any medications until the issue can be resolved.

43. c: A refill-too-soon error occurs when a patient attempts to get their prescription refilled before the insurance company permits a scheduled fill.

44. c: DAW 2 is the code when a prescriber indicates generic is permitted, but the patient requests brand name product.

45. c: DUR is a drug utilization review. This process consists of an evaluation of the prescribed medication against specific criteria that helps to ensure drug safety, and help reduce unnecessary costs.

46. a: Prior authorization is a special approval needed before an insurance company will cover a specific medication for a patient, generally an expensive brand name drug that is not present on the formulary.

47. a: Medicare Part A provides coverage for patients eligible for Medicare for inpatient hospital stays, nursing facilities, home healthcare services and hospice care.

48. d: Medicare Part D is voluntary and must be enrolled in during a designated time frame. All pharmacy technicians should be familiar with Part D plans.

49. d: A contraindication is when a medication should not be given to a specific patient for some sort of condition or factor, such as pregnancy.

50. b: DAW 1 is the code used when the prescriber indicates he or she wants the brand name dispensed.

NINE

1. b: Pharmacy automation includes robots, barcode scanners, and tabletop tablet counters.

2. d: Patient Handout Information References include patient counseling information.

3. a: A computer mouse is used for double clicking.

4. d: Drug information resources are written and electronic references, and available for patients and pharmacists.

5. d: CDSS over- or underutilization will help identify patient adherence.

6. c: Telepharmacy allows a pharmacist to counsel a patient in a different location.

7. d: Clinical information systems may include electronic orders, medication administration records, and patient information.

8. a: MAR stands for medication administration record.

9. a: *Drug Facts and Comparisons* is a general pharmacy reference that would contain storage requirements of a medication.

10. c: The patient profile does not contain the patient's social security number.

11. d: Computers, automated tablet counters, and barcode scanners are often used in the pharmacy.

12. b: A monitor is an output device, while a mouse, USB, and light pen can all input information into a computer.

13. a: During a power outage down-time procedures should be used.

14. d: A keyboard, mouse, and touch screen monitor can update a patient profile.

15. b: Patient allergy information should be reviewed frequently with patients.

16. a: An inventory report would be used to identify a product's availability.

17. c: Medication doses given to patients are recorded on the MAR.

18. b: The barcode scanner may not be able to read some bar codes.

19. d: The patient's current medications should include OTCs, other prescription medications, and nutritional supplements.

20. a: If a patient has limited vision the patient profile should contain a note.

21. c: Drug dosage information can be found in a General Drug Information Reference.

22. d: A patient's insurance card does not contain contracted pricing structure information.

23. a: State Law Books will contain information regarding record keeping requirements for prescriptions.

24. a: A modem allows a computer to communicate over a network.

25. b: *Natural Standard* would contain information regarding the recommended dose of ginkgo.

26. a: The poison control center number is 1-800-222-1222.

27. b: ADM stands for automated dispensing machine.

28. d: Allergy information should include food, medication, and environmental allergies.

29. d: General Drug Information and Patient Handout Information Reference will contain drug-food interactions.

30. d: Address, phone number, and allergies should be on the patient profile.

31. a: Amoxicillin prescribed for a penicillin allergic patient is an example of a drug-allergy interaction.

32. d: A Federal Law Book and General Drug Information Reference would contain information about DEA classification.

33. b: A patient's insurance card would not contain information about height and weight.

34. a: A MAR would help determine when a dose of medication is due.

35. d: A robot, dispensing cabinet, and barcode scanner are all examples of pharmacy automation.

36. c: A State Law Book would contain information regarding the requirements of prescription label.

37. b: A mainframe is used to house and process large amounts of data.

38. a: A disk drive is an output device.

39. b: Electronic health records (EHRs) are costly investments.

40. c: E-prescribing decreases handwriting errors.

41. a: The patient's name is found on a MAR.

42. d: Password, biometric fingerprint, and hard token generators are all secure identifiers.

43. d: CDSS may provide drug-allergy, therapeutic duplication, and pharmacokinetic monitoring.

44. b: Automated dispensing cabinets store medications on a nursing unit.

45. d: Robots, tabletop tablet counters, and automated dispensing cabinets may increase the speed of prescription dispensing.

46. c: The *Orange Book* is used to obtain equivalency information.

47. b: Usage reports would identify a fast-moving product.

48. b: Amoxicillin prescribed for a patient on Augmentin would be an example of a drug-drug interaction.

49. c: Stability information would be found in a General Drug Information Reference.

50. c: A patient's insurance card does not contain diagnosis information.

Practice Exam
MATH REVIEW

1. You receive a prescription written for pheno-barbital gr i. Which strength of phenobarbital tablets (in milligrams) should be dispensed?
   a. 15 mg
   b. 30 mg
   c. 60 mg
   d. 90 mg

2. The manufacturer produces dopamine intrave-nous solution in the concentration 1600 µg/mL. How many milligrams of dopamine are in the 250-mL stock bag?
   a. 160 mg
   b. 400 mg
   c. 800 mg
   d. 1600 mg

3. What is the weight in pounds of a 14-kg child?
   a. 6.4 lb
   b. 12.6 lb
   c. 26.4 lb
   d. 30.8 lb

4. What number does the Roman numeral xlv represent?
   a. 40
   b. 45
   c. 50
   d. 55

5. How many teaspoons are in 4 tablespoons?
   a. 1.3
   b. 2
   c. 8
   d. 12

6. $\dfrac{15}{20} \times \dfrac{2}{20} =$
   a. 17/23
   b. 40/45
   c. 45/40
   d. 30/60

7. Express your answer to #6 as a decimal (round to 1 decimal place).
   a. 0.7
   b. 0.9

   c. 1.1
   d. 0.5

8. How many fluid ounces are in 360 mL?
   a. 8 fl oz
   b. 12 fl oz
   c. 16 fl oz
   d. 36 fl oz

9. A patient comes to your pharmacy needing help. She received a prescription from a phar-macy across town. Her prescription label says "Metoclopramide 5 mg/5 mL solution—take 20 mL every 8 hours." She does not know how to measure out 20 mL. How many teaspoons should you tell her to take per dose?
   a. 1.5
   b. 2
   c. 4
   d. This amount cannot be measured in tea-spoons

10. How many milligrams of clindamycin are in a 30-g tube of 1% clindamycin topical gel?
    a. 0.3 mg
    b. 30 mg
    c. 300 mg
    d. 3000 mg

11. The concentration of what type of product is expressed in w/w percentage?
    a. Oral solution
    b. Topical ointment
    c. Injectable solution
    d. Oral suspension

12. How many milliliters does an 8-dram amber vial hold?
    a. 24 mL
    b. 32 mL
    c. 40 mL
    d. 80 mL

13. What types of drugs are typically expressed in milliequivalent?
   a. Insulin
   b. Narcotics
   c. Electrolytes
   d. Topical preparations

14. You receive an order for fentanyl 12 μg/h transdermal patch: replace patch every 72 hours. The physician is concerned about the potential for abuse and only wants you to dispense enough for 2 weeks. How many patches should you dispense?
   a. 4 patches
   b. 5 patches
   c. 6 patches
   d. 12 patches

Use the following scenario for questions 16 to 20:

You are given a prescription for azithromycin 1% ophthalmic solution. The directions are to use a dose of 0.2 mL in each eye twice daily for 2 days, then 0.2 mL in each eye once daily for an additional 5 days.

15. How many milligrams are in each dose of azithromycin 1% ophthalmic solution?
   a. 0.2 mg
   b. 2 mg
   c. 20 mg
   d. 200 mg

16. How many milligrams will the patient instill over the entire course of treatment?
   a. Not enough information
   b. 18 mg
   c. 36 mg
   d. 180 mg

17. Azithromycin 1% ophthalmic solution is available from the manufacturer in 2.5-mL bottles. How many doses will be in each bottle?
   a. 12 doses
   b. 13 doses
   c. 24 doses
   d. 26 doses

18. Will the 2.5-mL bottle be enough to last the entire course of treatment?
   a. Yes
   b. No
   c. Not enough information

19. The patient will not be able to measure out 0.2 mL to give himself each dose. How many drops should you tell the patient to instill in each eye in order to achieve the 0.2-mL dose?
   a. 1 drop
   b. 2 drops
   c. 3 drops
   d. 4 drops

20. $\dfrac{6}{7} \times \dfrac{3}{4} =$
   a. 24/21
   b. 21/24
   c. 28/18
   d. 18/28

21. Express your answer to #21 as a decimal (round to 2 decimal places).
   a. 1.14
   b. 0.86
   c. 1.56
   d. 0.64

22. You receive a prescription written as "ampicillin 0.5 g PO qid × 10 days." You only have ampicillin 250-mg capsules in stock. How many 250-mg capsules should you dispense?
   a. 40
   b. 60
   c. 80
   d. 160

23. What types of drugs are typically expressed in units?
   a. Electrolytes
   b. Chemotherapy
   c. Intravenous medications
   d. Insulin

24. A patient's total daily dose of diltiazem is 120 mg. The dose is to be divided q6h. How many milligrams of diltiazem should be given for each dose?
   a. 20 mg
   b. 30 mg
   c. 60 mg
   d. 480 mg

25. How many 30-mL individual prescriptions can you dispense from a 1-pint stock bottle?
   a. 16
   b. 32
   c. 50
   d. 100

26. Grains and drams are examples of measurements used in which system?
   a. Metric
   b. Apothecary
   c. Avoirdupois
   d. English

27. Express 25 as a Roman numeral.
   a. xxv
   b. vt
   c. xl
   d. vvvvv

28. The concentration of what type of product can be expressed in w/v percentage?
   a. Injectable solution
   b. Powder
   c. Topical ointment
   d. Tablets

29. You receive a prescription from a veterinarian for a 1:200 solution of furosemide. You only have 20-mg furosemide tablets in stock. How many tablets do you need in order to compound 60 mL of the furosemide solution?
   a. 10
   b. 15
   c. 30
   d. This solution cannot be made with 20-mg tablets

30. gr 1/4 = ____ mg
   a. 12.5
   b. 15
   c. 60
   d. 240

31. How many milliliters are in an 8-fl oz stock bottle of milk of magnesia?
   a. 120 mL
   b. 240 mL
   c. 360 mL
   d. 480 mL

32. You receive a prescription for insulin lispro 14 units with meals tid. Your pharmacy stocks insulin lispro 100 U/mL 3-mL vials. How many full days will 1 vial last if used as directed?
   a. 5 days
   b. 7 days
   c. 14 days
   d. 28 days

33. What is the abbreviation for units (as in, insulin glargine 10 units qhs)?
   a. U
   b. u
   c. un
   d. Units should not be abbreviated

34. $8 \times \dfrac{3}{4} =$
   a. 32/3
   b. 12/4
   c. 24/4
   d. 24/3

35. Express your answer to #34 as a whole number.
   a. 0
   b. 3
   c. 6
   d. 8

36. How many milligrams of lorazepam are required to prepare 30 mL of a 5% solution?
   a. 150 mg
   b. 500 mg
   c. 1000 mg
   d. 1500 mg

37. 23°C = ____°F
   a. −9
   b. −5
   c. 44.8
   d. 73.4

38. The pediatric dose of IV morphine is 0.1 mg/kg. How many milligrams of morphine sulfate should a child weighing 28 lb receive? (Round to 1 decimal point.)
   a. 0.6 mg
   b. 1.3 mg
   c. 6.2 mg
   d. 13 mg

39. You receive a prescription for cephalexin 250 mg. The prescription states to dispense xiv. How many capsules should be dispensed?
    a. 7
    b. 14
    c. 28
    d. None. Prescription instructions must be written in Arabic numerals.

40. Tablespoon and teaspoon are examples of measurements used in which system?
    a. Metric
    b. Avoirdupois
    c. Intravenous
    d. Apothecary

41. Convert 560 µg to mg.
    a. 56,000 mg
    b. 5600 mg
    c. 5.6 mg
    d. 0.56 mg

42. How many grams of ketoconazole are in a 30-g tube of 2% ketoconazole cream?
    a. 0.6 g
    b. 6 g
    c. 60 g
    d. 6000 g

43. $15 \times \dfrac{5}{6} =$
    a. 20/6
    b. 90/6
    c. 90/5
    d. 75/6

44. Express your answer to #43 as a decimal.
    a. 3.3
    b. 12.5
    c. 15.2
    d. 33.3

45. How many milligrams of drug are in 20 mL of a 1:100 solution?
    a. 0.2 mg
    b. 2 mg
    c. 20 mg
    d. 200 mg

46. You receive a prescription written for phenobarbital gr 1/2. Which strength of phenobarbital tablets (in milligrams) should be dispensed?

    a. 15 mg
    b. 30 mg
    c. 60 mg
    d. 90 mg

47. The manufacturer produces dopamine intravenous solution in the concentration of 3200 µg/mL. How many milligrams of dopamine are in the 250-mL stock bag?
    a. 160 mg
    b. 400 mg
    c. 800 mg
    d. 1600 mg

48. What is the weight in pounds of a 12-kg child?
    a. 6.4 lb
    b. 12.6 lb
    c. 26.4 lb
    d. 30.8 lb

49. What number does the Roman numeral xl represent?
    a. 40
    b. 45
    c. 50
    d. 55

50. How many teaspoons are in 3 tablespoons?
    a. 1.3
    b. 3
    c. 12
    d. 15

51. $\dfrac{10}{20} \times \dfrac{2}{3} =$
    a. 12/23
    b. 30/40
    c. 40/30
    d. 20/60

52. Express your answer to #51 as a decimal (round to 1 decimal place).
    a. 0.7
    b. 0.8
    c. 1.3
    d. 0.3

53. How many fluid ounces are in 480 mL?
    a. 8 fl oz
    b. 12 fl oz
    c. 16 fl oz
    d. 36 fl oz

54. A patient comes to your pharmacy needing help. She received a prescription from a pharmacy across town. Her prescription label says "Metoclopramide 5 mg/5 mL solution—take 10 mL in every 8 hours." She does not know how to measure out 10 mL. How many teaspoons should you tell her to take per dose?
   a. 1.5
   b. 2
   c. 4
   d. This amount cannot be measured in teaspoons

55. How many milligrams of clindamycin are in a 60-g tube of 1% clindamycin topical gel?
   a. 0.6 mg
   b. 60 mg
   c. 600 mg
   d. 6000 mg

56. The concentration of what type of product is expressed in w/w percentage?
   a. Codeine sulfate oral solution
   b. Lidocaine topical ointment
   c. Digoxin injectable solution
   d. Amoxicillin oral suspension

57. How many milliliters does a 16-dram amber vial hold?
   a. 24 mL
   b. 32 mL
   c. 40 mL
   d. 80 mL

58. The strength of which of the following medications is expressed in milliequivalent?
   a. Insulin glargine
   b. Morphine sulfate
   c. Potassium chloride
   d. Tetracaine

59. You receive an order for fentanyl 12 μg/h transdermal patch: replace patch every 72 hours. The physician is concerned about the potential for abuse and only wants you to dispense enough for 1 week. How many patches should you dispense?
   a. 2 patches
   b. 3 patches
   c. 5 patches
   d. 7 patches

Use the following scenario for questions 60-64:

You are given a prescription for azithromycin 1% ophthalmic solution. The directions are to use a dose of 0.1 mL in the right eye twice daily for 2 days, then 0.1 mL in the right eye daily for an additional 7 days.

60. How many milligrams are in each dose of azithromycin 1% ophthalmic solution?
   a. 0.1 mg
   b. 1 mg
   c. 10 mg
   d. 100 mg

61. How many milligrams will the patient instill over the entire course of treatment?
   a. Not enough information
   b. 6 mg
   c. 9 mg
   d. 11 mg

62. Azithromycin 1% ophthalmic solution is available from the manufacturer in 2.5-mL bottles. How many doses will be in each bottle?
   a. 12 doses
   b. 13 doses
   c. 25 doses
   d. 30 doses

63. Will the 2.5-mL bottle be enough to last the entire course of treatment?
   a. Yes
   b. No
   c. Not enough information

64. The patient will not be able to measure out 0.1 mL to give himself each dose. How many drops should you tell the patient to instill in each eye in order to achieve the 0.1-mL dose?
   a. 1 drop
   b. 2 drops
   c. 3 drops
   d. 4 drops

65. $\dfrac{6}{7} \times \dfrac{3}{5} =$
   a. 30/21
   b. 9/12
   c. 35/18
   d. 18/35

66. Express your answer to #65 as a decimal (round to 2 decimal places).
    a. 1.43
    b. 0.75
    c. 1.94
    d. 0.51

67. You receive a prescription written as "ampicillin 0.5 g PO tid × 7 days." You only have ampicillin 250-mg capsules in stock. How many 250-mg capsules should you dispense?
    a. 24
    b. 42
    c. 84
    d. 168

68. In which unit of measure is a dose of insulin expressed?
    a. Milliequivalent
    b. Milligram
    c. Grains
    d. Units

69. A patient's total daily dose of diltiazem is 180 mg. The dose is to be divided q6h. How many milligrams of diltiazem should be given for each dose?
    a. 15 mg
    b. 45 mg
    c. 90 mg
    d. 180 mg

70. How many 60-mL individual prescriptions can you dispense from a 1-pt stock bottle?
    a. 8
    b. 16
    c. 32
    d. 60

71. Which of the following are units used in the apothecary system?
    a. Milligrams
    b. Drams
    c. Teaspoons
    d. Liters

72. Express 40 as a Roman numeral.
    a. xxv
    b. vt
    c. xl
    d. vvvvv

73. The concentration of which of the following medications can be expressed in w/v percentage?
    a. Famotidine injectable solution
    b. Ketoconazole powder
    c. Ketoconazole cream
    d. Famotidine tablets

74. You receive a prescription from a veterinarian for a 1:200 solution of furosemide. You only have 20-mg furosemide tablets in stock. How many tablets do you need in order to compound 120 mL of the furosemide solution?
    a. 10
    b. 15
    c. 30
    d. This solution cannot be made with 20-mg tablets

75. gr iv = _____ mg
    a. 12.5
    b. 15
    c. 60
    d. 240

76. How many milliliters are in a 4-fl oz prescription bottle of magnesium citrate?
    a. 120 mL
    b. 240 mL
    c. 360 mL
    d. 480 mL

77. You receive a prescription for insulin glargine 30 units qhs. Your pharmacy stocks insulin glargine 100 U/mL 3-mL vials. How many full days will 1 vial last if used as directed?
    a. 5 days
    b. 10 days
    c. 15 days
    d. 30 days

78. What is the abbreviation for units (as in, insulin glargine 30 units qhs)?
    a. U
    b. u
    c. un
    d. Units should not be abbreviated

79. $4 \times \dfrac{3}{4} =$
    a. 7/4
    b. 16/4
    c. 12/4
    d. 12/3

80. Express your answer to #79 as a whole number.
    a. 0
    b. 3
    c. 4
    d. 6

81. How many milligrams of hydromorphone are required to prepare 10 mL of a 5% solution?
    a. 150 mg
    b. 500 mg
    c. 1000 mg
    d. 1500 mg

82. −14°C = ____°F
    a. −9
    b. −5
    c. 7
    d. 12

83. The pediatric dose of IV morphine is 0.1 mg/kg. How many milligrams of morphine sulfate should a child weighing 14 lb receive? (Round to 1 decimal point.)
    a. 0.6 mg
    b. 1.3 mg
    c. 6.3 mg
    d. 14 mg

84. You receive a prescription for pregabalin 75-mg capsules. The prescription states to dispense xxviii. How many capsules should be dispensed?
    a. 7
    b. 14
    c. 28
    d. None. Prescription instructions must be written in Arabic numerals.

85. Which of the following units of measure is used in the Avoirdupois system?
    a. Liter
    b. Tablespoon
    c. Kilogram
    d. Grain

86. Convert 850 µg to mg.
    a. 85,000 mg
    b. 8500 mg
    c. 8.5 mg
    d. 0.85 mg

87. How many grams of ketoconazole are in a 15-g tube of 2% ketoconazole cream?
    a. 0.3 g
    b. 3 g
    c. 30 g
    d. 3000 g

88. $15 \times \frac{5}{8} =$
    a. 20/8
    b. 90/8
    c. 90/5
    d. 75/8

89. Express your answer to #88 as a decimal (round to 1 decimal place).
    a. 3.3
    b. 9.4
    c. 18.8
    d. 33.3

90. How many milligrams of drug are in 20 mL of a 4:100 solution?
    a. 0.8 mg
    b. 4 mg
    c. 400 mg
    d. 800 mg

91. You receive a prescription written for Armour thyroid gr 1/2. Which strength of thyroid tablets (in milligrams) should be dispensed?
    a. 15 mg
    b. 30 mg
    c. 60 mg
    d. 90 mg

92. The manufacturer produces dopamine intravenous solution in the concentration of 1600 µg/mL. How many milligrams of dopamine are in the 500-mL stock bag?
    a. 160 mg
    b. 400 mg
    c. 800 mg
    d. 1600 mg

93. What is the weight in pounds of a 24-kg child?
    a. 6.4 lb
    b. 10.9 lb
    c. 52.8 lb
    d. 62.8 lb

94. What number does the Roman numeral xvii represent?
   a. 7
   b. 17
   c. 27
   d. 37

95. How many tablespoons are in 6 teaspoons?
   a. 1
   b. 2
   c. 3
   d. 4

96. $\dfrac{7}{20} \times \dfrac{2}{3} =$
   a. 9/23
   b. 21/40
   c. 40/60
   d. 14/60

97. Express your answer to #96 as a decimal (round to 1 decimal place).
   a. 0.8
   b. 0.7
   c. 0.4
   d. 0.2

98. How many fluid ounces are in 1 pt?
   a. 8
   b. 12
   c. 16
   d. 36

99. A patient comes to your pharmacy needing help. She received a prescription from a pharmacy across town. Her prescription label says "Metoclopramide 5 mg/5 mL solution—take 3 mL every 8 hours." She does not know how to measure out 3 mL. How many teaspoons should you tell her to take per dose?
   a. 1.5
   b. 2
   c. 4
   d. This amount cannot be accurately measured in teaspoons

100. How many milligrams of diphenhydramine are in a 60-g tube of 1% diphenhydramine topical ointment?
   a. 0.6 mg
   b. 60 mg
   c. 600 mg
   d. 6000 mg

101. The concentration of what type of product is expressed in w/w percentage?
   a. Lindane shampoo
   b. Calcium citrate oral chews
   c. Ranitidine injectable solution
   d. Cefaclor oral suspension

102. How many milliliters does a 13-dram amber vial hold?
   a. 35
   b. 45
   c. 55
   d. 65

103. A dose of which of the following medications is expressed in milliequivalent?
   a. Insulin aspart
   b. Metformin
   c. Sodium bicarbonate
   d. Ergocalciferol (vitamin D)

104. You receive an order for fentanyl 75 µg/h transdermal patch: replace patch every 72 hours, dispense quantity sufficient for 4 weeks. How many patches should you dispense?
   a. 7 patches
   b. 10 patches
   c. 20 patches
   d. 30 patches

Use the following scenario for questions 105 to 109:

You are given a prescription for prednisolone 1% ophthalmic solution. The directions are to use a dose of 0.1 mL in the right eye q4h for 2 days.

105. How many milligrams are in each dose of prednisolone 1% ophthalmic solution?
   a. 0.1 mg
   b. 1 mg
   c. 10 mg
   d. 100 mg

106. How many milligrams will the patient instill over the entire course of treatment?
   a. Not enough information
   b. 6 mg
   c. 12 mg
   d. 24 mg

107. Prednisolone 1% ophthalmic solution is available from the manufacturer in 5-mL bottles. How many doses will be in each bottle?
a. 5 doses
b. 10 doses
c. 25 doses
d. 50 doses

108. Will the 5-mL bottle be enough to last the entire course of treatment?
a. Yes
b. No
c. Not enough information

109. The patient will not be able to measure out 0.1 mL to give himself each dose. How many drops should you tell the patient to instill in each eye in order to achieve the 0.1-mL dose?
a. 1 drop
b. 2 drops
c. 3 drops
d. 4 drops

110. $\dfrac{9}{7} \times \dfrac{3}{5} =$
a. 12/12
b. 9/12
c. 35/27
d. 27/35

111. Express your answer to #110 as a decimal (round to 2 decimal places).
a. 1
b. 0.75
c. 1.29
d. 0.77

112. You receive a prescription written as "cephalexin 0.5 g PO q6h × 7 days." You only have cephalexin 250-mg capsules in stock. How many 250-mg capsules should you dispense?
a. 28
b. 56
c. 100
d. 112

113. Which unit of measure is the most common in expressing strengths of medications?
a. Milliequivalent
b. Milligram
c. Grains
d. Units

114. A patient's total daily dose of nifedipine is 60 mg. The dose is to be divided q8h. How many milligrams of nifedipine should be given for each dose?
a. 10 mg
b. 15 mg
c. 20 mg
d. 30 mg

115. How many 15-mL individual prescriptions can you dispense from a 1-pt stock bottle?
a. 8
b. 16
c. 32
d. 60

116. Which of the following are units used in the apothecary system?
a. Grams
b. Grains
c. Ounces
d. Teaspoons

117. Express 14 as a Roman numeral.
a. xiv
b. xiiii
c. ivxx
d. ivvv

118. The concentration of which of the following medications can be expressed in w/v percentage?
a. Diltiazem injectable solution
b. Ketoconazole powder
c. Ketoconazole cream
d. Diltiazem tablets

119. You receive a prescription from a veterinarian for a 1:400 solution of furosemide. You only have 20-mg furosemide tablets in stock. How many tablets do you need in order to compound 120 mL of the furosemide solution?
a. 10
b. 15
c. 30
d. This solution cannot be made with 20-mg tablets.

120. gr i = _____ mg?
a. 15
b. 30
c. 60
d. 120

121. How many milliliters are in a 12-fl oz prescription bottle of guaifenesin?
    a. 120 mL
    b. 240 mL
    c. 360 mL
    d. 480 mL

122. You receive a prescription for insulin NPH 12 units bid. Your pharmacy stocks insulin NPH 100 U/mL 3-mL vials. How many full days will 1 vial last if used as directed?
    a. 7 days
    b. 12 days
    c. 14 days
    d. 28 days

123. What is the abbreviation for units (as in, insulin NPH 12 units bid)?
    a. U
    b. u
    c. un
    d. Units should not be abbreviated

124. $4 \times \dfrac{7}{4} =$
    a. 11/4
    b. 16/7
    c. 28/4
    d. 28/7

125. Express your answer to #124 as a whole number.
    a. 1
    b. 7
    c. 11
    d. 16

126. How many milligrams of epinephrine are required to prepare 20 mL of a 2.5% solution?
    a. 150 mg
    b. 500 mg
    c. 1000 mg
    d. 1500 mg

127. $35°C = \underline{\hspace{1cm}} °F$
    a. 1.6
    b. 19
    c. 59
    d. 95

128. The pediatric dose of ibuprofen is 5 mg/kg. How many milligrams of ibuprofen should a child weighing 30 lb receive? (Round to the nearest milligram.)
    a. 68 mg
    b. 86 mg

c. 200 mg, since that is the adult dose
d. 330 mg

129. You receive a prescription for diphenoxylate/atropine capsules. The prescription states to dispense lx. How many capsules should be dispensed?
    a. 15
    b. 30
    c. 60
    d. None. Prescription instructions must be written in Arabic numerals

130. Which of the following units of measure is used in the avoirdupois system?
    a. Milliequivalent
    b. Teaspoon
    c. Grain
    d. Dram

131. Convert 1250 µg to mg.
    a. 12,500 mg
    b. 1250 mg
    c. 12.5 mg
    d. 1.25 mg

132. How many grams of hydrocortisone are in a 60-g tube of 2% hydrocortisone cream?
    a. 0.12 g
    b. 1.2 g
    c. 12 g
    d. 120 g

133. $15 \times \dfrac{7}{8} =$
    a. 22/8
    b. 120/8
    c. 120/5
    d. 105/8

134. Express your answer to #133 as a decimal (round to 1 decimal place).
    a. 2.7
    b. 13.1
    c. 26.2
    d. 33.3

135. How many milligrams of drug are in 5 mL of a 8:100 solution?
    a. 0.8 mg
    b. 4 mg
    c. 400 mg
    d. 800 mg

Practice Exam
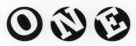

1. Who may recommend an over-the-counter (OTC) medication to a patient?
   a. Pharmacy technician
   b. Certified pharmacy technician
   c. Certified pharmacy technician with OTC training
   d. None of the above

2. What is the drip rate in mL/h of the continuous 10 μg/h infusion?
   a. 0.2 mL/h
   b. 0.4 mL/h
   c. 2 mL/h
   d. 5 mL/h

3. Which of the following prevention strategies should be utilized to decrease medication errors?
   a. Two-person independent check of medication calculation
   b. Tall-man lettering
   c. Shelf separators
   d. All of the above

4. Which organization is solely dedicated to medication error prevention?
   a. OSHA
   b. FDA
   c. TJC
   d. ISMP

5. Which of the following juices may interact with medications?
   a. Orange juice
   b. Apple juice
   c. Grapefruit juice
   d. Grape juice

6. Which of the following is an example of a schedule-III medication?
   a. Heroin
   b. Morphine
   c. Lorazepam
   d. Codeine with acetaminophen

7. Which of the following recalls is related to serious health problems from dangerous or defective products?
   a. Class I
   b. Class II
   c. Class III
   d. Market withdrawal

8. If a medication is taken qod, this means when should it be taken?
   a. Every day
   b. Four times daily
   c. Every other day
   d. Once a week

9. Which of the following is not required on a valid prescription?
   a. Date of issue
   b. Name and address of the practitioner
   c. Name of the patient
   d. The recommended pharmacy for a patient to use

10. A patient is instructed to take 1 tsp qid. How many milliliters will the patient take daily?
    a. 20 mL
    b. 40 mL
    c. 60 mL
    d. 80 mL

11. Which of the following is not a side effect of Augmentin?
    a. Diarrhea
    b. Allergic reaction
    c. Constipation
    d. Rash

12. What is another term for TPN?
    a. Hypercalcemia
    b. Hypomagnesemia
    c. Hyperalimentation
    d. Sustaination

13. Which organization requires that material safety data sheets be available?
    a. FDA
    b. OSHA
    c. P&T
    d. DEA

14. When can a medication that is scheduled III to V be refilled?
    a. Never
    b. As many times as the patient needs
    c. Up to 5 times within 6 months
    d. Up to 6 times within a year

15. Which of the following are high-alert medications?
    a. Morphine, heparin
    b. Potassium chloride, warfarin
    c. Hydromorphone, insulin
    d. All of the above

16. Compulsive gambling is a side effect of which medication?
    a. Carbidopa/levodopa
    b. Donepezil
    c. Ropinirole
    d. Memantine

17. Drugs are intended for use in which of the following?
    a. Prevention of disease
    b. Treatment of disease
    c. Diagnosis of disease
    d. All of the above

18. Which of the following medications can become toxic after its expiration date?
    a. Aspirin
    b. Vicodin
    c. Tetracycline
    d. Lorazepam

19. If a drug is not covered on the approved list of medications, it is not on which of the following?
    a. HMO
    b. Formulary
    c. Facilitator
    d. NCPDP

20. Which of the following is not a biometric identifier?
    a. Fingerprint
    b. Face recognition
    c. Password
    d. DNA

21. If a medication should be taken after meals, which sig code should be used?
    a. ac
    b. pc
    c. bid
    d. qd

22. Fentanyl transdermal is in which DEA class?
    a. I
    b. II
    c. III
    d. IV

23. What basic information is not contained in the patient profile?
    a. Patient's name
    b. Medication allergies
    c. Social security number
    d. Insurance information

24. How many digits are in an NDC?
    a. 10
    b. 12
    c. 14
    d. 16

25. What type of medications can easily be cut in half?
    a. Scored
    b. Capsules
    c. Controlled release
    d. Enteric coated

26. What do the first 4 or 5 digits of the NDC code represent?
    a. The product code
    b. The labeler code
    c. The package code
    d. The bar code

27. When a medication is given to a patient, it must be indicated on which of the following?
    a. Unit dose system
    b. Medication order
    c. Computer physician order entry
    d. Medication administration record

28. Which of the following antibiotics may be used for acne?
    a. Chlorhexidine gluconate
    b. Clindamycin
    c. Mupirocin
    d. Nitrofurantoin

29. Which of the following is a not an advantage of an electronic health record?
    a. Quickly track prescriptions
    b. Low cost
    c. Trigger patient care reminders
    d. Prompt allergy warnings

30. What is the term used to describe a bill of sale of products ordered?
    a. Invoice
    b. Purchase order
    c. MSDS
    d. Formulary

31. Which of the following policies would a patient not be billed any fees for services?
    a. Point-of-service
    b. HMO
    c. Workers' compensation insurance
    d. PPO

32. Which of the following is available as an injection?
    a. Acyclovir
    b. Oseltamivir
    c. Valacyclovir
    d. Zanamivir

33. Which of the following medications is permitted to be dispensed in nonchildproof containers?
    a. Ibuprofen
    b. Oxycodone
    c. Atenolol
    d. Sublingual nitroglycerin

34. Which form is used to document loss or theft of C-II medications?
    a. DEA 41
    b. DEA 106
    c. DEA 222
    d. None of the above

35. Which is an example of a drug–drug interaction?
    a. Bactrim prescribed for a penicillin-allergic patient
    b. Amoxicillin prescribed for a patient on Augmentin
    c. Acyclovir prescribed for a patient with a bacterial infection
    d. Oxycodone prescribed for a patient by a dentist

36. If a patient is eligible for Medicare Part A, they also have the option of enrolling in which part of Medicare?
    a. B
    b. C
    c. D
    d. None of the above

37. When is the effective date on an insurance card?
    a. Coverage is expired for the patient
    b. Coverage has started for the patient
    c. Prescriptions should be refilled
    d. None of the above

38. Lisinopril can potentially increase which electrolyte?
    a. Glucose
    b. Potassium
    c. Sodium
    d. Chloride

39. Which of the following organizations is devoted entirely to medication error prevention?
    a. Agency for Healthcare Research and Quality
    b. Food and Drug Administration
    c. Institute of Safe Medication Practices
    d. The Joint Commission

40. HIPAA sets standards to protect which of the following?
    a. USP
    b. PHI
    c. NF
    d. OTC

41. A patient's insurance card is likely to include all of the following except which one?
    a. Member's ID number
    b. Member's group number
    c. Billing identification number (BIN)
    d. Contracted pricing structure

42. The middle (green) copy of a DEA Form 222 is retained by which of the following?
    a. Supplier
    b. Manufacturer
    c. DEA
    d. Pharmacy

43. Which of the following needles is the smallest?
    a. 16 gauge
    b. 18 gauge
    c. 22 gauge
    d. 25 gauge

44. Which of the following strategies can help prevent illegible handwriting errors?
   a. Handwriting classes
   b. Verbal orders
   c. Telephone orders
   d. Preprinted order sets

45. Which of the following information is not required on the label of the medication vial?
   a. Pharmacy's name and address
   b. Patient's social security number
   c. Date when prescription was filled
   d. Prescription number

46. Which of the following is the amount a patient must pay each year before their benefits begin?
   a. Premium
   b. Copayment
   c. Deductible
   d. Coinsurance

47. Which of the following would be an example of a unit-of-use package?
   a. A 100-count bottle of a medication
   b. A 500-count bottle of a medication
   c. A pack of 30 tablets for a medication taken daily
   d. A vial of a medication to be reconstituted

48. Which patient should not be taking metformin?
   a. A 24-year-old woman with seizures
   b. A 56-year-old man with renal failure
   c. A 55-year-old woman with hypertension
   d. A 78-year-old man with heart failure

49. How many capsules should be dispensed for the following prescription: cephalexin 250 mg 1 PO qid × 10 days?
   a. 10 capsules
   b. 20 capsules
   c. 30 capsules
   d. 40 capsules

50. The liquid in which a solute is dissolved is known as which of the following?
   a. Precipitant
   b. Suspension
   c. Solution
   d. Solvent

51. What is the temperature range for storage of refrigerated products?
   a. −20 to −10°C
   b. 2 to 8°C
   c. −20 to −10°F
   d. 2 to 8°F

52. Which of the following is an example of the therapeutic substitution?
   a. Protonix-prevacid
   b. Norvasc-amlodipine
   c. Prozac-fluoxetine
   d. Ventolin-albuterol

53. You are filling a prescription for a patient who insists on getting the brand name medication. What dispense as written (DAW) code would this be?
   a. DAW 0
   b. DAW 1
   c. DAW 2
   d. DAW 3

54. The Pure Food and Drug Act passed in which year?
   a. 1906
   b. 1926
   c. 2006
   d. 1900

55. How many refills can a physician write for Adderall XR?
   a. 0
   b. 1
   c. 6
   d. 12

56. Medication labels must contain which of the following at the very least?
   a. The name, address, and phone number of the pharmacy
   b. Name of the patient
   c. Date of dispensing
   d. All of the above

57. You receive a prescription for ketoconazole 5% ointment, apply to affected area twice daily, dispense 120 g. You check the pharmacy shelves and find that you have ketoconazole 1% and 10% ointments. How many grams of each ointment do you need to mix together to dispense the prescription as written?

a. 66.6 g of 1% and 53.4 g of 10%
b. 53.4 g of 1% and 66.6 g of 10%
c. 60 g of 1% and 60 g of 10%
d. You cannot make 5% ointment with the products you have in stock

58. Which of the following abbreviations is on The Joint Commission's (TJCs) "Do Not Use" list?
    a. U
    b. mL
    c. cc
    d. L

59. In which reference book would you find detailed patient counseling information?
    a. State Law Book
    b. Federal Law Book
    c. Natural Product Reference
    d. Patient Handout Information Reference

60. How would the following prescription be interpreted: 1 gtt AU qd?
    a. Instill 1 gtt in the right eye 4 times daily
    b. Instill 1 gtt in both ears 4 times daily
    c. Instill 1 gtt in both ears once daily
    d. Instill 1 gtt in both eyes once daily

61. You extemporaneously compounded Magic Mouthwash on January 1, 2014. Your pharmacy's recipe for Magic Mouthwash contains viscous lidocaine (expiration date September 2014), diphenhydramine oral solution (expiration date February 2015), and Maalox (expiration date March 2014). What is the beyond-use date of your compounded Magic Mouthwash?
    a. January 15, 2014
    b. January 31, 2014
    c. March 31, 2014
    d. January 1, 2015

62. What is a common side effect of Zyprexa?
    a. Weight loss
    b. Depression
    c. Weight gain
    d. Constipation

63. Which OTC medication does the "Combat Methamphetamine Epidemic Act" restricts the sale of?
    a. Acetaminophen
    b. Ibuprofen
    c. Guaifenesin
    d. Pseudoephedrine

64. Which of the following is a technician permitted to do?
    a. Refill prescriptions
    b. Take transfers over the phone
    c. Take new prescriptions over the phone
    d. Counsel patients

65. Per the DEA, how many years must records of receipt for C-III, C-IV, and C-V drugs be kept on file?
    a. 1 year
    b. 2 years
    c. 5 years
    d. 7 years

66. An elderly patient with liver failure is prescribed a medication by a physician. If the dose is not adjusted accordingly, what drug utilization review (DUR) rejection could occur?
    a. Drug–drug interaction
    b. Allergy
    c. Therapeutic duplication
    d. Contraindication

67. Which of the following patients are at the highest risk of a calculation error?
    a. A 3 year-old girl
    b. A 15 year-old adolescent boy
    c. A 31 year-old woman
    d. A 70 year-old woman

68. Who issues a medication recall?
    a. TJC
    b. FDA
    c. DEA
    d. P&T

69. Which is a valid DEA number for Dr. John Smith?
    a. BS1234562
    b. MS1234564
    c. AS1234563
    d. All of the above could be correct

70. Which of the following is an expectorant?
    a. Dextromethorphan
    b. Pseudoephedrine
    c. Guaifenesin
    d. Codeine

71. Which of the following organizations accredits hospitals?
    a. Institute for Safe Medication Practices (ISMP)
    b. National Patient Safety Foundation
    c. The Joint Commission (TJC)
    d. The American Heart Association

72. Which of the following books is used to obtain equivalency information?
    a. *NeoFax*
    b. *Brigg's Drugs in Pregnancy and Lactation*
    c. *Orange Book*
    d. *Handbook for Nonprescription Drugs*

73. Which of the following routes has the fastest onset of action?
    a. Oral
    b. Intravenous injection
    c. Transdermal
    d. Intramuscular

74. What is an example of a drug-disease alert?
    a. Elevated international normalized ratio (INR) for a patient on warfarin
    b. Cephalexin being prescribed for a patient with a penicillin allergy
    c. Lisinopril being prescribed for a pregnant patient
    d. Pantoprazole being ordered for a patient on esomeprazole

75. Medications typically expire how many years after manufacturing?
    a. 1 to 5 years
    b. 5 to 10 years
    c. 1 to 5 months
    d. 5 to 10 months

76. AS is the abbreviation for which of the following?
    a. Right ear
    b. Left eye
    c. Both ears
    d. Left ear

77. What should the technician use on the stock bottle to verify the correct medication was pulled for the filling process?
    a. Expiration date
    b. Lot number
    c. Drug strength
    d. NDC number

78. What did the Controlled Substances Act define?
    a. Labeling requirements
    b. Drug schedules
    c. Privacy laws
    d. Purity standards

79. What are used to triturate solid ingredients in nonsterile compounding?
    a. Ointment slabs
    b. Oral syringes
    c. Analytical balances
    d. Mortar and pestles

80. The OBRA '90 required pharmacies to do which of the following?
    a. Perform a prospective drug utilization review on all prescriptions
    b. Provide drive-through service
    c. Therapeutically substitute brand to generic drugs
    d. Protect private information

81. Which committee determines the formulary?
    a. FDA
    b. Executive hospital committee
    c. P&T
    d. Medical executive council

82. Which of the following methods is preferred for prescription generation?
    a. Telephone
    b. E-prescribing
    c. Handwritten
    d. Faxed copy

83. The inscription is the part of the prescription that contains which of the following?
    a. Directions to the pharmacist
    b. Directions to the patient
    c. The Rx symbol
    d. The medication prescribed, quantity, and strength

84. When is the last day that a medication can be safely used if it has an expiration date of 9/16/2017?
    a. 9/1/2017
    b. 9/15/2017
    c. 9/16/2017
    d. 9/17/2017

85. Which type of medication order would be issued for a medication needed immediately?
    a. STAT order
    b. Discharge order
    c. PRN order
    d. Admitting order

86. A spouse or child who is also covered on the member's insurance policy is known as which of the following?
    a. Deductible
    b. Dependent
    c. Premium
    d. Subscriber

87. What is the number for the Poison Control Center?
    a. 1-800-222-1222
    b. 1-888-111-2111
    c. 1-800-111-2111
    d. 1-800-POISONC

88. Who sets standards for medications, biologics, medical devices, and compounded products?

    a. OSHA
    b. TJC
    c. USP
    d. P&T

89. Calculate the last digit of the DEA number AS258382_.
    a. 5
    b. 7
    c. 8
    d. 9

90. You receive a prescription for ketoconazole 4% powder, sprinkle on left foot q8h × 21 days. Ketoconazole powder is available from the manufacturer in 2% and 5% strengths. How much of each strength do you need to mix together to get 60 g of your final product?
    a. 20 g of 2% and 40 g of 5%
    b. 40 g of 2% and 20 g of 5%
    c. 15 g of 2% and 45 g of 5%
    d. 45 g of 2% and 15 g of 5%

Practice Exam

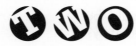

1. What is the Drug Enforcement Administration (DEA) electronic program used for ordering C-II medications?
   a. FDAS
   b. DEAS
   c. CSOS
   d. CMOS

2. Which of the following numbers could lead to a medication error due to a decimal point error?
   a. 1.5
   b. 0.5
   c. 3.4
   d. 6.0

3. The third 1 or 2 digits of the NDC code represent which of the following?
   a. The product code
   b. The labeler code
   c. The package code
   d. The bar code

4. A lot number is a unique identifying code assigned to each _____ of medication produced at a given time.
   a. Unit
   b. Brand
   c. Batch
   d. Strength

5. If a medication is available as a 20 mg/5 mL suspension, how many milliliters would be needed to give a dose of 40 mg?
   a. 5 mL
   b. 10 mL
   c. 15 mL
   d. 20 mL

6. Which of the following third party plans requires the patient to designate a primary care physician (PCP)?
   a. Health Maintenance Organization (HMO)
   b. Preferred Provider Organization (PPO)
   c. Medicare Part D
   d. TRICARE

7. The act of reconstituting or otherwise preparing a medication into a dosage form usable by a patient is defined as which of the following?
   a. Dispensing
   b. Graduating
   c. Compounding
   d. Trituration

8. Which of the following is *not* a type of pharmacy automation?
   a. Robot
   b. Ointment slab and spatula
   c. Barcode scanner
   d. Tabletop tablet counter

9. Which of the following abbreviations is on The Joint Commission's (TJCs) "Do Not Use" list?
   a. qd
   b. qid
   c. bid
   d. tid

10. Which of the following may a technician be responsible for in the retail pharmacy setting?
    a. Entering prescriptions into the computer
    b. Updating the patient profile
    c. Counting medications on a counting tray
    d. All of the above

11. Rotating stock is a process in which products with the shortest expiration dates are moved to which part of the shelf when stocking?
    a. Side
    b. Back
    c. Front
    d. Bottom

12. Which of the following drugs is indicated for the treatment of influenza?
    a. Augmentin
    b. Tamiflu
    c. Levaquin
    d. Valtrex

13. Which of the following organizations accredits hospitals?
    a. Institute of Safe Medication Practices (ISMP)
    b. National Patient Safety Foundation
    c. The Joint Commission (TJC)
    d. The American Heart Association

14. A drug company is required to remove their medication from market due to the risk of death. What type of recall is this?
    a. Class I
    b. Class II
    c. Class III
    d. Market withdrawal

15. If a patient picks up 60 tablets of a medication with the directions, 1 tablet PO qid, how long will this last the patient?
    a. 15 days
    b. 20 days
    c. 30 days
    d. 45 days

16. The abbreviation USP refers to which of the following?
    a. United States Pharmacopeia
    b. United States Pharmacists
    c. Universal Sales Program
    d. United Service Plan

17. Which clinical decision support system (CDSS) function helps identify patient adherence?
    a. Therapeutic duplication
    b. Drug-allergy
    c. Drug-laboratory
    d. Over- or underutilization

18. When is the last day that a medication can be safely used if it has an expiration date of January 2017?
    a. December 31, 2016
    b. January 1, 2017
    c. January 31, 2017
    d. December 31, 2017

19. Which organization oversees Medwatch?
    a. FDA
    b. DEA
    c. USP
    d. TJC

20. How many patient identifiers should be used to verify a patient's identity?
    a. 1
    b. 2
    c. 3
    d. 4

21. Costs that a member pays which are sometimes limited by the insurance policy are known as which of the following?
    a. Out-of-pocket expenses
    b. Member services
    c. Dependents
    d. Subscribers

22. The DEA Form 222 is a(n) _____ form designed specifically for the sale of C-II medications.
    a. Duplicate
    b. Triplicate
    c. Electronic
    d. Optional

23. The inscription is the part of the prescription that contains which of the following?
    a. Directions to the pharmacist
    b. Directions to the patient
    c. The Rx symbol
    d. The medication prescribed, quantity, and strength

24. Which of the following strategies can help prevent illegible handwriting errors?
    a. Verbal orders
    b. Telephone orders
    c. Computerized physician order entry (CPOE)
    d. Handwriting classes

25. What is the temperature range for storage of frozen products?
    a. −20 to −10°C
    b. 2 to 8°C
    c. −20 to −10°F
    d. 2 to 8°F

26. Fluconazole is indicated for the treatment of which of the following?
    a. Candidiasis
    b. Influenza
    c. Bacterial infection
    d. Herpes

27. In which reference book would you find information regarding the storage requirements of a medication?
    a. *Drug Facts and Comparisons*
    b. *Natural Standard*
    c. *Federal Law Book*
    d. *NeoFax*

28. A patient is ordered 25 mg of hydroxyzine to be taken tid for 20 days. How many capsules should be dispensed for this order, if the pharmacy stocks 25-mg capsules?
    a. 30 capsules
    b. 40 capsules
    c. 50 capsules
    d. 60 capsules

29. Which of the following is a solid ingredient dissolved in a liquid?
    a. Solvent
    b. Solution
    c. Solute
    d. Suspension

30. Which of the following medications has a narrow therapeutic range?
    a. Esomeprazole
    b. Insulin
    c. Ibuprofen
    d. Albuterol

31. Which organization is solely dedicated to medication error prevention?
    a. OSHA
    b. FDA
    c. TJC
    d. ISMP

32. What does the DEA enforce?
    a. State-specific dispensing laws
    b. Pharmacist licensing
    c. Controlled substance laws of the United States
    d. OTC product labeling

33. Where should the medications that must be protected from light be stored until use?
    a. In the refrigerator
    b. In a cabinet
    c. In their original containers
    d. In the basement

34. Which of the following patients are at the highest risk of a calculation error?
    a. A 2 year-old girl
    b. A 16 year-old adolescent girl
    c. A 34 year-old man
    d. A 66 year-old woman

35. Which of the following is true about patient's allergy information?
    a. Is not necessary
    b. Should be reviewed frequently with patients
    c. Should include *only* drug-allergy information
    d. May not be collected by technicians

36. Which of the following is a COX-2 selective anti-inflammatory?
    a. Celebrex
    b. Cambia
    c. Cataflam
    d. Caldolor

37. Which part of Medicare covers durable medical equipment (DME) and physician services or outpatient hospital visits?
    a. Part A
    b. Part B
    c. Part C
    d. Part D

38. Which of the following medications is in schedule III?
    a. Pregabalin
    b. Buprenorphine
    c. Zolpidem
    d. Temazepam

39. What is identifying, analyzing, assessing, and controlling risk?
    a. CQI
    b. PSO
    c. Risk management
    d. Productivity

40. A lot of Tylenol has been determined to contain only 160 mg per tablet rather than the labeled 325 mg. In which class would this product be recalled?
    a. Class I
    b. Class II
    c. Class III
    d. This product would not be recalled

41. tid is the sig code for which of the following?
   a. Twice daily
   b. Three times daily
   c. Four times daily
   d. Five times daily

42. Which of the following organizations is devoted entirely to medication error prevention?
   a. Agency for Healthcare Research and Quality
   b. Food and Drug Administration
   c. Institute of Safe Medication Practices
   d. The Joint Commission

43. In which reference book would you find information regarding dosage forms available for a specific medication?
   a. Natural Product Reference
   b. Federal Law Book
   c. General Drug Information Reference
   d. Patient Handout Information Reference

44. Sumatriptan is indicated for which of the following?
   a. Hypertension
   b. Back pain
   c. Migraine
   d. Parkinson disease

45. What did the Pure Food and Drug Act of 1906 require?
   a. That drugs not be mislabeled
   b. Industry purity and strength standards
   c. Therapeutic benefit documentation
   d. Both a and b

46. Which of the following products are medications administered by any route other than oral?
   a. Intravenous
   b. Subcutaneous
   c. Parenteral
   d. Nonsterile

47. When should Pravachol be taken?
   a. Before breakfast
   b. With lunch
   c. After dinner
   d. Prior to going to bed

48. Which of the following is not an important part of a patient profile?
   a. Address
   b. Phone number

   c. Allergies
   d. All are important in a patient profile

49. Which of the following are high-alert medications?
   a. Insulin, heparin
   b. Insulin, citalopram
   c. Heparin, citalopram
   d. Morphine, pantoprazole

50. When a sentinel event occurs in a hospital, which organization is this information reported to?
   a. FDA
   b. DEA
   c. USP
   d. TJC

51. Which of the following is the abbreviation for both eyes?
   a. AU
   b. OU
   c. AD
   d. AS

52. Which of the following is a correct DEA number for a resident at University Hospital?
   a. AU2866626
   b. AU2866626-2132
   c. BH2866626
   d. BH2866626-2132

53. When a patient has multiple insurance providers, and one is selected as primary and billed first, to ensure there is not a duplication of payments, this is known as which of the following?
   a. Point-of-service
   b. Coordination of benefits
   c. Pharmacy benefit manager
   d. Third party resolution

54. What is the primary indication of angiotensin-converting enzyme inhibitors (ACEIs)?
   a. Hypertension
   b. Hyperlipidemia
   c. Hypertriglyceridemia
   d. Hyperactivity attention disorder

55. Which of the following pharmacy personnel can counsel a patient on how to use a fluticasone inhaler?
    a. Cashier
    b. Pharmacy technician
    c. Certified pharmacy technician
    d. Pharmacist

56. Drugs are intended for use in which of the following?
    a. Prevention of disease
    b. Treatment of disease
    c. Diagnosis of disease
    d. All of the above

57. What should the technician use on the stock bottle to verify the correct medication was pulled for the filling process?
    a. Expiration date
    b. Lot number
    c. Drug strength
    d. NDC number

58. You extemporaneously compounded Magic Mouthwash on January 1, 2014. Your pharmacy's recipe for Magic Mouthwash contains viscous lidocaine (expiration date September 2014), diphenhydramine oral solution (expiration date February 2015), and Maalox (expiration date March 2014). What is the beyond-use date of your compounded Magic Mouthwash?
    a. January 15, 2014
    b. January 31, 2014
    c. March 31, 2014
    d. January 1, 2015

59. Which of the following methods is preferred for prescription generation?
    a. Telephone
    b. E-prescribing
    c. Handwritten
    d. Faxed copy

60. How many refills are permitted on a schedule-II medication?
    a. Five times in 6 months
    b. Zero
    c. One
    d. Six times in 5 months

61. Which of the following committees manages the formulary system?
    a. Medical Executive Committee
    b. Nursing Council
    c. Pharmacy and Therapeutics Committee
    d. Pharmacy Administration Board

62. Which of the following may be provided by a clinical decision support system (CDSS)?
    a. Drug-allergy
    b. Therapeutic duplication
    c. Pharmacokinetic monitoring
    d. All of the above

63. What fee is usually paid monthly to an insurance company by the policy holder?
    a. Deductible
    b. Copayment
    c. Premium
    d. Coinsurance

64. Nitrates should not be given concurrently with which medication?
    a. Aspirin
    b. Diltiazem
    c. Sildenafil
    d. Valsartan

65. Which type of medication order is given at the same time every day?
    a. STAT order
    b. Discharge order
    c. PRN order
    d. Scheduled order

66. Calculate the last digit of the DEA number BE214855_.
    a. 0
    b. 9
    c. 8
    d. 7

67. Which of the following medication is a short-acting β_2 agonist (rescue inhaler)?
    a. Proventil
    b. Foradil
    c. Flovent
    d. Spiriva

68. Which of the following is not a biometric identifier?
a. Fingerprint
b. Face recognition
c. Password
d. DNA

69. How many schedules of medications were defined by the Controlled Substances Act?
a. 4
b. 5
c. 2
d. 1

70. Calculate the number of tablets needed to fill the following prescription: metformin 500 mg 1 PO bid.
a. 15 tablets
b. 30 tablets
c. 45 tablets
d. 60 tablets

71. A spouse of the card holder would be a person code of which of the following?
a. 1
b. 2
c. 3
d. 4

72. What is an example of a drug-laboratory alert?
a. Elevated international normalized ratio (INR) for a patient on warfarin
b. Bactrim being prescribed for a patient with a sulfa allergy
c. Lisinopril being prescribed for a pregnant patient
d. Pantoprazole being ordered for a patient on omeprazole

73. Which of the following is the process in which unused or expired medications are returned to the manufacturer?
a. Geometric dilution
b. Hazardous waste
c. Reverse distribution
d. DEA Form 222

74. If a prescription order calls for 2 tbsp tid dispense 450 mL, how long will this last the patient?
a. 5 days
b. 15 days
c. 20 days
d. 30 days

75. Which of the following is used for constipation?
a. Lomotil
b. Zofran
c. Imodium
d. Miralax

76. A physician orders gentamicin 70 mg q12h. Gentamicin is available as an injectable 40 mg/mL solution. How much gentamicin must be drawn up in order to dispense the ordered dose?
a. 0.6 mL
b. 1.75 mL
c. 2.5 mL
d. 3.5 mL

77. Medications with a high abuse potential and with acceptable uses are considered as which of the following?
a. Schedule II
b. Schedule III
c. Schedule I
d. OTC

78. If a patient was taking a medication q8h, how many times daily would this medication be taken?
a. 2
b. 3
c. 4
d. 5

79. What time of the day should bisphosphonates be taken?
a. Before breakfast
b. With lunch
c. Before dinner
d. At bedtime

80. Assuming all are available, which of the following size syringes should be used to withdraw 8 mL of solution from a vial?
    a. 5 mL
    b. 10 mL
    c. 20 mL
    d. 30 mL

81. Which of the following is an example of a schedule-II medication?
    a. Heroin
    b. Morphine
    c. Lorazepam
    d. Pregabalin

82. Which of the following would Medicare Part D not cover?
    a. DME
    b. Lipitor
    c. Lisinopril
    d. Zetia

83. A patient is ordered to take 4 mL of medication that is stocked as 200 mg/5 mL. How many milligrams are contained in 1 dose?
    a. 125 mg
    b. 150 mg
    c. 160 mg
    d. 200 mg

84. Where would a buccal tablet be placed?
    a. Orally
    b. Rectally
    c. Between the cheek and gums
    d. Under the tongue

85. When must an offer to counsel a patient be made?
    a. Prior to dispensing the finished product
    b. Via phone call 1 week after dispensing

c. On dispensing the finished product to the patient
d. None of the above

86. Which of the following routes has the fastest onset of action?
    a. Oral
    b. Intravenous injection
    c. Transdermal
    d. Intramuscular

87. Which of the following is an example of a medication that does not require child-resistant packaging?
    a. Ovcon
    b. Zyrtec
    c. Protonix
    d. Zocor

88. Which of the following is the abbreviation for nitroglycerin?
    a. NS
    b. mL
    c. $FeSO_4$
    d. NTG

89. Which chapter of USP defines guidelines for sterile compounding?
    a. 795
    b. 797
    c. 979
    d. 959

90. If a patient has a 5-fl oz bottle of medication, how many 1-tsp doses can they get from this bottle?
    a. 10 doses
    b. 15 doses
    c. 20 doses
    d. 30 doses

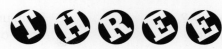
1. Which DEA form is used to document the destruction of controlled substances?
   a. Form 41
   b. Form 106
   c. Form 222
   d. Form 224

2. In which reference book would you find detailed patient counseling information?
   a. State Law Book
   b. Federal Law Book
   c. Natural Product Reference
   d. Patient Handout Information Reference

3. What is an NDC?
   a. An optical machine-readable representation of information related to the object to which it is attached
   b. A unique, 3-segment number which identifies drug products
   c. Issued by the DEA
   d. Issued by the State Board of Pharmacy

4. Which of the following is a required information sheet that instructs proper storage, handling, and containment procedures for hazardous substances?
   a. Formulary
   b. NDC
   c. MSDS
   d. PAR

5. Calculate the last digit of the DEA number AH318825_.
   a. 6
   b. 4
   c. 3
   d. 1

6. Which of the following is a combination of a Health Maintenance Organization (HMO) and Preferred Provider Organization (PPO) plan where patients pay more for services when they are needed?
   a. CHAMPVA
   b. Medicare Part B

c. Point-of-service (POS)
d. Deductible

7. Which of the following numbers could lead to a medication error due to a decimal point error?
   a. .6
   b. 0.6
   c. 1.6
   d. 6

8. Which of the following may a technician *never* do?
   a. Enter prescriptions into the computer
   b. Counsel patients
   c. Update insurance information
   d. Take a refill over the phone

9. What is another term for a wholesaler?
   a. Distributor
   b. Manufacturer
   c. Formulary manager
   d. Pharmacy benefit manager

10. Which of the following is a solid ingredient dissolved in a liquid?
    a. Solvent
    b. Solution
    c. Solute
    d. Suspension

11. An elevation of which of the following can lead to gout?
    a. Potassium
    b. Magnesium
    c. Uric acid
    d. Iron

12. Which of the following abbreviations is on The Joint Commission's (TJCs) "Do Not Use" list?
    a. qd
    b. qid
    c. bid
    d. tid

13. Which of the following refers to DEA?
   a. Drug Enforcement Administration
   b. Drug Enforcement Agency
   c. Drug Elimination Administration
   d. Drug Evaluation Agency

14. What is the benefit of having a prime vendor for a pharmacy?
   a. Discounts are offered
   b. Markups are offered
   c. Reverse distributor status
   d. Use of CSOS is allowed

15. Which of the following is not a side effect of anticholinergic drugs?
   a. Dry eyes
   b. Constipation
   c. Diarrhea
   d. Dry mouth

16. Who created patient safety organizations?
   a. The FDA
   b. The Department of Health and Human Services
   c. The DEA
   d. The State Board of Pharmacy

17. Which of the following is the superscription?
   a. Rx symbol
   b. Refill(s) amount
   c. Directions given to the patient
   d. Medication prescribed, quantity, and strength

18. Which of the following individuals may be responsible for a medication error?
   a. Nurse
   b. Physician
   c. Pharmacist
   d. All of the above

19. The bottom (blue) copy of a DEA Form 222 is retained by whom?
   a. Supplier
   b. Manufacturer
   c. DEA
   d. Pharmacy

20. When a patient is responsible for a percentage of the cost of services, instead of a flat fee, this is known as which of the following?
   a. Copayment
   b. Coinsurance
   c. Premium
   d. Point-of-service

21. What pharmacy system allows a pharmacist to counsel a patient in a different location?
   a. CPOE
   b. E-prescribing
   c. Telepharmacy
   d. EHR

22. The Pure Food and Drug Act passed in which year?
   a. 1906
   b. 1926
   c. 2006
   d. 1900

23. If a prescriber writes an order for a liquid medication, but does not specify a quantity and instead writes qs on the prescription. Which of the following means the same?
   a. Quantity sufficient
   b. Dispense as written
   c. Quality standards
   d. Quinapril suspension

24. Which of the following medications is injected directly into the fatty layer below the skin's surface?
   a. Intramuscular
   b. Subcutaneous
   c. Intravenous
   d. Epidural

25. What basic information is *not* contained in the patient profile?
   a. Patient's name
   b. Medication allergies
   c. Social security number
   d. Insurance information

26. Which of the following procedures helps eliminate errors during medication administration to hospital patients?
   a. Single patient identifier
   b. Barcode technology
   c. Tall-man letters
   d. Shelf separators

27. What is the temperature range for storage of refrigerated products?
    a. −20 to −10°C
    b. 2 to 8°C
    c. −20 to −10°F
    d. 2 to 8°F

28. Which of the following Medicare plans was originally known as the Medicare + Choice plan?
    a. Part A
    b. Part B
    c. Part C
    d. Part D

29. Which segment of the NDC code represents the labeler code?
    a. The first 4 or 5 digits
    b. The second 3 or 4 digits
    c. The third 1 or 2 digits
    d. Both a and c

30. What is the generic name of Adipex-P?
    a. Lorcaserin
    b. Orlistat
    c. Phentermine
    d. Topiramate

31. Which of the following reports is most useful to identify a product's availability?
    a. Inventory report
    b. Usage report
    c. Override report
    d. Diversion report

32. If a medication is dispensed in a gtt, it is given as which of the following?
    a. Tablet
    b. Capsule
    c. Ointment
    d. Drop

33. Which of the following strategies can help prevent illegible handwriting errors?
    a. Handwriting classes
    b. Verbal orders
    c. Telephone orders
    d. Preprinted order sets

34. In which schedule are medications with a low abuse potential and acceptable medical use?
    a. Schedule II
    b. Schedule III
    c. Schedule IV
    d. OTC

35. Sterile powders for injection and powders for reconstitution must be protected from which of the following?
    a. Theft
    b. Pyrogens
    c. Light
    d. Humidity

36. Name the process to ensure programs are intentionally improving service and increasing positive outcomes.
    a. Risk management
    b. Productivity
    c. Entrepreneurship
    d. Continuous quality improvement

37. Which of the following is used to treat fungal infections?
    a. Lidoderm
    b. Clobex
    c. Lotrisone
    d. Temovate

38. Which of the following would *not* be needed to process a patient's insurance claim?
    a. Member's ID number
    b. Member's birthdate
    c. Medication prescribed, dose, and quantity
    d. Member's social security number

39. A patient's insurance card is likely to include all of the following *except* which one?
    a. Member's ID number
    b. Member's group number
    c. Billing identification number (BIN)
    d. Contracted pricing structure

40. A manufacturer has determined that the rubber stopper in several lots of their furosemide IV vials has a tendency to core easily. In which class would this product be recalled?
    a. Class I
    b. Class II
    c. Class III
    d. This product would not be recalled

41. Compounding should always take place how many inches from the front and sides of a laminar flow hood?
    a. 3
    b. 6
    c. 9
    d. 12

42. Which of the following is an example of a schedule-III medication?
    a. Heroin
    b. Morphine
    c. Lorazepam
    d. Codeine with acetaminophen

43. Which of the following should not be used during prescribing in order to minimize errors?
    a. Milligram
    b. Grain
    c. Milliliter
    d. Gram

44. A patient takes 1 tablet tid ac and hs. How many tablets will the patient need for a 30-day supply?
    a. 90 tablets
    b. 120 tablets
    c. 150 tablets
    d. 200 tablets

45. Which of the following information is *not* required on the label of the medication vial?
    a. Pharmacy's name and address
    b. Patient's social security number
    c. Date when prescription was filled
    d. Prescription number

46. What is the most common adverse effect of Zithromax?
    a. Gastrointestinal (GI) toxicity
    b. Rash
    c. Hearing loss
    d. Visual changes

47. Which code is used for the third party to determine if the proper brand or generic medication was used to fill the prescription?
    a. USAN
    b. DAW
    c. Adjudication
    d. Trade

48. What type of recall would be there in a situation in which use or exposure to a product is not likely to cause adverse health consequences?
    a. Class I
    b. Class II
    c. Class III
    d. Class IV

49. Which of the following patients is at the highest risk of a calculation error?
    a. A 3 year-old girl
    b. A 15 year-old adolescent boy
    c. A 31 year-old woman
    d. A 70 year-old woman

50. Which is an example of a drug–allergy interaction?
    a. Amoxicillin prescribed for a penicillin-allergic patient
    b. Amoxicillin prescribed for a patient on Augmentin
    c. Amoxicillin prescribed for a patient with a bacterial infection
    d. Amoxicillin prescribed for a patient by a dentist

51. If a patient is ordered 1 g of Valtrex to be taken daily, and the pharmacy only has the 500-mg tablets in stock, how many tablets will the patient receive with each dose?
    a. 1 tablet
    b. 1½ tablets
    c. 2 tablets
    d. 3 tablets

52. The Poison Prevention Act created which pharmacy dispensing standard?
    a. Patient counseling
    b. Child-resistant container use
    c. Counting tray use
    d. All of the above

53. Which of the following organizations is devoted entirely to medication error prevention?
    a. The Joint Commission
    b. Institute for Safe Medication Practices
    c. Food and Drug Administration
    d. Centers for Disease Control and Prevention

54. What is the beyond-use date of products prepared at a patient's bedside in an emergent situation?
    a. Immediate use only
    b. 48 hours
    c. 30 hours
    d. 24 hours

55. Which of the following books is used to obtain equivalency information?
    a. *NeoFax*
    b. *Brigg's Drugs in Pregnancy and Lactation*
    c. *Orange Book*
    d. *Handbook for Nonprescription Drugs*

56. A patient brings in a prescription for Relafen. How many months may the prescription be refilled?
    a. None
    b. 3 months
    c. 6 months
    d. 12 months

57. If a patient is taking metoclopramide 5-mg tablets, 1 tid × 15 days, how many tablets will be needed to fill the order?
    a. 30 tablets
    b. 45 tablets
    c. 60 tablets
    d. 90 tablets

58. Which of the following is an example of a medication that does *not* require child-resistant packaging?
    a. Reglan
    b. Levothyroxine
    c. Seroquel
    d. Cholestyramine powder (canister)

59. After an error has occurred, what type of analysis may be performed?
    a. FMEA
    b. Productivity report
    c. RCA
    d. Efficiency report

60. Which of the following are high-alert medications?
    a. Morphine, heparin
    b. Potassium chloride, warfarin
    c. Hydromorphone, insulin
    d. All of the above

61. Which of the following medications is indicated for type 1 diabetes?
    a. Glipizide
    b. Metformin
    c. Insulin glargine
    d. Pioglitazone

62. Which of the following would be an example of a unit-of-use package?
    a. A 100-count bottle of a medication
    b. A 500-count bottle of a medication
    c. A pack of 30 tablets for a medication taken daily
    d. A vial of a medication to be reconstituted

63. Which organization requires that material safety data sheets be available?
    a. FDA
    b. OSHA
    c. P&T
    d. DEA

64. What type of filter is used in laminar flow hoods and clean rooms to ensure 99.97% removal of air particles?
    a. LEPA
    b. HVAC
    c. HEPA
    d. EPA

65. What is an example of a portable computer?
    a. Mainframe
    b. Minicomputer
    c. Tablet computer
    d. Desktop computer

66. Which of the following is a list of medications covered under a patient's insurance plan?
    a. DAW
    b. HMO
    c. Deductible
    d. Formulary

67. Which of the following pharmacy personnel can counsel a patient on how to use an insulin pen?
    a. Cashier
    b. Pharmacy technician
    c. Certified pharmacy technician
    d. Pharmacist

68. The "Combat Methamphetamine Epidemic Act" restricts the sale of which OTC medication?
    a. Acetaminophen
    b. Ibuprofen
    c. Guaifenesin
    d. None of the above

69. The number of days a medication should last if used correctly is known as which of the following?
    a. Sig code
    b. Days supply
    c. Superscription
    d. Medication order

70. Which USP chapter defines guidelines for nonsterile compounding?
    a. 795
    b. 797
    c. 979
    d. 959

71. If a patient is instructed to take a medication 1 tsp tid for 30 days, how many milliliters would the pharmacy need to give this patient for the entire order?
    a. 150 mL
    b. 300 mL
    c. 450 mL
    d. 600 mL

72. Which medication cannot treat seizures?
    a. Neurontin
    b. Keppra
    c. Wellbutrin
    d. Topamax

73. What is an example of a drug-disease alert?
    a. Elevated INR for a patient on warfarin
    b. Cephalexin being prescribed for a patient with a penicillin allergy
    c. Lisinopril being prescribed for a pregnant patient
    d. Pantoprazole being ordered for a patient on esomeprazole

74. A patient brings in a prescription for buspirone 5 mg #90—1 PO tid. What is the indication?
    a. Depression
    b. Bipolar disorder
    c. Anxiety
    d. Insomnia

75. Calculate the days supply for a medication given 1 PO qid #40.
    a. 10 days
    b. 15 days
    c. 20 days
    d. 40 days

76. DEA Form 106 is used to report which of the following?
    a. Order C-II medications
    b. Document destruction of C-II medications
    c. Document theft or loss of C-II medications
    d. None of the above

77. Which of the following medications requires a package insert every time it is dispensed?
    a. Warfarin
    b. Ethinyl estradiol and norgestrel
    c. Pantoprazole
    d. None of the above

78. Which of the following is required to submit an insurance claim?
    a. RxBin number
    b. RxGroup number
    c. Patient's ID number
    d. All of the above

79. How would the following prescription be interpreted: 1 gtt AU qd?
    a. Instill 1 gtt in the right eye 4 times daily
    b. Instill 1 gtt in both ears 4 times daily
    c. Instill 1 gtt in both ears once daily
    d. Instill 1 gtt in both eyes once daily

80. Pregnant women should not handle which of the following?
    a. Avodart
    b. Detrol
    c. Flomax
    d. Cardura

81. If a patient takes 1 tablet tid for 14 days, how many tablets will the pharmacy need to fill this order?
    a. 28 tablets
    b. 36 tablets
    c. 42 tablets
    d. 48 tablets

82. A physician orders an abciximab infusion of 8 mg/250 mL NS at a rate of 19 mL/h. Abciximab is available as a 10 mg/5 mL injectable solution. What volume of this solution should be drawn up to provide the requested dosage?
    a. 5 mL
    b. 4 mL
    c. 3 mL
    d. 2 mL

83. Which of the following should be avoided in neonates?
    a. Syrup
    b. Elixir
    c. Suspension
    d. Emulsion

84. When can a patient purchase 9 g of pseudoephedrine?
    a. Every month
    b. Every 3 months
    c. Every 6 months
    d. Every 12 months

85. A patient is instructed to take 1 tablet before breakfast, 2 tablets with lunch, 1 tablet with dinner, and 1 tablet before bedtime. If the pharmacy is requested to dispense a 30-day supply, how many tablets should be dispensed?
    a. 45 tablets
    b. 90 tablets
    c. 150 tablets
    d. 200 tablets

86. Which of the following is a cylindrical or conical-shaped container with clearly defined measurement calibrations used in nonsterile compounding?

    a. Graduate
    b. Analytical balance
    c. Ointment slab
    d. Meniscus

87. What should patients be instructed to do after using a Flovent inhaler?
    a. Brush teeth
    b. Rinse out mouth
    c. Chew a piece of gum
    d. Eat a meal

88. Which of the following is a correct DEA number for a resident at Methodist Hospital?
    a. BM2866626
    b. AH2866626-3884
    c. AH2866626-6626
    d. BM2866626-3884

89. In order to be enrolled in Medicare Part C, a patient must be enrolled in which of the following?
    a. Parts A and B
    b. Parts A and D
    c. Parts B and D
    d. None of the above

90. If a prescription calls for a medication to be given PV, how should it be administered?
    a. Rectally
    b. Orally
    c. Optically
    d. Vaginally

Practice Exam

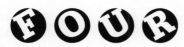

1. Medications that are used frequently ("fast movers") should have which of the following PAR levels?
   a. Small
   b. Large
   c. Varying
   d. None of the above

2. Which of the following strategies can help decrease handwriting errors?
   a. Verbal orders
   b. CPOE
   c. Tall-man letters
   d. Bar code

3. What is the unique 3-segment number which identifies drug products?
   a. The bar code
   b. The NDC
   c. The federal legend
   d. The schedule

4. Which of the following is a medication that requires a prescription for use?
   a. Legend drug
   b. Over-the-counter drug
   c. Behind-the-counter drug
   d. None of the above

5. The curve is the surface of a liquid that occurs around the edge of a container due to surface tension and must be taken into account when reading volume level is known as which of the following?
   a. Levigate
   b. Precipitant
   c. Solvent
   d. Meniscus

6. Which beverage should not be consumed with metronidazole?
   a. Water
   b. Grapefruit juice
   c. Wine
   d. Orange juice

7. Which of the following are drug information resources?
   a. Written references used to find answers to questions
   b. Electronic references used to find answers to questions
   c. Available for patients and pharmacists to read and review
   d. All of the above

8. Calculate the last digit of the DEA number FH133957_.
   a. 4
   b. 5
   c. 6
   d. 7

9. The middle (green) copy of a DEA Form 222 is retained by whom?
   a. Supplier
   b. Manufacturer
   c. DEA
   d. Pharmacy

10. The cost of the coverage of an insurance policy is known as which of the following?
    a. Deductible
    b. Copayment
    c. Coinsurance
    d. Premium

11. Which of the following numbers could lead to a medication error due to a decimal point error?
    a. 1.00
    b. 1.01
    c. 0.11
    d. 0.01

12. Tendon rupture can occur with which class of medications?
    a. Quinolones
    b. Penicillins
    c. Cephalosporins
    d. Tetracyclines

13. A clinical information system may contain which of the following information?
   a. Electronic orders
   b. Medication administration records
   c. Patient information
   d. All of the above

14. If a prescriber wanted a medication not be substituted with generic, he or she would indicate which of the following?
   a. No refills
   b. DAW
   c. Superscription
   d. Inscription

15. Which of the following is a correct DEA number for a resident at City Wide Hospital?
   a. AC2866626-262
   b. AC2866626
   c. BH2866626-626
   d. BH2866626-262

16. The label on a blood pressure monitor indicates the product must be stored at controlled room temperature. What is the appropriate temperature range?
   a. 15 to 30°C
   b. 30 to 40°C
   c. 15 to 30°F
   d. 30 to 40°F

17. Which of the following abbreviations is on The Joint Commission's (TJCs) "Do Not Use" list?
   a. U
   b. mL
   c. cc
   d. L

18. A patient is taking a medication PRN. Which of the following is the route of administration?
   a. Rectally
   b. As needed
   c. Every 6 hours
   d. None of the above

19. Which of the following is the amount a patient must pay each year before their benefits begin?
   a. Premium
   b. Copayment
   c. Deductible
   d. Coinsurance

20. Humidity decreases which of the following of powders for reconstitution.
   a. Sterility
   b. Stability
   c. Effectiveness
   d. Bioavailability

21. This agency in the Department of Health and Human Services is responsible for improving quality, safety, and efficiency in the health care system.
   a. PSO
   b. CQI
   c. AHRQ
   d. DEA

22. Which of the following is not used to input information into a computer?
   a. Mouse
   b. Monitor
   c. USB
   d. Light pen

23. IV piggybacks are a small volume of medication, typically less than _____, which is infused through the same lines as a primary IV fluid.
   a. 50 mL
   b. 250 mL
   c. 500 mL
   d. 1000 mL

24. Which of the following is not a side effect of methadone?
   a. Diarrhea
   b. Constipation
   c. Sedation
   d. Miosis

25. Medications, medical equipment, devices, and medical supplies are regulated by which of the following?
   a. CSOS
   b. AWP
   c. FDA

26. Which of the following health care professionals may be responsible for a medication error?
   a. Pharmacy technician
   b. Pharmacist
   c. Nurse
   d. All of the above

27. Which of the following stands for MDI?
    a. Multivitamin
    b. Metered-dose inhaler
    c. Multidrug inspection
    d. Multidrug inhalation

28. How many milligrams of codeine are in Tylenol #4?
    a. 15 mg
    b. 30 mg
    c. 45 mg
    d. 60 mg

29. Where should recalled medications be stored?
    a. In the refrigerator
    b. On the shelf in alphabetical order
    c. Segregated from normal stock
    d. In the narcotic cabinet

30. Which Medicare part, known as the Medicare Advantage plan, can private companies offer Medicare benefits through their own policies?
    a. Part A
    b. Part B
    c. Part C
    d. Part D

31. Medication doses given to patients are recorded on which of the following?
    a. CIS
    b. Monitor
    c. MAR
    d. Barcode scanner

32. During medication administration, what can help elimination medication errors?
    a. Drug utilization review
    b. Single patient identifier
    c. Barcode technology
    d. Tall-man letters

33. Who licenses wholesalers?
    a. The State Board of Pharmacy
    b. The USP
    c. The FDA
    d. The DEA

34. The stock label on the bottle of medication will *not* include which of the following?
    a. Lot number
    b. Expiration date

c. Bar code
d. Pharmacy address

35. What is the proper procedure for cleaning a horizontal laminar flow hood?
    a. Wipe with isopropyl alcohol from back to front
    b. Wipe with isopropyl alcohol from top to bottom
    c. Wipe with soap and water from back to front
    d. Wipe with soap and water from top to bottom

36. Which of the following patients should not be prescribed Lotensin?
    a. A 34 year-old pregnant woman
    b. A 7 year-old girl
    c. A 65 year-old man
    d. A 95 year-old man

37. When a physician is able to enter into the pharmacy system directly, this is known as which of the following?
    a. Medication administration record
    b. Medication order
    c. DEA number
    d. Computer physician order entry (CPOE)

38. Which organization is in charge of licensing pharmacists?
    a. DEA
    b. FDA
    c. BOP
    d. TJC

39. Which law sets standards for sharing patient information?
    a. Poison Prevention Act
    b. Controlled Substances Act
    c. HIPAA
    d. All of the above

40. Handwriting errors can be minimized by using which of the following strategy?
    a. Handwriting classes
    b. Verbal orders
    c. Telephone orders
    d. Computerized physician order entry

41. In which reference book would you find information regarding recordkeeping requirements for prescriptions?
  a. State Law Book
  b. Natural Product Reference
  c. Drug Information Reference
  d. Patient Handout Information Reference

42. Which of the following may be used for migraine prophylaxis?
  a. Sumatriptan
  b. Propranolol
  c. Oxycodone
  d. Ramipril

43. A patient has a prescription for 3 mg of a suspension that is available 2 mg/5 mL. How many teaspoonsful will the patient need to take for each dose?
  a. 1 tsp
  b. 1½ tsp
  c. 2 tsp
  d. 2½ tsp

44. What is the room temperature of beyond-use date of a TPN prepared in a horizontal laminar flow hood?
  a. 24 hours
  b. 30 hours
  c. 36 hours
  d. 48 hours

45. Which of the following is an example of a schedule-III medication?
  a. Buprenorphine
  b. Morphine
  c. Hydromorphone
  d. All of the above

46. Which of the following should not be used during prescribing in order to minimize errors?
  a. 7 mg
  b. 1/200 grain
  c. 3 mL
  d. 17 g

47. A medication that is prepackaged for a single dose administration is known as which of the following?
  a. Unit-of-use
  b. STAT order
  c. Unit dose
  d. ADC

48. Which of the following steps is not part of infection control in sterile compounding?
  a. Remove all personal outer garments
  b. Take off shoes
  c. Remove all cosmetics
  d. Put on hair cover

49. Which of the following computers is used to house and process large amounts of data?
  a. Desktop
  b. Mainframe
  c. Laptop
  d. Tablet

50. A third party administrator of prescription drug programs for a large group of employers is known as which of the following?
  a. Formulary
  b. PCN
  c. Pharmacy benefit manager (PBM)
  d. Coordination of benefits

51. Calculate the amount to dispense in the following prescription: Bactrim suspension 2 tsp bid × 10 days, dispense qs.
  a. 100 mL
  b. 150 mL
  c. 200 mL
  d. 250 mL

52. Diuretics can cause a decrease in which of the following?
  a. Electrolytes
  b. Cholesterol
  c. Blood sugar
  d. Serotonin

53. Which of the following patients are at the highest risk of a calculation error?
  a. A 7-week old
  b. A 14-year old
  c. A 28-year old
  d. A 56-year old

54. A patient's insurance card is likely to include all of the following *except* which one?
a. Member's ID number
b. Member's group number
c. Patient's diagnosis
d. Billing identification number (BIN)

55. A patient is instructed to apply 1 nitroglycerin patch each week. How many patches will a month's supply contain?
a. 1 patch
b. 2 patches
c. 3 patches
d. 4 patches

56. The "Combat Methamphetamine Epidemic Act" restricts the sale of ephedrine and pseudoephedrine to which of the following?
a. 9 g every 30 days
b. 2.4 g every 30 days
c. 3.6 g every 30 days
d. 5 g every 30 days

57. Calculate how much to dispense for the following medication: amoxicillin suspension 125 mg/5 mL 1 tsp tid × 10 days qs.
a. 80 mL
b. 100 mL
c. 125 mL
d. 150 mL

58. What is methimazole is indicated for?
a. Hypothyroidism
b. Hypoglycemia
c. Hyperthyroidism
d. Hyperglycemia

59. Which of the following is an example of a medication that does *not* require child-resistant packaging?
a. Atenolol
b. Aleve
c. Albuterol HFA inhaler
d. Atorvastatin

60. What characteristics describe a MAR?
a. Permanent and legal record of medication administration
b. Optional for medication administration documentation
c. Legal record of medication dispensing
d. Temporary record of medication ordering

61. Which of the following organizations is devoted entirely to medication error prevention?
a. Institute of Safe Medication Practices
b. National Patient Safety Foundation
c. The Joint Commission
d. The American Heart Association

62. A patient is ordered Zofran 2 teaspoonsful twice daily. If the medication is available 4 mg/5 mL, how many milligrams are in 1 dose?
a. 8 mg
b. 16 mg
c. 24 mg
d. 32 mg

63. Atypical antipsychotics can increase which of the following?
a. Electrolytes
b. Cholesterol
c. Blood sugar
d. Blood pressure

64. A patient has an order to take 2 capsules qid × 10 days. How many capsules should be dispensed?
a. 20 capsules
b. 30 capsules
c. 40 capsules
d. 80 capsules

65. Which of the following DAW codes would be submitted when a generic drug is dispensed or a brand name product that does not have a generic available?
a. DAW 0
b. DAW 1
c. DAW 2
d. DAW 3

66. If a medication is given pc daily, when should it be given?
a. Every morning
b. After meals
c. Before meals
d. At bedtime

67. Which of the following is an example of a schedule-IV medication?
a. Heroin
b. Morphine
c. Lorazepam
d. Hydrocodone with acetaminophen

68. Which of the following pharmacy personnel can counsel a patient on how to use a medication device?
    a. Cashier
    b. Pharmacy technician
    c. Certified pharmacy technician
    d. Pharmacist

69. What is the term for a company that carries a selection of medications, medical devices, and supplies from which a pharmacy may order?
    a. Wholesaler
    b. Manufacturer
    c. Reverse distributor
    d. AWP

70. Lidoderm patch should be removed after how many hours?
    a. 6
    b. 12
    c. 24
    d. 48

71. Who sets standards for medications, biologics, medical devices, and compounded products?
    a. OSHA
    b. TJC
    c. USP
    d. P&T

72. If a pharmacy manager wanted to evaluate insurance reimbursement, what type of report could be run?
    a. Productivity report
    b. Controlled substance use report
    c. Financial report
    d. Medication usage report

73. If a patient has coinsurance that pays 90% of services, and their prescription costs $50, how much will they owe the pharmacy?
    a. $5
    b. $10
    c. $15
    d. $25

74. Which of the following contributes to medication errors?
    a. Poor lighting
    b. Cluttered work space
    c. Loud noise
    d. All of the above

75. In which schedule are medications with a low abuse potential and limited physical and psychological dependence potential?
    a. Schedule II
    b. Schedule V
    c. Schedule I
    d. OTC

76. PCN stands for which of the following?
    a. Patient controlled narcotics
    b. Processor control number
    c. Pharmacy control number
    d. Patient centered number

77. Which of the following is the rapid administration of a small volume of medication into the vein?
    a. IV piggyback
    b. IV push
    c. Epidural
    d. Subcutaneous injection

78. When a prescriber writes qs on a prescription, this is to indicate which of the following?
    a. The pharmacy should calculate a quantity sufficient to be dispensed
    b. The patient should always get a month's supply
    c. The prescriber will call in the amount to be dispensed
    d. The pharmacy should only dispense enough for 1 week

79. Which of the following therapeutic equivalence codes means that the drug is not equivalent?
    a. AB
    b. BX
    c. AN
    d. AA

80. What is the Agency for Healthcare Research and Quality (AHRQ)?
    a. An agency in the Department of Health and Human services
    b. An agency dedicated to improve quality, safety, and efficiency of health care
    c. Both a and b
    d. None of the above

81. What was the purpose of the Food, Drug, and Cosmetic Act of 1938?
    a. Officially defined drugs
    b. Established policies to determine drug safety
    c. Created childproof cap laws
    d. a and c

82. What is a common side effect of SlowFE?
    a. Diarrhea
    b. Constipation
    c. Cough
    d. Dry mouth

83. What is the term for the DEA-regulated process in which all unwanted, recalled, or outdated controlled substances are returned to a distributor for disposal?
    a. Rotating stock
    b. Inventory management
    c. Markup
    d. Reverse distribution

84. Which segment of the NDC code represents the package code?
    a. The first 4 or 5 digits
    b. The second 3 or 4 digits
    c. The third 1 or 2 digits
    d. a and c

85. If a patient has an order to take 2 capsules bid for 5 days, how many capsules should be given for this order?
    a. 10 capsules
    b. 14 capsules
    c. 20 capsules
    d. 28 capsules

86. What does FDA stand for?
    a. Federal Drug Administration
    b. Food and Drug Administration
    c. Food and Dental Agency
    d. Federal Drug Agency

87. Medicare Part C is also known as which of the following?
    a. Medicaid
    b. Prescription drug plan
    c. DME
    d. Medicare Advantage plan

88. Which DEA form is used for the purchase and sale of C-II medications?
    a. Form 41
    b. Form 106
    c. Form 222
    d. Form 224

89. A physician orders a labetalol 100 mg/100 mL infusion. Labetalol is available from the manufacturer as a 5 mg/mL injectable solution. How many milliliters of the solution must be drawn up to compound the requested IV infusion?
    a. 100 mL
    b. 80 mL
    c. 60 mL
    d. 20 mL

90. Which of the following intravenous medications is a high-alert medication?
    e. Heparin
    f. Insulin
    g. Potassium chloride
    h. All of the above

Answers to Practice Exams

MATH REVIEW

1. c: There are 60 mg per grain.

2. b: $\dfrac{1600\ \mu g}{mL} \times \dfrac{1\ mg}{1000\ \mu g} \times 250\ mL = 400\ mg$

3. d: There are 2.2 lb per kg.

4. b: x = 10; l = 50; v = 5. Since the x is first and smaller than the l, it is 50 − 10 + 5 = 45.

5. d: There are 3 teaspoons per tablespoon.

6. d: 30/60

7. d: 0.5

8. b: There are approximately 30 mL per fluid ounce.

9. c: There are 5 mL per teaspoon.

10. c: $\dfrac{1}{100\ g} = \dfrac{X}{30\ g}$

    X = 0.3 g or 300 mg

11. b: Ointments and other solids are expressed in w/w.

12. c: There are approximately 5 mL per dram.

13. c: Electrolytes are typically expressed in milliequivalent.

14. b: Each patch will last 3 days. (72 hours = 3 days); 5 patches will last 15 days (2 weeks = 14 days).

15. b: $\dfrac{1\ g}{100\ mL} = \dfrac{X}{0.2\ mL}$

    X = 0.002 g or 2 mg.

16. c: 2 mg twice daily in each eye for 2 days = 16 mg

    2 mg once daily for 5 days = 20 mg

    20 mg + 16 mg = 36 mg.

17. a: 2.5 mL/0.2 mL per dose = 12 doses.

18. b: No—the patient will need

    0.2 mL twice daily in each eye for 2 days = 1.6 mL

    0.2 mL once daily for 5 days = 2 mL

    2 mL + 1.6 mL = 3.6 mL.

19. d: One drop is approximately 0.05 mL.

20. d: 18/28.

21. d: 0.64.

22. c: 0.5 g = 500 mg. Thus, 250 mg × 2 caps × 4 times per day × 10 days = 80.

23. d: Insulin is expressed in units.

24. b: 120 mg divided by 4 doses is 30 mg.

25. a: There are approximately 480 mL per pint.

26. b: Apothecary is the system using grains and drams.

27. a: x = 10, v = 5. Thus, xxv = 25.

28. a: Injectable solutions are expressed as weight per volume.

29. b: $\dfrac{1\,g}{200\ mL} = \dfrac{X}{60\ mL}$

    X = 0.3 g = 300/20 mg = 15 tabs.

30. b: There are 60 mg per grain.

31. a: There are approximately 30 mL per fluid ounce.

32. b: 14 units × 3 times per day = 42 U/d

    100 U/mL × 3 mL = 300 units

    300/42 units = 7 days.

33. d: Units should not be abbreviated.

34. c: 24/4.

35. c: 6.

36. d: $\dfrac{5\,g}{100\ mL} = \dfrac{X}{30\ mL}$

    X = 1.5 g = 1500 mg.

37. d: °F = °C × (9/5) + 32. Thus, 23 × (9/5) + 32 = 73.4.

38. b: 28 lb/2.2 lb/kg = 13 kg

    13 kg × 0.1 mg/kg = 1.3 mg.

39. b: x = 10; i = 1; v = 5. Since the i is smaller than the v, it is 5 − 1 = 4 + 10 = 14.

40. b: The avoirdupois system uses tablespoon and teaspoon.

41. d: 1000 µg = 1 mg, so 560 µg/1000 µg = 0.56 mg.

42. a: $\dfrac{2\ g}{100\ g} = \dfrac{X}{30\ g}$

    X = 0.6 g.

43. d: 75/6.

44. b: 12.5.

45. d: $\dfrac{1\ g}{100\ mL} = \dfrac{X}{20\ mL}$

    X = 0.2 g or 200 mg.

46. b: There are 60 mg per grain.

47. c: $\dfrac{3200\ \mu g}{mL} \times \dfrac{1\ mg}{1000\ \mu g} \times 250\ mL = 800\ mg$

48. c: There are 2.2 lb/kg.

49. a: x = 10; l = 50. Since the x is first and smaller than the l, it is 50 − 10 = 40.

50. d: There are 5 mL per tablespoon.

51. d: 20/60

52. d: 0.3

53. c: There are approximately 30 mL per fluid ounce.

54. b: There are approximately 5 mL per teaspoon. 10/5 mL = 2 teaspoons.

55. c: $\dfrac{1\ g}{100\ g} = \dfrac{X}{60\ g}$

    X = 0.6 g or 600 mg.

56. b: Ointment is a solid in a solid, thus expressed as weight/weight or w/w.

57. d: There are approximately 5 mL per dram.

58. c: Potassium chloride is expressed in milliequivalent.

59. b: Each patch will last 3 days. (72 hours = 3 days); 3 patches will last 9 days (1 week = 7 days).

60. b: $\dfrac{1\,g}{100\,mL} = \dfrac{X}{0.1\,mL}$

X = 0.001 g or 1 mg.

61. d: Twice daily × 2 days = 4 doses, then once daily × 7 days = 7 doses; thus 4 + 7 = 11 × 1 mg = 11 mg total treatment course.

62. c: $\dfrac{1\,dose}{0.1\,mL} = \dfrac{X\,doses}{2.5\,mL}$

x = 25 doses.

63. a: Yes, the patient needs 11 doses and the bottle contains 25 doses.

64. b: Each drop contains 0.05 mL. So, 0.1 mL/0.05 = 2 drops.

65. d: 18/35.

66. d: 0.51.

67. b: 0.5 g = 500 mg. Thus, 250 mg × 2 caps × 3 times per day × 7 days = 42.

68. d: Insulin is expressed in units.

69. b: 180 mg divided by 4 doses = 45 mg per dose.

70. a: There are approximately 480 mL per pint.

71. b: Drams are used in the apothecary system.

72. c: x = 10; l = 50. Since the x is first and smaller than the l, it is 50 − 10 = 40.

73. a: Solutions can be expressed as w/v percentage.

74. c: $\dfrac{1\,g}{200\,mL} = \dfrac{X}{120\,mL}$

X = 0.6 g = 600/20 mg = 30 tabs.

75. d: There are 60 mg per grain. iv = 4.

76. a: There are 30 mL per fluid ounce.

77. b: 30 units × 1 time per day = 30 U/d
100 U/mL × 3 mL = 300 units
300/30 units = 10 days.

78. d: Units should not be abbreviated.

79. c: 12/4.

80. b: 3.

81. b: $\dfrac{5\text{ g}}{100\text{ mL}} = \dfrac{X}{10\text{ mL}}$

   $X = 0.5\text{ g} = 500\text{ mg}.$

82. c: $°F = °C \times (9/5) + 32.$ Thus, $-14 \times (9/5) + 32 = 7.$

83. b: $14\text{ lb}/2.2\text{ lb/kg} = 6\text{ kg}$

   $6\text{ kg} \times 0.1\text{ mg/kg} = 0.6\text{ mg}.$

84. c: $x = 10; v = 5; i = 1.$ So, $xxviii = 10 + 10 + 5 + 1 + 1 + 1 = 28.$

85. b: The avoirdupois system uses tablespoon and teaspoon.

86. d: $\dfrac{850\ \mu g}{X} = \dfrac{1000\ \mu g}{1\text{ mg}}$

   $X = 0.85\text{ mg}.$

87. a: $\dfrac{2}{100\text{ g}} = \dfrac{X}{15\text{ g}}$

   $X = 0.3\text{ g}.$

88. d: 75/8.

89. b: 9.4.

90. d: $\dfrac{4\text{ g}}{100\text{ mL}} = \dfrac{X}{20\text{ mL}}$

   $X = 0.8\text{ g} = 800\text{ mg}.$

91. b: $1\text{ gr} = 60\text{ mg}.$ Thus $1/2\text{ gr} = 30\text{ mg}.$

92. c: $\dfrac{1600\ \mu g}{\text{mL}} \times \dfrac{1\text{ mg}}{1000\ \mu g} \times 500\text{ mL} = 800\text{ mg}$

93. c: $24\text{ kg} \times 2.2\text{ lb/kg} = 52.8\text{ lb}.$

94. b: $x = 10; v = 5; i = 1.$ So, $xvii = 10 + 5 + 1 + 1 = 17.$

95. b: There are 3 teaspoons (tsp) per tablespoon (tbsp).

96. d: 14/60.

97. d: 0.2.

98. c: There are 16 fl oz in 1 pt.

99. d: A teaspoon contains approximately 5 mL. Most household teaspoons do not have calibrations to measure portions of a teaspoon.

100. c: $\dfrac{1}{100\ g} = \dfrac{X}{60\ g}$

     X = 0.6 g = 600 mg.

101. b: Solids are expressed as w/w percentage.

102. d: There are 5 mL per dram. So, 5 × 13 = 65.

103. c: Sodium bicarbonate is an electrolyte expressed in milliequivalent.

104. b: Each patch will last 3 days. (72 hours = 3 days); 10 patches will last 28 days (4 weeks = 28 days).

105. b: $\dfrac{1\ g}{100\ mL} = \dfrac{X}{0.1\ mL}$

     X = 0.001 g or 1 mg.

106. d: Every 4 hours × 2 days = 12 doses × 1 mg/dose = 12 mg.

107. c: $\dfrac{1\ dose}{0.1\ mL} = \dfrac{X\ doses}{5\ mL}$

     X = 50 doses.

108. a: Yes, the patient needs 12 doses and the bottle contains 50 doses.

109. b: Each drop contains 0.05 mL. So, 0.1 mL/0.05 = 2 drops.

110. b: 27/35.

111. d: 0.77.

112. b: 0.5 g = 500 mg. Thus, 250 mg × 2 capsules × 4 times per day × 7 days = 56.

113. b: Medications are most commonly expressed in milligram.

114. c: 60 mg divided by 3 doses is 20 mg.

115. c: There are approximately 480 mL per pint. 480/15 mL = 32.

116. b: Grains are a part of the apothecary system.

117. a: x = 10, v = 5, i = 1; 10 + (5 − 1) = 14. Since the i is before and smaller than the v, it is 5 − 1 = 4.

118. a: Solutions are expressed as w/v or v/v.

119. b: $\dfrac{1\ g}{400\ mL} = \dfrac{X}{120\ mL}$

     X = 0.3 g = 300/20 mg = 15 tabs.

120. c: 1 gr = 60 mg.

121. c: There are 30 mL per fluid ounce.

122. b: 12 units × 2 times per day = 24 U/d
100 U/mL × 3 mL = 300 units
300/24 units = 12 days.

123. d: Units should not be abbreviated.

124. c: 28/4.

125. b: 7.

126. b: $\dfrac{2.5\ g}{100\ mL} = \dfrac{X}{20\ mL}$
X = 0.5 g = 500 mg.

127. d: °F = °C × (9/5) + 32. Thus, 35 × (9/5) + 32 = 95.

128. a: 30 lb/2.2 lb/kg = 13.6 kg × 5 mg/kg = 68 mg.

129. c: l = 50, x = 10; Thus, 50 + 10 = 60.

130. b: Teaspoons are used in the avoirdupois system.

131. d: $\dfrac{1250\ \mu g}{X} = \dfrac{1000\ \mu g}{1\ mg}$
X = 1.25 mg.

132. b: $\dfrac{2}{100\ g} = \dfrac{X}{60\ g}$
X = 1.2 g.

133. d: 105/8.

134. b: 13.1.

135. c: $\dfrac{8\ g}{100\ mL} = \dfrac{X}{5\ mL}$
X = 0.4 g = 400 mg.

ONE

1. d: Only a pharmacist may recommend an OTC medication to a patient.

2. a: $\dfrac{10\ \mu g}{h} \times \dfrac{mL}{50\ \mu g} = 0.2\ mL/h$

3. d: Independent checks, tall-man lettering, and shelf separators help decrease medication errors.

4. d: The Institute of Safe Medication Practices (ISMP) only focuses on medication safety.

5. c: Grapefruit juice contains a compound not found in other citrus juices that increased the absorption of some medications. The increased absorption can enhance the effects and increase the risk of adverse effects.

6. d: Codeine with acetaminophen is a schedule-III medication because of its moderate-to-low abuse potential and acceptable medical use.

7. a: A class I recall is when a drug company is required to remove their medication from market due to the risk of death.

8. c: qod means every other day.

9. d: A valid prescription requires the date of issue, name and address of the practitioner, and the name of the patient.

10. a: 1 tsp qid = 1 × 5 mL × 4 daily = 20 mL.

11. c: The most common side effects of Augmentin (amoxicillin/clavulanate) are diarrhea, allergic reaction, and rash.

12. c: Another term for TPN is hyperalimentation.

13. b: Occupational Safety and Health Administration (OSHA) requires material safety data sheets.

14. c: Schedule-III and -IV medications can only be refilled up to 5 times within 6 months.

15. d: Morphine, heparin, potassium chloride, warfarin, hydromorphone, and insulin are all high-alert medications.

16. c: Ropinirole (Requip) has been associated with compulsive gambling.

17. d: Drugs are intended to diagnosis, prevent, or treat a disease.

18. c: Tetracycline can become toxic after its expiration date.

19. b: A formulary is a list of approved medications on an insurance plan.

20. c: Fingerprints, face recognition, and DNA are all biometric identifiers.

21. b: pc = after meals, ac = before meals, bid = twice daily, qd = once daily.

22. b: Fentanyl transdermal is in DEA class II.

23. c: The patient profile does not contain the patient's social security number.

24. a: The NDC is a 10-digit product identifying code used for all drugs marketed in the United States.

25. a: Scored tablets have a line or crevice through the center which makes dividing the tablet in half easier and more accurate.

26. b: The NDC consists of the labeler code (4 or 5 digits), the product code (3 or 4 digits), and the package code (1 or 2 digits).

27. d: The medication administration record (MAR) is a record of each time a medication is administered to a patient; it also shows what time the dose was given and who administered the dose.

28. b: Clindamycin may be taken orally or applied topically for acne.

29. b: Electronic health records are costly investments.

30. a: An invoice is a bill of sale for products ordered.

31. c: Under workers' compensation insurance, the patient provides the pharmacy or other provider with the workers' compensation information and the patient is not billed any fees for services.

32. a: Acyclovir (Zovirax) is available as an injection formulation.

33. d: Certain medications are permitted to be dispensed with a nonchildproof lid, such as oral contraceptives, inhalation aerosols, and sublingual nitroglycerin. Nitroglycerin should always be dispensed with an easy off cap so that it is easily accessible during emergencies.

34. b: DEA 106 is used to document loss or theft of C-II medications.

35. b: Amoxicillin prescribed for a patient on Augmentin would be an example of a drug-drug interaction.

36. a: Any patient eligible for Part A has the option of enrolling in Medicare Part B.

37. b: An effective date is the date when coverage is effective for a patient.

38. b: Lisinopril which is an angiotensin-converting enzyme inhibitor (ACEI) can increase potassium.

39. c: The Institute for Safe Medication Practices is devoted entirely to medication error prevention.

40. b: Health Insurance Portability and Accountability Act (HIPAA) protects protected health information (PHI).

41. d: A patient's insurance card does not contain contracted pricing structure information.

42. c: The middle (green) copy of a DEA Form 222 is retained by the DEA.

43. d: 25 gauge is the smallest needle.

44. d: Preprinted order sets can help prevent illegible handwriting errors.

45. b: The pharmacy's name and address, date when prescription was filled, and prescription number are all required on the pharmacy label.

46. c: A deductible must be paid before benefits will kick in.

47. c: Unit-of-use packaging is provided by the manufacturer in the most commonly dispensed unit so the pharmacy only has to label the drug and not count any individual drugs.

48. b: Metformin (Glucophage, Fortamet, Glucophage, Glumetza, Riomet) is contraindicated in renal failure.

49. d: 1 PO qid = 1 capsule 4 times daily = 4 capsules per day for 10 days = 4 × 10 = 40 total capsules.

50. d: A solvent is the liquid in which the solute is dissolved.

51. b: The temperature range for storage of refrigerated products is 2 to 8°C.

52. a: Protonix-prevacid would be a therapeutic substitution since they are in the same therapeutic class.

53. c: DAW 2 is the code when a prescriber indicates generic is permitted, but the patient requests brand name product.

54. a: The Pure Food and Drug Act passed in 1906.

55. a: Adderall XR is a DEA class II and can have no refills.

56. d: At a minimum medication labels must contain the name, address, and phone number of the pharmacy, name of the patient, and date of dispensing.

57. a: 66.6 g of 1% and 53.4 g of 10%.

58. a: U should be spelled out as units.

59. d: *Patient Handout Information References* include patient counseling information.

60. c: gtt = drop, AU = both ears, qd = once daily.

61. a: Oral preparations have a beyond-use date of no greater than 14 days.

62. c: A common side effect of Zyprexa (olanzapine) is weight gain.

63. d: The "Combat Methamphetamine Epidemic Act" restricts the sale of pseudoephedrine.

64. a: A technician can refill prescriptions if a patient has already filled a prescription at that location.

65. b: Per the DEA, records of receipt for C-III, C-IV, and C-V drugs must be kept on file for 2 years.

66. d: Liver failure is contraindicated in medications if dosage is not adjusted.

67. a: Pediatric patients are at the highest risk for a calculation error due to their small size.

68. b: The Food and Drug Administration (FDA) issues a medication recall.

69. c: 1 + 3 + 5 = 9, 2 + 4 + 6 = 12 × 2 = 24 + 9 = 33. The letter A is a letter that is used for physicians and the physician's last name begins with the letter S.

70. c: Guaifenesin is an expectorant.

71. c: The Joint Commission (TJC) accredits hospitals.

72. c: The *Orange Book* is used to obtain equivalency information.

73. b: Intravenous injection has the fastest onset of action.

74. c: A drug-disease alert would be for a pregnant patient being prescribed lisinopril.

75. a: Medications typically expire 1 to 5 years after manufacturing.

76. d: A is the abbreviation for ear, S is the abbreviation for left, AS is the abbreviation for left ear.

77. d: The NDC number can be used to verify the medication pulled with what drug is on the label to be filled.

78. b: The Controlled Substances Act defined drug schedules.

79. d: Mortar and pestles are used to triturate solid ingredients in nonsterile compounding.

80. a: OBRA '90 required pharmacists to perform a prospective drug utilization review on all prescriptions.

81. c: A formulary is a list of medications that are approved by the P&T Committee.

82. b: E-prescribing is preferred for prescription generation.

83. d: The inscription is the part of the prescription that contains the name and strength of the medication and the amount prescribed.

84. c: When the actual day is listed, that is the day it expires.

85. a: STAT means immediately; so a STAT order would be for a medication needed immediately.

86. b: A dependent is generally a spouse or child(ren) of the subscriber.

87. a: The Poison Control Center number is 1-800-222-1222.

88. c: The United States Pharmacopeia (USP) sets standards for medications, biologics, medical devices, and compounded products.

89. c: $2 + 8 + 8 = 18, 5 + 3 + 2 = 10 \times 2 = 20 + 18 = 38$.

90. a: 20 g of 2% and 40 g of 5%.

TWO

1. c: The Controlled Substance Ordering System (CSOS) is the DEA electronic program used for ordering C-II medications.

2. d: Trailing zeros should be avoided.

3. d: The National Drug Code (NDC) consists of the labeler code (4 or 5 digits), the product code (3 or 4 digits), and the package code (1 or 2 digits).

4. c: A lot number is a unique identifying code assigned to each batch of medication produced at a given time.

5. b: $\dfrac{X \text{ mg}}{2.5 \text{ mL}} = \dfrac{5 \text{ mL}}{20 \text{ mg}}$

$X = 10$ mL

6. a: Health Maintenance Organizations (HMOs) require the designation of a primary care physician (PCP).

7. c: Compounding is the act of reconstituting or otherwise preparing a medication into a dosage form usable by a patient.

8. b: Pharmacy automation includes robots, barcode scanners, and tabletop tablet counters.

9. a: qd should be spelled out as daily or once daily.

10. d: Pharmacy technicians have many responsibilities in a retail pharmacy setting including entering prescriptions into the computer, updating the patient profile, and counting medications on a counting tray.

11. c: Rotating stock is a process in which products with the shortest expiration dates are moved to the front of the shelf when stocking.

12. b: Tamiflu (oseltamivir) is indicated for the treatment of influenza.

13. c: The Joint Commission (TJC) accredits hospitals.

14. a: A class I recall is when a drug company is required to remove their medication from market due to the risk of death.

15. a: 1 tablet PO qid = 1 tablet· × 4 times = 4 daily, 60 total tablets = 60/4 = 15 days.

16. a: USP stands for United States Pharmacopeia.

17. d: CDSS over- or underutilization will help identify patient adherence.

18. c: When an expiration date lists only month and year, the product expires on the last day of the listed month.

19. a: The Food and Drug Administration (FDA) oversees Medwatch.

20. b: At least 2 unique patient identifiers should be used to verify a patient's identity.

21. a: An expense paid by the member is known as an out-of-pocket expense. Insurance companies generally limit this to a designated maximum amount.

22. b: The DEA Form 222 is a triplicate form designed specifically for the sale of C-II medications.

23. d: The inscription is the part of the prescription that contains the name and strength of the medication and the amount prescribed.

24. c: Computerized physician order entry (CPOE) can decrease handwriting errors.

25. a: The temperature range for the storage for frozen products is −20 to −10°C.

26. a: Fluconazole is indicated for the treatment of candidiasis (fungal) infections.

27. a: *Drug Facts and Comparisons* is a general pharmacy reference that would contain storage requirements of a medication.

28. d: 1 capsule tid for 20 days = 1 capsule· × 3 times × 20 days = 60 capsules.

29. c: A solute is a solid ingredient dissolved in a liquid.

30. b: Insulin has a narrow therapeutic range and is a high-alert medication.

31. d: ISMP is dedicated solely to medication error prevention.

32. c: The DEA enforces the controlled substance laws of the United States.

33. c: Medications that must be protected from light should be stored in their original container until use.

34. a: Pediatric patients are at the highest risk for a calculation error due to their small size.

35. b: Patient's allergy information should be reviewed frequently with patients.

36. a: Celebrex (celecoxib) is a COX-2 selective anti-inflammatory drug.

37. b: Medicare Part B provides coverage for patients eligible for Medicare for durable medical equipment (DME), outpatient services from hospitals, and physician services.

38. b: Buprenorphine is a schedule-III medication.

39. c: Risk management is identifying, analyzing, assessing, and controlling risk.

40. b: Class II recalls include medications that contain less active ingredient than intended.

41. b: tid is the sig code for 3 times daily.

42. c: The Institute of Safe Medication Practices is devoted entirely to medication error prevention.

43. c: Drug dosage information can be found in a *General Drug Information Reference*.

44. c: Sumatriptan (Imitrex) is indicated for the treatment of migraine.

45. a: The Pure Food and Drug Act of 1906 required that drugs not be mislabeled.

46. c: Parenteral products are medications administered by any route other than oral.

47. d: Pravachol (pravastatin) should be taken prior to going to bed.

48. d: Address, phone number, and allergies should be on the patient profile.

49. a: Insulin and heparin are high-alert medications.

50. d: Sentinel events are reported to The Joint Commission (TJC).

51. b: O is the abbreviation for eye, U is the abbreviation for both, and OU is the abbreviation for both eyes.

52. b: The first letter of the hospital's name is the second letter, and each resident is also given a suffix code to attach to the end to identify the resident.

53. b: Coordination of benefits occurs if a patient has multiple insurance providers, one is selected as primary and is billed first. The second insurance company is not billed unless there are still unpaid claims remaining, then they are billed only the remainder of the costs so that there is not a duplication of payment.

54. a: The primary indication of ACEIs is hypertension.

55. d: Only a pharmacist can counsel a patient on how to use a fluticasone inhaler.

56. d: Drugs are intended to prevent, treat, and diagnose disease. Any product that claims to do one of those things is considered a drug.

57. d: The NDC number can be used to verify the medication pulled with what drug is on the label to be filled.

58. a: Oral preparations have a beyond-use date of no greater than 14 days.

59. b: E-prescribing is preferred for prescription generation.

60. b: C-II medications cannot be refilled.

61. c: The Pharmacy and Therapeutics (P&T) Committee manages the formulary system.

62. d: CDSS may provide drug-allergy, therapeutic duplication, and pharmacokinetic monitoring.

63. c: A premium is the cost of the insurance coverage that a patient must pay to be eligible for services and is usually deducted from the card member's paycheck or paid monthly by the member.

64. c: Nitrates should not be given with sildenafil (Viagra, Revatio) which are phosphodiesterase-5 enzyme inhibitors due to decreasing blood pressure.

65. d: A scheduled order is a type of medication order given at the same time every day.

66. b: $2 + 4 + 5 = 11$, $1 + 8 + 5 = 14 \times 2 = 28 + 11 = 39$.

67. a: Proventil (albuterol) is a short-acting β_2 agonist.

68. c: Fingerprints, face recognition, and DNA are all biometric identifiers.

69. b: There are 5 schedules of medications defined by the Controlled Substances Act.

70. d: 1 PO bid = 1 twice daily = 2 tablets per day for 1 month = $2 \times 30 = 60$ total tablets.

71. b: A member would have a person code of 1, a spouse would be 2, and then a child could be 3 or 4.

72. a: A drug-laboratory alert would be for an elevated INR for a patient on warfarin.

73. c: Reverse distribution is the process in which unused or expired medications are returned to the manufacturer.

74. a: 2 tbsp = 30 mL. tid = 3 times daily. = 30 × 3 = 90 mL daily, dispense 450 mL = 450/90 = 5 total days.

75. d: Miralax (polyethylene glycol) is indicated for constipation.

76. b: $\dfrac{40\ mg}{mL} = \dfrac{70\ mg}{X}$

$X = 1.75\ mL$

77. a: Medications with a high-abuse potential and with acceptable uses are considered as schedule II.

78. b: q8h = every 8 hours, 24 hours/8 = 3 times daily.

79. a: Bisphosphonates should be taken 30 minutes prior to the first food of the day.

80. b: Always use the smallest size available that will hold the volume required.

81. b: Morphine is considered as a schedule-II medication because it has a high abuse potential and with acceptable use.

82. a: Medicare Part D provides coverage for prescription drugs; Medicare Part B provides coverage for DME.

83. c: $\dfrac{X}{4\ mL} = \dfrac{200\ mg}{5\ mL}$

$X = 160\ mg$

84. c: A buccal tablet would be placed between the cheek and gums.

85. c: An offer to counsel a patient must be made on dispensing the finished product to the patient.

86. b: Intravenous injection has the fastest onset of action.

87. a: Oral contraceptives do not require child-resistant packaging.

88. d: NTG stands for nitroglycerin, NS stands for normal saline, mL stands for milliliter, and $FeSO_4$ stands for ferrous sulfate.

89. b: USP Chapter 797 defines guidelines for sterile compounding.

90. d: First convert to metric units: 5 fl oz = 5 × 30 mL = 150 mL, 1-tsp dose = 5 mL. 150/5 mL = 30 doses.

THREE

1. a: Form 41 is used to document the destruction of controlled substances.

2. d: Patient Handout Information References include patient counseling information.

3. b: The National Drug Code (NDC) is a unique, 3-segment number which identifies drug products.

4. c: The material safety data sheet (MSDS) contains instructions for proper storage, handling, and containment procedures for a hazardous substance.

5. d: 3 + 8 + 2 = 13, 1 + 8 + 5 = 14 × 2 = 28 + 13 = 41.

6. c: Point-of-service (POS) is a type of plan which combines qualities of both HMO and PPO. Patients do not make a choice about type of service until it is needed.

7. a: Always use leading zeros when writing numbers less than 1.

8. a: A prescription is an order written for outpatient purposes by a licensed prescriber.

9. a: Distributor is another term for a wholesaler.

10. c: A solute is a solid ingredient dissolved in a liquid.

11. c: An elevation of uric acid can lead to gout.

12. a: qd should be spelled out as daily or once daily.

13. a: DEA refers to Drug Enforcement Administration.

14. a: The benefit of having a prime vendor is having discounts.

15. c: Anticholinergic drugs cause dry eyes, constipation, and dry mouth.

16. b: The Department of Health and Human Services created patient safety organizations.

17. a: The superscription is the Rx symbol.

18. d: All health care professionals may be responsible for a medication error.

19. d: The bottom (blue) copy of a DEA Form 222 is retained by the pharmacy.

20. b: Coinsurance differs from a copayment in that it requires patients to pay a percentage of the cost of services instead of a flat fee.

21. c: Telepharmacy allows a pharmacist to counsel a patient in a different location.

22. a: The Pure Food and Drug Act passed in 1906.

23. a: qs means quantity sufficient to fill the order.

24. b: Subcutaneous medications are injected directly into the fatty layer below the skin's surface.

25. c: The patient profile does not contain the patient's social security number.

26. b: Barcode technology helps eliminate errors during medication administration to hospital patients.

27. b: The temperature range for storage of refrigerated products is 2 to 8°C.

28. c: Medicare Part C was known as the Medicare + Choice plan.

29. a: The NDC consists of the labeler code (4 or 5 digits), the product code (3 or 4 digits), and the package code (1 or 2 digits).

30. c: The generic name of Adipex-P is phentermine.

31. a: An inventory report would be used to identify a product's availability.

32. d: gtt stands for drop.

33. d: Preprinted order sets can help prevent illegible handwriting errors.

34. c: Medications with a low abuse potential and acceptable medical use are considered as schedule IV.

35. d: Sterile powders for injection and powders for reconstitution must be protected from humidity. Humid air contains water that may leach into the product and limit its stability.

36. d: Continuous quality improvement ensures that programs are intentionally improving service and increasing positive outcomes.

37. c: Lotrisone (betamethasone/clotrimazole) is used to treat fungal infections.

38. d: A social security number is not needed to process a patient's insurance claim from the pharmacy, but a patient's birthdate, member ID number, and medication prescribed *are* necessary to process a claim.

39. d: A patient's insurance card does not contain contracted pricing structure information.

40. c: Class III recalls include products with minor container defects.

41. b: Aseptic technique dictates compounding should occur 6 in from the front and sides of the laminar flow hood.

42. d: Codeine with acetaminophen is a schedule-III medication because of its moderate-to-low abuse potential and acceptable medical use.

43. b: Grain—The use of the apothecary system should be minimized.

44. b: 1 tablet tid ac and hs = 1×4 times daily $\times 30$ days = 120 tablets.

45. b: The pharmacy's name and address, date when prescription was filled, and prescription number are all required on the pharmacy label.

46. a: The most common adverse effect of Zithromax (azithromycin) is gastrointestinal (GI) toxicity.

47. b: The dispense as written (DAW) code is used for third parties to determine if the proper brand or generic medication was used to fill the prescription.

48. c: A class III recall is there when exposure to a product is not likely to cause adverse health consequences.

49. a: Pediatric patients are at the highest risk for a calculation error due to their small size.

50. a: Amoxicillin prescribed for a penicillin-allergic patient is an example of a drug-allergy interaction.

51. c: $\dfrac{X \text{ tablets}}{1000 \text{ mg}} = \dfrac{1 \text{ tablet}}{500 \text{ mg}}$

    $X = 2$ tablets

52. b: The Poison Prevention Act created child-resistant container use.

53. b: The Institute for Safe Medication Practices is devoted entirely to medication error prevention.

54. a: Products prepared at a patient's bedside in an emergent situation are for immediate use only.

55. c: The *Orange Book* is used to obtain equivalency information.

56. d: Relafen (nabumetone) is an nonsteroidal anti-inflammatory drug (NSAID) and may be refilled for 12 months.

57. b: 1 tid × 15 days = 1 tablet × 3 times × 15 days = 45 tablets.

58. d: Since cholestyramine powder is in a canister it does not require a child-resistant packaging.

59. c: RCA occurs *after* an error has occurred.

60. d: Morphine, heparin, potassium chloride, warfarin, hydromorphone, and insulin are all high-alert medications.

61. c: Only insulin may be used to treat type 1 diabetes.

62. c: Unit-of-use packaging is provided by the manufacturer in the most commonly dispensed unit so the pharmacy only has to label the drug and not count any individual drugs.

63. b: Occupational Safety and Health Administration (OSHA) requires material safety data sheets.

64. c: HEPA filters are used in laminar flow hoods and clean rooms to ensure 99.97% removal of air particles.

65. c: Tablet computers are portable.

66. d: A formulary is a list of approved drugs.

67. d: Only a pharmacist can counsel a patient on how to use an insulin pen.

68. d: The "Combat Methamphetamine Epidemic Act" restricts the sale of pseudoephedrine.

69. b: Days supply is the days calculated a medication should last if it is taken correctly.

70. a: USP Chapter 795 defines guidelines for nonsterile compounding.

71. c: 1 tsp tid for 30 days = 5 mL × 3 daily × 30 = 450 mL.

72. c: Neurontin (gabapentin), Keppra (levetiracetam), and Topamax (topiramate) are all indicated to treat seizures.

73. c: A drug-disease alert would be for a pregnant patient being prescribed lisinopril.

74. c: Buspirone (Buspar) is indicated for the treatment of anxiety.

75. a: 1 PO qid = 1 capsule 4 times daily = 4 capsules per day, dispense total 40 = 40/4 = 10 total days.

76. c: DEA Form 106 is used to document the theft or loss of C-II medications.

77. b: Oral contraceptives require a package insert to be dispensed to the patient every time.

78. d: The RxBin, RxGroup, and member's ID number are all required to submit an insurance claim properly.

79. c: gtt = drop, AU = both ears, qd = once daily.

80. a: Pregnant women should not handle Avodart (dutasteride); it is of category X.

81. c: 1 tablet tid for 14 days = 1 tablet × 3 daily × 14 days = 42 tablets.

82. b: $\dfrac{10 \text{ mg}}{5 \text{ mL}} = \dfrac{8 \text{ mg}}{X}$

$X = 4 \text{ mL}$

83. b: A neonate should not be given elixir due to the high alcohol content.

84. a: The "Combat Methamphetamine Epidemic Act" restricts the sale of ephedrine and pseudoephedrine to 9 g every 30 days.

85. c: Add up the total number of tablets taken per day and multiply this by 30: 1 breakfast + 2 lunch + 1 dinner + 1 bedtime = 5 tablets per day × 30 days = 150 tablets total.

86. a: A graduate is a cylindrical or conical-shaped container with clearly defined measurement calibrations used in nonsterile compounding.

87. b: Patients should be instructed to rinse out their mouth after using Flovent (fluticasone) inhalers in order to prevent oral thrush.

88. d: The first letter of the hospital's name is the second letter and each resident is also given a suffix code to attach to the end to identify the resident.

89. a: Medicare Part C is a Medicare plan in which patients must be enrolled in both Medicare Parts A and B to receive Part C benefits through a separate provider.

90. d: PV means per vagina or vaginally.

FOUR

1. b: Medications that are used frequently ("fast movers") should have large PAR levels and more medication should be stocked.

2. b: Computerized physician order entry (CPOE) can decrease handwriting errors.

3. b: National Drug Code (NDC) is the unique 3-segment number which identifies a drug product.

4. a: Legend drugs require prescriptions whereas over-the-counter (OTC) medications can be obtained without a prescription.

5. d: A meniscus is the curve in the surface of a liquid that occurs around the edge of a container due to surface tension.

6. c: Metronidazole should not be taken with alcohol as it can cause a disulfiram reaction.

7. d: Drug information resources are written and electronic references, and available for patients and pharmacists.

8. d: $1 + 3 + 5 = 9$, $3 + 9 + 7 = 19 \times 2 = 38 + 9 = 47$.

9. c: The middle (green) copy of a DEA Form 222 is retained by the Drug Enforcement Administration (DEA).

10. d: Patients must pay a premium to have insurance coverage.

11. a: Trailing zeros should be avoided.

12. a: Tendon rupture is a rare, but serious complication of quinolones.

13. d: Clinical information systems may include electronic orders, medication administration records, and patient information.

14. b: DAW is dispensed as written which is what a prescriber would indicate if he or she wanted the patient to be given the brand name medication.

15. a: The first letter of the hospital's name is the second letter and each resident is also given a suffix code to attach to the end to identify the resident.

16. a: The controlled room temperature range is 15 to 30°C.

17. a: U should be spelled out as units.

18. b: PRN means as needed.

19. c: A deductible must be paid before benefits will kick in.

20. b: Humidity decreases the stability of powders for reconstitution. Humid air contains water that may leach into the product and limit its stability.

21. c: The Agency for Healthcare Research and Quality (AHRQ) is in the Department of Health and Human Services and dedicated to improve quality, safety, and efficiency of health care.

22. b: A monitor is an output device, while a mouse, USB, and light pen can all input information into a computer.

23. b: IV piggybacks are a small volume of medication, typically less than 250 mL, which is infused through the same lines as a primary IV fluid.

24. a: Methadone causes constipation, sedation, and miosis (pupil constriction).

25. c: Medications, medical equipment, devices, and medical supplies are regulated by the Food and Drug Administration (FDA).

26. d: All health care professionals may be responsible for a medication error.

27. b: MDI stands for metered-dose inhaler.

28. d: Tylenol #4 contains 60 mg of codeine.

29. c: Recalled medications should be stored segregated from normal stock.

30. c: Medicare Part C is also known as Medicare Advantage plan; patients must be enrolled in both Medicare Parts A and B to receive Part C benefits through a separate provider.

31. c: Medication doses given to patients are recorded on the medication administration record (MAR).

32. c: Barcode technology helps eliminate errors during medication administration to hospital patients.

33. a: Wholesalers are licensed by the State Board of Pharmacy.

34. d: A stock bottle of medication has a label which contains the lot number and expiration date of the medication, as well as a bar code.

35. a: Horizontal flow hoods should be cleaned with isopropyl alcohol in the direction of clean air flow, from back to front.

36. a: Lotensin (benazepril) which is an angiotensin-converting enzyme (ACE) inhibitor is contraindicated in pregnancy.

37. d: CPOE stands for computer physician order entry; a physician can enter orders directly into the hospital system.

38. c: Individual State Boards of Pharmacy are in charge of licensing pharmacists.

39. c: The Health Insurance Portability and Accountability Act (HIPAA) sets standards for sharing patient information.

40. d: Computerized physician order entry can decrease handwriting errors.

41. a: *State Law Book* will contain information regarding recordkeeping requirements for prescriptions.

42. b: Propranolol may be used for migraine prophylaxis.

43. b:
$$\frac{X\,mL}{3\,mg} = \frac{5\,mL}{2\,mg}$$
$$X = 7.5\,mL$$
$$5\,mL = 1\,tsp$$
$$7.5\,mL/5\,mL = 1.5\,tsp$$

44. b: TPNs are medium-risk sterile products, which have a beyond-use date of 30 hours.

45. a: Buprenorphine is a schedule-III medication.

46. b: 1/200 grain—The use of the apothecary system should be minimized.

47. c: Unit doses are used in the hospital and are medications that have been prepackaged for a single dose administration.

48. b: In sterile compound, infection control steps include removing all personal outer garments, cosmetics, and putting on hair cover.

49. b: A mainframe is used to house and process large amounts of data.

50. c: A pharmacy benefit manager (PBM) is a third party administrator of prescription drug programs; they also process and pay for the drug claims and maintain the formulary for each plan.

51. c: 2 tsp = 10 mL, bid = twice daily, 10 × 2 = 20 mL daily for 10 days, 10 × 20 = 200 total mL.

52. a: Diuretics can cause a decrease in electrolytes.

53. a: Infants are at the highest risk for a calculation error due to their small size.

54. c: A patient's insurance card does not contain diagnosis information.

55. d: 1 patch per week, assume 4 weeks in 1 month = 4 patches.

56. a: The "Combat Methamphetamine Epidemic Act" restricts the sale of ephedrine and pseudoephedrine to 9 g every 30 days.

57. d: 1 tsp = 5 mL tid = 3 times daily = 5 × 3 = 15 mL daily × 10 days = 150 mL.

58. c: Methimazole (Tapazole) is indicated for the treatment of hyperthyroidism.

59. c: Albuterol HFA inhalers do not require child-resistant packaging.

60. a: MARs are permanent and legal records of medication administration.

61. a: The Institute of Safe Medication Practices (ISMP) is devoted entirely to medication error prevention.

62. a:
$$1 = \text{dose} = 2 \text{ tsp} = 5 \text{ mL} \times 2 = 10 \text{ mL}$$
$$\frac{X \text{ mg}}{10 \text{ mL}} = \frac{4 \text{ mg}}{5 \text{ mL}}$$
$$X = 8 \text{ mg}$$

63. c: Atypical antipsychotics can increase blood sugar.

64. d: 2 qid = 2 four times daily × 10 days = 2 capsules × 4 × 10 days = 80 capsules total.

65. a: DAW 0 is the default code used when dispensing a generic drug or when dispensing a brand name product that does not have a generic available.

66. b: ac means before meals, pc means after meals.

67. c: Lorazepam is a schedule-IV medication because it has low abuse potential and acceptable medical use.

68. d: Only a pharmacist can counsel a patient on how to use a medication device.

69. a: A wholesaler, or distributor, is a company that carries a selection of medications, medical devices, and supplies.

70. b: A Lidoderm (lidocaine) patch should be removed after 12 hours.

71. c: The United States Pharmacopeia (USP) sets standards for medications, biologics, medical devices, and compounded products.

72. c: Financial reports evaluate insurance reimbursement.

73. a: The patient's insurance will pay 90%, so 90% of 50 = (0.9) × (50) = 45. This is the amount the insurance will pay. To determine the amount the patient must pay, subtract this amount from the total billed: $50 – $45 = $5. The patient owes the pharmacy $5.

74. d: Poor lighting, cluttered work space, and loud noise can contribute to medication errors.

75. b: Medications with a low abuse potential and limited physical and psychological dependence potential are considered as schedule V.

76. b: The PCN, or processor control number, helps direct the electronic claim to the proper location.

77. b: IV push is the rapid administration of a small volume of medication into the vein.

78. a: qs means pharmacy determines a sufficient quantity to dispense to fill the patient's prescription.

79. b: BX—The "B" code means that drug is not therapeutically equivalent to the reference drug.

80. c: The AHRQ is in the Department of Health and Human Services and dedicated to improve quality, safety, and efficiency of health care.

81. d: The Food, Drug, and Cosmetic Act of 1938 officially defined drugs and created childproof cap laws.

82. b: The most common side effect of SlowFE (ferrous sulfate) is constipation.

83. d: Reverse distribution is the term for the DEA-regulated process in which all unwanted, recalled, or outdated controlled substances are returned to a distributor for disposal.

84. c: The NDC consists of the labeler code (4 or 5 digits), the product code (3 or 4 digits), and the package code (1 or 2 digits)

85. c: 2 capsules bid for 5 days = 2 capsules × 2 daily × 5 days = 20 capsules.

86. b: FDA stands for Food and Drug Administration.

87. d: Medicare Part C is known as the Medicare Advantage plan.

88. c: DEA Form 222 is used for the purchase and sale of C-II medications.

89. d: $\dfrac{5 \text{ mg}}{\text{mL}} = \dfrac{100 \text{ mg}}{X}$

$X = 20 \text{ mL}$

90. d: Heparin, insulin, and potassium chloride are high-alert medications.

Pharmacy Technician Certification Board Guidelines and Requirements

APPENDIX

A

CERTIFICATION OVERVIEW

The Pharmacy Technician Certification Board (PTCB) is a national certification program that enables pharmacy technicians to work more effectively with pharmacists to offer safe and effective care and service. The Pharmacy Technician Certification Examination (PTCE) was developed by the PTCB to determine whether individuals have mastered the knowledge and skills needed to practice as a pharmacy technician.

PTCB certification is valid nationwide; however, regulations to work in a pharmacy vary from state to state. For more information regarding working as a pharmacy technician in your state contact your local board of pharmacy or visit the National Association of Boards of Pharmacy for more information.

Those who meet eligibility requirements and pass the PTCE may use the designation certified pharmacy technician (CPhT). Please refer to the PTCB regarding recertification and continuing education requirements (www.ptcb.org).

Applying for Certification

The PTCB accepts applications for the PTCE continually on a year round basis. Candidates are encouraged to apply for the PTCE online. Online applications require payment with a check or credit card. A paper application is only available to individuals who are able to document a disability or hardship that would prevent the use of the online application.

Eligibility

To be eligible for PTCB certification, a candidate must satisfy all of the following requirements:

- High school diploma or equivalent diploma (eg, a GED or foreign diploma)
- Full disclosure of all criminal and State Board of Pharmacy registration or licensure actions
- Compliance with all applicable PTCB certification policies
- Passing score on the PTCE

An individual may be disqualified for PTCB certification upon the disclosure or discovery of the following:

- Criminal conduct involving the candidate
- State Board of Pharmacy registration or licensure action involving the candidate
- Violation of a PTCB certification policy, including but not limited to the code of conduct

The PTCB may investigate criminal background, verify candidate eligibility, and deny certification to any individual. Once certified, CPhTs must report any felony conviction, drug or pharmacy-related violations, or State Board of Pharmacy action taken against their license or registration at the occurrence and at the time of recertification, to PTCB for review. Disqualification determinations are made on a case-by-case basis.

Applying for the Test

Individuals apply for the examination on the PTCB's website (www.ptcb.org). Candidates must register for a PTCB account prior to applying for the test. The cost to apply for the certification and take the PTCE is $129. Those who require special accommodations should request those during the application process.

Authorization Period

After an application is approved, individuals will be authorized to schedule and take the PTCE. The authorization to schedule lasts 90 days. If a candidate cannot schedule and take the examination within 90 days, they must withdraw their application to avoid forfeiting the application fee.

Scheduling

Candidates may schedule examination appointments online at www.pearsonvue.com/ptcb or call Pearson VUE at (866) 902-0593. Once you have scheduled an appointment, a confirmation e-mail will be sent within 24 hours. Candidates with special testing accommodations should call (800) 466-0450 to schedule examination appointments.

Withdrawing an Application

If one decides not to take the test within the 90-day test period, they can withdraw from their PTCB account. Candidates with scheduled examination appointments must first cancel the appointment with Pearson VUE. Candidates who withdraw will receive a refund, less an administrative fee. Individuals may withdraw on or before the last day of the authorization period.

Updated Pharmacy Technician Certification Examination Blueprint

APPENDIX

KNOWLEDGE DOMAINS AND AREAS

Pharmacology for Technicians 13.75%*

1.1 Generic and brand names of pharmaceuticals

1.2 Therapeutic equivalence

1.3 Drug interactions (eg, drug–disease, drug–drug, drug–dietary supplements, drug-OTC, drug–laboratory, and drug–nutrient)

1.4 Strengths or dose, dosage forms, physical appearance, routes of administration, and duration of therapy*

1.5 Common and severe side or adverse effects, allergies, and therapeutic contraindications associated with medications

1.6 Dosage and indication of legend, over-the-counter (OTC) medications, herbal and dietary supplements

Pharmacy Law and Regulations 12.5%*

2.1 Storage, handling, and disposal of hazardous substances and wastes (eg, material safety data sheet [MSDS])

2.2 Hazardous substances exposure, prevention, and treatment (eg, eyewash, spill kit, and MSDS)

2.3 Controlled substances transfer regulations (Drug Enforcement Administration [DEA])

2.4 Controlled substance documentation requirements for receiving, ordering, returning, loss or theft, and destruction (DEA)

2.5 Formula to verify the validity of a prescriber's DEA number (DEA)

2.6 Record keeping, documentation, and record retention (eg, length-of-time prescriptions are maintained on file)

2.7 Restricted drug programs and related prescription-processing requirements (eg, thalidomide, isotretinoin, and clozapine)

2.8 Professional standards related to data integrity, security, and confidentiality (eg, The Health Insurance Portability and Accountability Act [HIPAA], backing up, and archiving)

2.9 Requirement for consultation (eg, OBRA'90)

2.10 Food and Drug Administration's (FDA's) recall classification

2.11 Infections control standards (eg, laminar air flow, clean room, hand washing, cleaning counting trays, countertop, and equipment) (Occupational Safety and Health Administration [OSHA], The United States Pharmacopeia [USP] 795 and 797)

2.12 Record keeping for repackaged and recalled products and supplies (The Joint Commission [TJC], The State Boards of Pharmacy [BOP])

2.13 Professional standards regarding the roles and responsibilities of pharmacists, pharmacy technicians, and other pharmacy employees (TJC, BOP)

2.14 Reconciliation between state and federal laws and regulations

2.15 Facility, equipment, and supply requirements (eg, space requirements, prescription file storage, cleanliness, and reference materials) (TJC, USP, BOP)

3.0 Sterile and Nonsterile Compounding 8.75%*

3.1 Infection control (eg, hand washing and personal protective equipment [PPE])

3.2 Handling and disposal requirements (eg, receptacles and waste streams)

3.3 Documentation (eg, batch preparation and compounding record)*

3.4 Determine product stability (eg, beyond-use dating, signs of incompatibility)*

3.5 Selection and use of equipment and supplies

3.6 Sterile compounding processes*

3.7 Nonsterile compounding processes*

4.0 Medication Safety 12.5%

4.1 Error prevention strategies for data entry (eg, prescription or medication order to correct patient)

4.2 Patient package insert and medication guide requirements (eg, special directions and precautions)

4.3 Identify issues that require pharmacist's intervention (eg, drug utilization review [DUR], adverse drug reaction [ADR], over-the-counter [OTC] recommendation, therapeutic substitution, misuse, and missed dose)

4.4 Look-alike-sound-alike medications

4.5 High-alert or risk medications

4.6 Common safety strategies (eg, tall-man lettering, separating inventory, leading and trailing zeros, and limit use of error-prone abbreviations)

5.0 Pharmacy Quality Assurance 7.5%

5.1 Quality assurance practices for medication and inventory control systems (eg, matching National Drug Code (NDC) number, bar code, and data entry)

5.2 Infection control procedures and documentation (eg, PPE, needle recapping)

5.3 Risk management guidelines and regulations (eg, error prevention strategies

5.4 Communication channels necessary to ensure appropriate follow-up and problem resolution (eg, product recalls and shortages)

5.5 Productivity, efficiency, and customer service measures

6.0 Medication Order Entry and Fill Process 17.5%

6.1 Order entry process*

6.2 Intake, interpretation, and data entry*

6.3 Calculate doses required*

6.4 Fill process (eg, select appropriate product, apply special handling requirements, measure, and prepare product for final check)

6.5 Labeling requirements (eg, auxiliary and warning labels, expiration date, and patient-specific information)

6.6 Packaging requirements (eg, type of bags, syringes, glass, pvc, child resistant, light resistant)*

6.7 Dispensing process (eg, validation, documentation, and distribution)

7.0 Pharmacy Inventory Management 8.75%*

7.1 Function and application of NDC, lot number, and expiration dates

7.2 Formulary or approved/preferred drug list

7.3 Ordering and receiving processes (eg, maintain par levels and rotate stock)*

7.4 Storage requirements (eg, refrigeration, freezer, and warmer)

7.5 Removal (eg, recalls, returns, outdates, and reverse distribution)

8.0 Pharmacy Billing and Reimbursement 8.75%*

8.1 Reimbursement policies and plans (eg, health maintenance organizations [HMOs], preferred provide organization [PPO], Centers for Medicare and Medicaid Services [CMS], and private plans)

8.2 Third party resolution (eg, prior authorization, rejected claims, and plan limitations)*

8.3 Third party reimbursement systems (eg, pharmacy benefit manager [PBM], medication assistance programs, coupons, and self-pay)

8.4 Health care reimbursement systems (eg, home health, long-term care, and home infusion)

8.5 Coordination of benefits

9.0 Pharmacy Information System's Usage and Application 10%

9.1 Pharmacy-related computer applications for documenting the dispensing of prescriptions or medication orders (eg, maintaining the electronic medical record, patient adherence, risk factors, alcohol use, drug allergies, and side effects)

9.2 Databases, pharmacy computer applications, and documentation management (eg, user access, drug database, interface, inventory report, usage reports, override reports, and diversion reports)

---

*Denotes content that includes calculations.

Top 200 Drugs

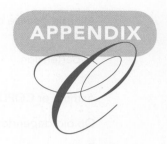

Generic Name	Brand Name	Indication(s)	Usual Dose
Acetaminophen/codeine	Tylenol with Codeine	Pain	30–60 mg PO every 4 hours (based on codeine)
Acyclovir	Zovirax	Herpes infection	200–800 mg PO 5 times per day
Albuterol	AccuNeb, ProAir, Proventil, Ventolin, VoSpire	Asthma/COPD	Inhaler: 1–2 puffs qid Nebulizer: 2.5 mg qid
Alendronate	Binosto, Fosamax	Osteoporosis	5–10 mg PO daily or 35–70 mg PO weekly
Allopurinol	Aloprim, Zyloprim	Gout	100–600 mg PO daily
Alprazolam	Niravam, Xanax, Xanax XR	Anxiety or panic disorder	0.25–0.5 mg PO tid
Amitriptyline	Elavil	Depression	50–150 mg PO qhs
Amlodipine	Norvasc	Angina or hypertension	5–10 mg PO daily
Amoxicillin	Amoxil, Moxatag	Infection	250–500 mg PO tid or 500–875 mg PO bid
Amoxicillin/clavulanate	Augmentin	Infection	250–500 mg PO tid or 875 mg PO bid
Aripiprazole	Abilify	Bipolar/schizophrenia/depression	Bipolar/schizophrenia: 15–30 mg PO daily Depression: 2–15 mg PO daily
Aspirin	Ascriptin, Bufferin, Ecotrin	Cardiovascular/analgesic/antipyretic	Cardiovascular: 81–325 mg PO daily Analgesic/antipyretic: 325–650 mg PO q4h
Atenolol	Tenormin	Angina or hypertension	25–100 mg PO daily
Atorvastatin	Lipitor	Hypercholesterolemia	10–80 mg PO qhs
Azithromycin	Zithromax, Zmax	Infection	250–500 mg PO daily
Baclofen	Gablofen, Lioresal	Muscle pain or spasms	5–10 mg PO tid
Benazepril	Lotensin	Hypertension	10–80 mg PO daily
Benzonatate	Tessalon, Zonatuss	Cough	100–200 mg PO tid
Benztropine	Cogentin	Parkinson disease or extrapyramidal symptoms	1–4 mg PO/IM/IV 1–2 times daily

Betamethasone/clotrimazole	Lotrisone	Allergic disease or tinea corporis	Apply bid
Bisoprolol/hydrochlorothiazide	Ziac	Hypertension	2.5/6.25 mg to 20/12.5 mg PO daily
Budesonide/formoterol	Symbicort	Asthma or COPD	2 puffs bid (all strengths)
Buprenorphine/naloxone	Suboxone	Opioid dependence	4–24 mg PO/SL daily
Bupropion	Aplenzin, Budeprion, Buproban, Forfivo, Wellbutrin, Zyban	Depression/seasonal affective disorder/smoking cessation	IR: 100 mg PO tid SR: 150 mg PO bid XL: 150 mg PO daily
Buspirone	Buspar	Anxiety	10–15 mg PO bid
Butalbital/acetaminophen/caffeine	Esgic, Fioricet	Headache	1–2 caps PO q4h
Carisoprodol	Soma	Muscle pain	250–350 mg PO tid
Carvedilol	Coreg	Hypertension or heart failure	IR: 3.125–50 mg PO bid ER: 20–80 mg PO daily
Cefdinir	Omnicef	Infection	300 mg PO bid
Celecoxib	Celebrex	Arthritis or pain	100–200 mg PO bid
Cephalexin	Keflex	Infection	250–1000 mg PO qid
Chlorhexidine gluconate	Peridex	Periodontitis	15-mL swish/spit bid
Ciprofloxacin	Cipro	Infection	250–500 mg PO bid
Citalopram	Celexa	Depression	20–40 mg PO daily
Clarithromycin	Biaxin	Infection	IR: 250–500 mg PO bid XR: 1000 mg PO daily
Clindamycin	Cleocin	Infection	150–450 mg PO qid
Clobetasol	Clobex, Cormax, Olux, Temovate	Dermatitis	Apply bid
Clonazepam	Klonopin	Panic disorder or seizure	0.25–1 mg PO tid
Clonidine	Catapres, Duraclon, Kapvay	Hypertension	0.1–0.4 mg PO bid
Clopidogrel	Plavix	Cardiovascular or stroke	75 mg PO daily
Colchicine	Colcrys	Gout	0.6–1.2 mg PO bid
Cyclobenzaprine	Amrix, Fexmid, Flexeril	Muscle spasm	5–10 mg PO tid
Desvenlafaxine	Pristiq	Depression	50 mg PO daily
Dextroamphetamine/amphetamine	Adderall	ADHD or narcolepsy	IR: 40 mg/day PO in 1–3 divided doses XR: 20 mg PO daily
Diazepam	Diastat, Valium	Anxiety/alcohol withdrawal/sedation/seizures	2–10 mg PO qid

Diclofenac	Voltaren	Arthritis or pain	50 mg PO tid
Dicyclomine	Bentyl	Irritable bowel	20–40 mg PO qid
Digoxin	Lanoxin	Atrial fibrillation or heart failure	125–250 µg PO/IV daily
Diltiazem	Cardizem, Cartia, Dilacor, Diltia, Diltzac, Matzim, Taztia, Tiazac	Angina/atrial fibrillation/heart failure	IR: 30–60 mg PO qid XR: 120–480 mg PO daily
Divalproex	Depakote	Mania/migraine prophylaxis/seizures	250–1000 mg PO bid-qid
Donepezil	Aricept	Dementia	5–23 mg PO daily
Doxazosin	Cardura	Benign prostatic hyperplasia or hypertension	4–8 mg PO daily
Doxycycline	Adoxa, Alodox, Doryx, Monodox, Ocudox, Oracea, Oraxyl, Periostat, Vibramycin	Infection	100 mg PO bid
Duloxetine	Cymbalta	Depression/anxiety/pain	30–60 mg PO daily
Dutasteride	Avodart	Benign prostatic hyperplasia	0.5 mg PO daily
Enalapril	Vasotec	Hypertension or heart failure	2.5–20 mg PO bid
Escitalopram	Lexapro	Anxiety or depression	10–20 mg PO daily
Esomeprazole	Nexium	Esophagitis/GERD/heartburn/ulcers	20–40 mg PO daily
Estradiol	Estrace, Femtrace	Menopause	1–2 mg PO daily
Estrogen, conjugated	Cenestin, Enjuvia, Premarin	Menopause	0.3–0.625 mg PO daily
Eszopiclone	Lunesta	Insomnia	1–3 mg PO qhs
Ethinyl estradiol/drospirenone	Ocella, Yasmin, Yaz	Contraception	1 tablet PO daily
Ethinyl estradiol/etonogestrel	NuvaRing	Contraception	1 ring vaginally every 3 weeks, then removed for 1 week
Ethinyl estradiol/norethindrone	Estrostep, Loestrin, Microgestin, Neocon, Ortho-Novum, Ovcon	Contraception	1 tablet PO daily
Ethinyl estradiol/norgestimate	MonoNessa, Ortho-Tri-Cyclen, Previfem, Sprintec, Tri-Previfem, Tri-Sprintec, TriNessa	Contraception	1 tablet PO daily
Ezetimibe	Zetia	Hyperlipidemia	10 mg PO daily
Ezetimibe/simvastatin	Vytorin	Hyperlipidemia	10 mg/10–80 mg PO daily
Famotidine	Pepcid	Esophagitis/GERD/heartburn/ulcers	10–20 mg PO bid

Fenofibrate	Antara, Fenoglide, Lipofen, Lofibra, TriCor, Triglide	Hypertriglyceridemia	40–200 mg PO daily
Fenofibric acid	Fibricor, Trilipix	Hypertriglyceridemia	35–135 mg PO daily
Fentanyl transdermal	Duragesic	Pain	25–100 µg topically q72h
Ferrous sulfate	Feosol, Fer-In-Sol, Fer-iron, SlowFE	Anemia	300 mg PO bid
Fexofenadine	Allegra	Allergic rhinitis	60 mg PO bid or 180 mg PO daily
Finasteride	Propecia, Proscar	Benign prostatic hyperplasia/baldness	1–5 mg PO daily
Fluconazole	Diflucan	Fungal infection	150–800 mg PO/IV daily
Fluoxetine	Prozac, Sarafem	Bulimia/depression/OCD/panic disorder/premenstrual dysphoric disorder	20–80 mg PO daily
Fluticasone	Flovent	Asthma	88–440 mg inhaled bid
Fluticasone nasal	Flonase, Veramyst	Rhinitis	2 sprays per nostril daily
Fluticasone/salmeterol	Advair	Asthma or COPD	Disk: 1 puff bid (all strengths) Inhaler: 2 puffs bid (all strengths
Folic acid	Folvite, Folacin	Anemia or pregnancy	400 µg to 4 mg PO daily
Furosemide	Lasix	Hypertension or heart failure	20–80 mg PO/IV daily to bid
Gabapentin	Gralise, Neurontin	Fibromyalgia/neuropathic pain/restless Legs syndrome/seizures	100–1200 mg PO tid
Gemfibrozil	Lopid	Hypertriglyceridemia	600 mg PO bid
Glimepiride	Amaryl	Diabetes	1–8 mg PO daily
Glipizide	Glucotrol	Diabetes	5–20 mg PO daily
Glyburide	DiaBeta, Glynase	Diabetes	2.5–10 mg PO daily
Glyburide/metformin	Glucovance	Diabetes	1.25/250 mg to 5/1000 mg PO bid
Guaifenesin/codeine	Cheratussin AC, Guaiatussin AC	Cough	5–15 mL PO q4h
Hydralazine	Apresoline	Hypertension or heart failure	25–100 mg PO bid
Hydrochlorothiazide	Microzide	Edema or hypertension	25–100 µg PO daily
Hydrochlorothiazide/triamterene	Dyazide, Maxzide	Hypertension	1–2 caps PO daily
Hydrocodone/acetaminophen	Lortab, Norco, Vicodin	Pain	5–10 mg PO qid (based on hydrocodone)
Hydroxychloroquine	Plaquenil	Malaria/systemic lupus erythematosus/rheumatoid arthritis	200–600 mg PO daily

Hydroxyzine	Atarax, Vistaril	Anxiety/insomnia/rhinitis/sedation/urticaria	25–100 mg PO qid
Ibandronate	Boniva	Osteoporosis	150 mg PO monthly
Ibuprofen	Advil, Motrin	Arthritis/fever/pain	200–800 mg PO qid
Insulin aspart	Novolog	Diabetes	Doses are patient specific
Insulin glargine	Lantus	Diabetes	Doses are patient specific
Ipratropium/albuterol	Combivent, Combivent Respimat	COPD	1–2 puffs qid
Irbesartan	Avapro	Hypertension	75–300 mg PO daily
Isosorbide mononitrate	Imdur	Angina	30–120 mg PO daily
Ketoconazole topical	Extina, Nizoral	Fungal infection	Apply daily
Lamotrigine	Lamictal	Bipolar or seizures	25–300 mg PO bid
Lansoprazole	Prevacid	Esophagitis/GERD/heartburn/ulcers	15–30 mg PO daily
Latanoprost	Xalatan	Glaucoma	1 drop in affected eye daily
Levetiracetam	Keppra	Seizures	500–1500 mg PO bid
Levofloxacin	Levaquin	Infection	250–750 mg PO daily
Levothyroxine	Levothroid, Levoxyl, Synthroid	Hypothyroidism	25–200 μg PO daily
Lidocaine topical	Lidoderm	Pain	Apply up to 3 patches for up to 12 hours per 24-hour period
Lisdexamfetamine	Vyvanse	ADHD	30–70 mg PO daily
Lisinopril	Prinivil, Zestril	Hypertension or heart failure	5–40 mg PO daily
Lisinopril/hydrochlorothiazide	Prinzide, Zestoretic	Hypertension	10/12.5 mg to 40/50 mg PO daily
Lorazepam	Ativan	Anxiety/alcohol withdrawal/sedation/seizures	0.5–2 mg PO bid-tid
Losartan	Cozaar	Hypertension	25–100 mg PO daily
Losartan/hydrochlorothiazide	Hyzaar	Hypertension	50/12.5 mg to 100/25 mg PO daily
Lovastatin	Altoprev, Mevacor	Hyperlipidemia	20–80 mg PO qhs
Meclizine	Antivert	Motion sickness or vertigo	25 mg PO qid
Meloxicam	Mobic	Arthritis	7.5–15 mg PO daily
Memantine	Namenda	Dementia	IR: 10 mg PO bid XR: 7–28 mg PO daily
Metformin	Fortamet, Glucophage, Glumetza, Riomet	Diabetes	IR: 500–1000 mg PO bid XR: 500–2000 mg PO daily

Methadone	Dolophine, Methadose	Pain or detoxification	2.5–10 mg PO tid (pain) 80–120 mg PO daily (detoxification)
Methocarbamol	Robaxin	Muscle spasm	750–1500 mg PO qid
Methotrexate	Rheumatrex, Trexall	Crohn disease/ectopic pregnancy/oncology/psoriasis/rheumatoid arthritis	Doses are patient specific
Methylphenidate	Concerta, Daytrana, Metadate, Methylin, Ritalin	ADHD/narcolepsy	IR: 5–20 mg PO BID XR: 20–60 mg PO daily
Methylprednisolone	Depo-Medrol, Medrol, Solu-Medrol	Anti-inflammatory	Doses are patient specific
Metoclopramide	Metozolv, Reglan	Gastroparesis/GERD/nausea	5–15 mg PO qid
Metoprolol succinate	Toprol XL	Angina/atrial fibrillation/heart failure/hypertension	25–400 mg PO daily
Metoprolol tartrate	Lopressor	Angina/atrial fibrillation/hypertension	25–200 mg PO bid
Metronidazole	Flagyl	Infection	250–500 mg PO qid
Minocycline	Dynacin, Minocin, Solodyn	Infection	100 mg PO bid
Mirtazapine	Remeron	Depression	15–45 mg PO qhs
Mometasone	Nasonex	Rhinitis	2 sprays per nostril daily
Montelukast	Singulair	Asthma or rhinitis	10 mg PO daily
Moxifloxacin ophthalmic	Vigamox	Bacterial conjunctivitis	1 drop in affected eye tid
Mupirocin	Bactroban, Centany	Infection	Apply tid
Nabumetone	Relafen	Arthritis	500–1000 mg PO bid
Naproxen	Aleve, Anaprox, Naprosyn	Arthritis or pain	250–500 mg PO bid
Nebivolol	Bystolic	Hypertension	5–40 mg PO daily
Niacin	Niacor, Niaspan	Hyperlipidemia	500–2000 mg PO qhs
Nifedipine	Adalat, Nifedical, Procardia	Angina or hypertension	IR: 10–30 mg PO tid XR: 30–180 mg PO daily
Nitrofurantoin	Furadantin, Macrobid, Macrodantin	Infection	Furadantin/Macrodantin: 50–100 mg PO qid Macrobid: 100 mg PO bid
Nitroglycerin	Minitran, Nitro-Bid, Nitro-Dur, NitroMist, Rectiv	Angina/heart failure/anal fissure (rectal ointment)	Doses are patient specific
Nortriptyline	Pamelor	Depression	25–50 mg PO qid

Olanzapine	Zyprexa	Bipolar/schizophrenia/depression	Bipolar/schizophrenia: 15–30 mg PO daily Depression: 2–15 mg PO daily
Olmesartan	Benicar	Hypertension	20–40 mg PO daily
Olmesartan/hydrochlorothiazide	Benicar HCT	Hypertension	20/12.5 mg to 40/25 mg PO daily
Omega-3-acid ethyl esters	Lovaza	Hypertriglyceridemia	4 g PO daily
Omeprazole	Prilosec	Esophagitis/GERD/heartburn/ulcers	20–40 mg PO daily
Ondansetron	Zofran, Zuplenz	Nausea	4–8 mg PO qid
Oxycodone	Oxecta, Oxycontin, Roxicodone	Pain	IR: 5–20 mg PO q4h CR: 10–40 mg PO bid
Oxycodone/acetaminophen	Endocet, Percocet, Roxicet, Tylox	Pain	2.5–10 mg PO q4h (based on oxycodone)
Pantoprazole	Protonix	Esophagitis/GERD/heartburn/ulcers	20–40 mg PO daily
Paroxetine	Paxil, Pexeva	Anxiety/depression/OCD/panic disorder/premenstrual dysphoric disorder	20–60 mg PO daily
Penicillin V potassium	Pen VK	Infection	250–500 mg PO qid
Phenazopyridine	Pyridium	Urinary analgesic	100–200 mg PO tid
Phentermine	Adipex-P, Suprenza	Obesity	15–37.5 mg PO daily
Phenytoin	Dilantin, Phenytek	Seizures	300–600 mg PO daily
Pioglitazone	Actos	Diabetes	15–30 mg PO daily
Polyethylene glycol	Miralax	Constipation	17 g PO daily
Potassium chloride	Epiklor, K-Tab, Kaon-CL, Klor-Con, microK	Hypokalemia	10–40 mEq PO daily
Pravastatin	Pravachol	Hyperlipidemia	10–80 mg PO daily
Prednisolone	Orapred, Pediapred	Anti-inflammatory	5–60 mg PO daily
Prednisone		Anti-inflammatory	5–60 mg PO daily
Pregabalin	Lyrica	Fibromyalgia/neuropathic pain/seizures	75–225 mg PO bid
Promethazine	Phenadoz, Phenergan, Promethegan	Nausea	12.5–25 mg PO q4h
Promethazine/codeine	Phenergan/Codeine	Cough	5 mL PO q4h
Propranolol	Inderal	Atrial fibrillation/hypertension/migraine prophylaxis	40–120 mg PO bid
Quetiapine	Seroquel	Bipolar/schizophrenia/depression	IR: 50–400 mg PO bid XR: 400–800 mg PO daily

Quinapril	Accupril	Hypertension or heart failure	5–20 mg PO bid
Raloxifene	Evista	Osteoporosis	60 mg PO daily
Ramipril	Altace	Hypertension or heart failure	2.5–20 mg PO daily
Ranitidine	Zantac	Esophagitis/GERD/ heartburn/ulcers	150 mg PO bid
Risperidone	Risperdal	Bipolar or schizophrenia	1–4 mg PO bid
Ropinirole	Requip	Parkinson disease or restless leg syndrome	IR: 0.25–3 mg PO tid XL: 2–24 mg PO daily
Rosuvastatin	Crestor	Hyperlipidemia	5–40 mg PO qhs
Sertraline	Zoloft	Depression/OCD/panic disorder/premenstrual dysphoric disorder	50–200 mg PO daily
Sildenafil	Revatio, Viagra	Erectile dysfunction or pulmonary artery hypertension	Revatio: 20 mg PO tid Viagra: 25–100 mg PO daily
Simvastatin	Zocor	Hyperlipidemia	10–80 mg PO qhs
Sitagliptin	Januvia	Diabetes	100 mg PO daily
Spironolactone	Aldactone	Edema/hypokalemia/ hypertension/heart failure	25–100 mg PO bid
Sulfamethoxazole/ trimethoprim	Bactrim, Septra	Infection	1–2 tabs PO bid
Sumatriptan	Alsuma, Imitrex, Sumavel DosePro	Migraine	25–100 mg PO PRN
Tadalafil	Adcirca, Cialis	Erectile dysfunction or pulmonary artery hypertension	Adcirca: 40 mg PO daily Cialis: 2.5–5 mg PO daily or 10–20 mg PO PRN
Tamsulosin	Flomax	Benign prostatic hyperplasia	0.4–0.8 mg PO daily
Temazepam	Restoril	Insomnia	7.5–30 mg PO qhs
Terazosin	Hytrin	Benign prostatic hyperplasia or hypertension	1–20 mg PO daily
Tiotropium	Spiriva	COPD	18 μg inhaled daily
Tizanidine	Zanaflex	Muscle spasm	4–8 mg PO tid
Tolterodine	Detrol	Overactive bladder	IR: 1–2 mg PO bid XR: 2–4 mg PO daily
Topiramate	Topamax	Diabetic neuropathy/ migraine prophylaxis/ neuropathic pain/seizures	IR: 25–200 mg PO bid XR: 50–400 mg PO daily
Tramadol	ConZip, Ultram, Ryzolt, Rybix	Pain	IR: 50–100 mg PO q4h XR: 100–300 mg PO daily

Trazodone	Desyrel, Oleptro	Depression	50–200 mg PO tid
Triamcinolone	Kenalog, Oralone, Pediaderm, Trianex, Triderm, Zytopic	Dermatitis	Apply bid-qid
Valacyclovir	Valtrex	Herpes infection	500–1000 mg PO bid
Valsartan	Diovan	Hypertension or heart failure	40–160 mg PO bid
Valsartan/ hydrochlorothiazide	Diovan HCT	Hypertension	80/12.5 mg to 320/25 mg PO daily
Venlafaxine	Effexor, Effexor XR	Anxiety/depression/panic disorder	IR: 25–100 mg PO tid XR: 37.5–225 mg PO daily
Verapamil	Calan, Calan SR, Covera, Isoptin, Verelan, Verelan PM	Angina/atrial fibrillation/ hypertension	IR: 40–120 mg PO tid XR: 180–480 mg PO daily
Warfarin	Coumadin, Jantoven	Atrial fibrillation/cardiac valve replacement/ clotting disorders/ myocardial infarction/ stroke	2–10 mg PO daily
Zolpidem	Ambien, Edluar, Intermezzo, Zolpimist	Insomnia	2.5–10 mg PO qhs

Top OTC Drugs

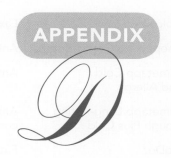

Generic Name	Brand Name	Pharmacologic Category
Acetaminophen	Tylenol	Analgesia, antipyretic
Acetaminophen/aspirin/caffeine	Excedrin	Antipyretic, analgesia or vasoconstrictor
Acetaminophen/caffeine/pyrilamine maleate	Midol	Antipyretic, analgesia/diuretic/antihistamine
Acetaminophen/chlorpheniramine	Coricidin HBP Cold and Flu	Analgesia, antipyretic/antihistamine combination
Acetaminophen/dextromethorphan/ doxylamine succinate	NyQuil	Analgesia, antipyretic/antitussive/antihistamine combination
Acetaminophen/dextromethorphan/ phenylephrine	Dayquil Cold and Flu	Analgesia, antipyretic/antitussive/decongestant combination
Acetaminophen/diphenhydramine	Excedrin PM	Analgesia, antipyretic/antihistamine combination
Acetaminophen/diphenhydramine	Tylenol PM	Analgesia, antipyretic/antihistamine combination
Acetaminophen/phenylephrine	Tylenol Sinus Congestion and Pain	Analgesia, antipyretic/decongestant combination
Acetaminophen/phenylephrine/ guaifenesin/dextromethorphan	Tylenol Cold Multi-Symptom	Analgesia, antipyretic/decongestant/ expectorant/antitussive combination
Aluminum hydroxide	Alternagel	Antacid
Aluminum hydroxide and magnesium carbonate	Gaviscon	Antacid
Aluminum hydroxide, magnesium hydroxide, and simethicone	Maalox	Antacid, antiflatulent
Aluminum/magnesium hydroxide/ simethicone	Mylanta, Maalox	Antacid
Artificial tears	Systane, Tears Naturale	Ocular lubricant
Aspirin, buffered	Bufferin	Antipyretic, analgesia
Aspirin, chewable	Bayer Children's Aspirin	Antipyretic, analgesia
Aspirin, enteric coated	Ecotrin	Antipyretic, analgesia
Bacitracin/polymyxin B	Polysporin	Topical antibiotic
Benzocaine	Anbesol, Orabase, Orajel	Topical anesthetic

Bisacodyl	Dulcolax	Laxative
Bismuth	Kaopectate, Pepto-Bismol	Antidiarrheal
Brompheniramine/phenylephrine	Dimetapp Cold and Allergy	Antihistamine/decongestant combination
Brompheniramine/pseudoephedrine/dextromethorphan	Dimetapp Long-Acting Cough Plus Cold	Antihistamine/decongestant/antitussive combination
Caffeine	NoDoz	Fatigue
Calcium carbonate	Rolaids, Tums	Antacid
Calcium polycarbophil	FiberCon, Fiber-Lax	Laxative
Capsaicin	Capzasin-P, Zostrix	Topical analgesic
Carbamide peroxide	Debrox	Cerumenolytic (ear wax removal)
Cetirizine	Zyrtec	Antihistamine
Cetirizine/pseudoephedrine	Zyrtec D	Antihistamine/decongestant combination
Chlorpheniramine	Chlor-Trimeton	Antihistamine
Chlorpheniramine/dextromethorphan	Coricidin HBP Cough and Cold	Antihistamine/antitussive combination
Cimetidine	Tagamet	Histamine-2 blocker
Clotrimazole	Lotrimin AF	Topical antifungal
Cromolyn	NasalCrom	Nasal antiallergy
Dextromethorphan	Dayquil Cough, Delsym	Antitussive
Dimenhydrinate	Dramamine	Antihistamine (motion sickness)
Diphenhydramine	Benadryl	Antihistamine
Docosanol	Abreva	Topical antiviral
Docusate sodium	Colace	Laxative
Doxylamine	Unisom	Antihistamine (insomnia)
Epinephrine	Asthmanefrin	Bronchodilator (asthma)
Famotidine	Pepcid AC	Histamine-2 blocker
Famotidine/calcium carbonate/magnesium hydroxide	Pepcid Complete	Histamine-2 blocker/antacid
Fexofenadine	Allegra OTC	Antihistamine
Fexofenadine/pseudoephedrine	Allegra D	Antihistamine/decongestant combination
Fructose, dextrose, and phosphoric acid	Emetrol	Antiemetic
Guaifenesin	Mucinex, Robitussin	Expectorant
Guaifenesin/pseudoephedrine	Mucinex D	Expectorant/decongestant combination
Guaifenesin/dextromethorphan	Robitussin DM, Mucinex DM	Expectorant/antitussive combination

Guaifenesin/phenylephrine/ dextromethorphan	Robitussin Cold Multi-Symptom	Expectorant/decongestant/antitussive combination
Hydrocortisone	Cortaid, Cortizone 10	Topical steroid
Ibuprofen	Advil, Motrin	Anti-inflammatory, analgesia, antipyretic
Ibuprofen/pseudoephedrine	Advil Cold and Sinus	Anti-inflammatory, analgesia, antipyretic/ decongestant combination
Ketoconazole	Nizoral AD	Topical antifungal
Ketotifen fumarate	Zaditor	Ocular antihistamine
Lactic acid and ammonium hydroxide	AmLactin	Topical lubricant/anti-itch
Lansoprazole	Prevacid 24 Hour	Proton pump inhibitor
Loperamide	Imodium AD	Antidiarrheal
Loratidine	Alavert, Claritin	Antihistamine
Loratidine	Alavert, Claritin	Antihistamine
Loratidine/pseudoephedrine	Claritin D	Antihistamine/decongestant combination
Magnesium citrate	Citrate of Magnesia	Laxative
Magnesium hydroxide	Milk of Magnesium (MOM)	Antacid
Meclizine	Bonine	Antihistamine (motion sickness, vertigo)
Methyl salicylate/menthol	Bengay	Topical analgesic
Miconazole	Baza Antifungal, Monistat	Topical antifungal
Mineral oil/white petrolatum	Lacri-Lube	Ocular lubricant
Minoxidil	Rogaine	Topical hair regrowth
Naphazoline	Naphcon	Ocular vasoconstrictor
Naproxen	Aleve	Anti-inflammatory, analgesia
Neomycin sulfate/polymyxin B/ bacitracin zinc	Neosporin	Topical antibiotic
Nicotine	Nicoderm CQ, Nicorette	Smoking cessation
Nizatidine	Axid AR	Histamine-2 blocker
Omeprazole	Prilosec OTC, Zegerid OTC	Proton pump inhibitor
Orlistat	Alli	Lipase inhibitor (weight loss)
Oxymetazoline	Afrin, Neo-Synephrine	Nasal decongestant
Permethrin	Nix	Topical pediculicide (lice)
Phenazopyridine	Azo Urinary Pain Relief	Urinary analgesia
Phenol	Chloraseptic	Topical anesthetic
Phenylephrine	Preparation H	Topical vasoconstrictor

Phenylephrine	Sudafed PE	Decongestant
Polyethylene glycol	Miralax	Laxative
Polymyxin B, neomycin, bacitracin	Triple Antibiotic Ointment	Topical antibiotic
Polyvinyl alcohol drops	Akwa Tears	Ocular lubricant
Pseudoephedrine	Sudafed	Decongestant
Psyllium seed	Metamucil	Laxative
Pyrethrins and piperonyl butoxide	RID	Topical pediculicide (lice)
Ranitidine	Zantac	Histamine-2 blocker
Salicylic acid	Compound W, Kerasal Foot Cream	Topical wart/corn/callus removal
Sennosides	Senokot	Laxative
Sennosides/docusate sodium	Peri-Colace/Senokot-S	Laxative
Simethicone	Mylicon, Gas X	Antiflatulent
Sodium chloride	Ocean, Sea Soft	Nasal lubricant
Sodium phosphate	Fleet Enema	Laxative
Terbinafine	Lamisil AT	Topical antifungal
Tetrahydrozoline	Visine	Ocular vasoconstrictor
Zinc oxide	Desitin	Topical skin protectant

Top 25 Herbal Products

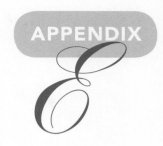

Common Name	Use
Aloe vera	Wound and burn healing
Bilberry	Diarrhea, mouth/throat inflammation, night vision
Black cohosh root	Menopause
Cayenne	Analgesic, used as an irritant in self-defense sprays
Cranberry	Urinary tract infection prevention
Echinacea	Common cold
Elderberry	Influenza, antioxidant
Evening primrose	Rheumatoid arthritis, diabetic neuropathy
Garlic	Cardiovascular health, common cold
Ginger	Nausea
Ginkgo	Memory
Ginseng	Increases mental and physical capability
Grape seed	Antioxidant
Green tea	Metabolic syndromes
Hawthorn	Heart failure, anxiolytic, analgesic
Horny goat week	Increases blood flow, kidney support
Kava kava	Sedative effects
Kelp	Nutritional support of minerals and elements
Milk thistle	Liver support
Saw palmetto	Benign prostatic hyperplasia
Soy	Menopause, osteoporosis, diabetes, heart disease
Spirulina	Nutritional support
St. John's wort	Depression, anxiety
Valerian root	Sedative, muscle spasms
Yohimbe	Sexual dysfunction, weight loss, dry mouth

Index